CW01368507

Colourful Semantics

This comprehensive resource pack, developed in conjunction with education staff, draws on the principles of Alison Bryan's original Colourful Semantics approach to provide professionals with an engaging, dynamic way to support children's language development. By coding sentences using colour, symbols and signs, this visual approach aims to:

- teach understanding of question words;
- develop vocabulary and increase sentence complexity;
- increase range and complexity of verbs (children with delayed or disordered spoken language skills often overuse simple verbs such as *do, go* or *get*);
- improve children's written language skills.

This practical resource consists of three parts: a printed book containing ready-made session plan ideas, black and white vocabulary cards and worksheets; an online version using the current Colourful Semantics colour coding system, and an online version using the colour coding system used by speech and language therapists from NHS Forth Valley.

This is an essential pack for teachers and professionals looking to work on language development with children aged four to nine. The flexible session plans can be used with individuals, small groups and whole classes, and can be easily adapted by speech and language therapists, teachers and other practitioners.

NHS Forth Valley would like to thank the following members of staff for their hard work and dedication in the design and development of this pack: Anna Blackburn, Glenn Carter, Cara Chalmers, Katie Clark, Mary Coleman, Louise Illingworth, Jen Keating, Ruth Kerr, Niamh Murphy and Stephanie Wood. Forth Valley would also like to thank Alison Bryan for developing the original idea and for suggesting improvements to the pack. Thank you to all the many teachers from across Forth Valley who were instrumental in designing a pack that can be effectively used in the context of education.

NHS Forth Valley provides a large number of health services across Central Scotland including Clackmannanshire, Falkirk and Stirling. The Children's Speech and Language Therapy team in Forth Valley are an innovative group of staff who understand the importance of transformational change, collaboration and compassionate, person-centred care in order to improve outcomes for the children and young people they serve.

Access your online resources:
Colourful Semantics is accompanied by two additional online versions designed to ensure this resource best supports your professional needs:

- A version using the current *Colourful Semantics* colours

- A version using the NHS Forth Valley colours

Activate your online resources:
Go to www.routledge.com/cw/speechmark and click on the cover of this book
Click the 'Sign in or Request Access' button and follow the instructions in order to access the resources

Colourful Semantics

A Resource for Developing Children's
Spoken and Written Language Skills

NHS Forth Valley

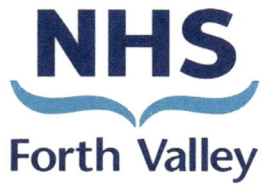

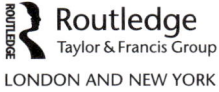
Routledge
Taylor & Francis Group

LONDON AND NEW YORK

First published 2020
by Routledge
2 Park Square, Milton Park, Abingdon, Oxon OX14 4RN

and by Routledge
52 Vanderbilt Avenue, New York, NY 10017

Routledge is an imprint of the Taylor & Francis Group, an informa business

© 2020 NHS Forth Valley

The right of NHS Forth Valley to be identified as author of this work has been asserted by it in accordance with sections 77 and 78 of the Copyright, Designs and Patents Act 1988.

All rights reserved. The purchase of this copyright material confers the right on the purchasing institution to photocopy pages which bear the photocopy icon and copyright line at the bottom of the page. No other parts of this book may be reprinted or reproduced or utilised in any form or by any electronic, mechanical, or other means, now known or hereafter invented, including photocopying and recording, or in any information storage or retrieval system, without permission in writing from the publishers.

Trademark notice: Product or corporate names may be trademarks or registered trademarks, and are used only for identification and explanation without intent to infringe.

British Library Cataloguing-in-Publication Data
A catalogue record for this book is available from the British Library

Library of Congress Cataloging-in-Publication Data
Names: Carter, Glenn, (Speech therapist), author. | Coleman, Mary, (Speech therapist).
Title: Colourful semantics : a resource for developing children's spoken and written language skills /
    [Glenn Carter and Mary Coleman ; foreword by Alison Bryan].
Other titles: Colorful semantics
Description: First Edition. | London ; New York : Routledge, 2020. | "NHS Forth Valley."
Identifiers: LCCN 2019038508 (print) | LCCN 2019038509 (ebook) | ISBN 9780367210502 (Paperback) |
    ISBN 9780429265112 (eBook)
Subjects: LCSH: Language arts (Early childhood)
Classification: LCC LB1139.5.L35 C365 2020 (print) | LCC LB1139.5.L35 (ebook) | DDC 372.6–dc23
LC record available at https://lccn.loc.gov/2019038508
LC ebook record available at https://lccn.loc.gov/2019038509

ISBN: 978-0-367-21050-2 (pbk)
ISBN: 978-0-429-26511-2 (ebk)

Typeset in Univers
by Servis Filmsetting Ltd, Stockport, Cheshire

Visit the companion website: www.routledge.com/cw/speechmark

Contents

Foreword

It is my great pleasure to write this foreword, recommending this comprehensive and effective resource for using Colourful Semantics in education and clinical contexts.

Colourful Semantics came into being in 1992 when I met a five-year-old boy called Gordon. I had worked with both children and adults in my job as a speech and language therapist. What struck me about Gordon was the marked similarity of his language difficulties to a stroke patient I had worked with. The worlds of adult and paediatric therapy were seen as completely separate disciplines. The idea of using as adult therapy approach with a child was a no-go area, but the similarities were too tempting to ignore!

In 1986 a speech and language therapist, Eirian Jones, had written about using a semantic approach with one of her stroke patients, in contrast to the grammatical approaches which dominated at that time. This 'mapping therapy' focused on the meaning relationships connected to the verb in the sentence: the '*Who* does *What* to *Whom*'. She used question words to help her patient chop up written sentences into chunks to show how that chunk related to the meaning of the verb, i.e. finding the words that showed 'WHO did the action', 'WHAT the action was done to' or 'WHERE the action was done'. Once the sentence had been chopped up to show these different 'meaning chunks', it was easier to see how each chunk was connected to, or mapped onto, the surface grammar of the sentence.

It was this approach that gave birth to Colourful Semantics. In a world of child language therapy that then focused heavily on developing grammar skills, I decided to try something new and focus on the meaning relationships. Like Eirian, I used the question words to find the meaning relationships around the verb in a sentence: 'verb semantics'. However, I added in a colour for each question word to make the different 'meaning chunks' stand out. Each question word was then always linked to that colour, as well as to a question word sign. After all, I was working with a five-year-old, so extra visual support was needed.

The impact of using this approach with Gordon was astounding and rapid. I was invited to present the new approach at a conference in 1996, which was later published as one chapter in the book *Language Disorders in Children and Adults*.[1]

My use of the Colourful Semantics approach has continued to develop and expand over the last 27 years, more often using symbols rather than written words to help the children recognise each 'meaning chunk' of the sentence. New colours have been also added, linked to other question words such as 'When', 'How' and 'Why', to help extend simple sentences with information not directly connected with the verb semantics.

Colourful Semantics can be used to support both spoken and written sentence development (understanding as well as expression), narrative and word/fact learning. One development that occurred nearly 20 years ago was a slight change in the colours from those originally published. This came about because I worked in Hertfordshire, where my Colourful Semantics was being used in the East and North Speech and Language bases and Susan Ebbels' Shape Coding was being used in the West bases. Therapists and children were crossing the border, so to enable easier transitions I changed 'Where' from red to blue (in line with the colour used for prepositions in shape coding) and changed 'What like' from blue to a cloud shape (in line with shape coding for adjectives).

Little did I know that therapists, both across the country and abroad, were using the published chapter to try the approach with their children, with the original colours. They too were extending and developing the approach.

So I come to this amazing Colourful Semantics Resource Pack. With just the original chapter as their source the authors, in conjunction with education staff, have developed a comprehensive resource which can be used both in schools and by therapists working in clinical contexts and is flexible for use with whole classes, small groups and individuals. You will find easy to apply session plans which gradually build up the children's spoken and written language skills. All the cue cards, sentence templates and worksheets to support the delivery of Colourful Semantics sessions can be found in the appendices of this pack. The authors have also come up with some great activities to engage the children, my particular favourite being silly sentence necklaces, referred to in the session plans!

I am particularly grateful to the authors for letting me have some input as this resource pack was being prepared for publication. This has enabled some very slight adaptations to the original pack which makes it compatible with the both the Colourful Semantics colours used by the authors and the updated colours I use in my own work and for my training courses. A black and white version also enables its use by practitioners who are using their colour system with Colourful Semantics principles. This makes the resource very flexible and so enables thousands of speech and language therapists, teaching staff and children to benefit from the hard work and commitment of those who contributed to the development of this pack.

I cannot praise this resource too highly. At its core it remains faithful to the original concept of Colourful Semantics, i.e. identifying the verb and the meaning relationships connected with it. After all, it is called 'Colourful Semantics' and not 'Colourful Grammar'. This is not the case with many resources I have come across online!

A huge well done to all those involved in developing this pack. Speech and language therapists, teaching staff and children across the UK and beyond will be extremely grateful. THANK YOU.

Alison Bryan
Developer of Colourful Semantics

Note

1 S. Chiat, J. Law and J. Marshall (eds) (1997) *Language Disorders in Children and Adults: Psycholinguistic Approaches to Therapy*, London, Whurr.

Introduction

Colourful Semantics is an approach, created by Alison Bryan, which was primarily devised to develop spoken language. However, the principles of the approach can easily be applied to support development of children's written language skills. There is a growing body of evidence as to the essential role of spoken language in supporting literacy development. If a child has difficulties with spoken language, such as a limited vocabulary, poor understanding of spoken language, short sentences and/or poor use of verbs, these difficulties will translate to the written word.

Colourful Semantics is a visual sentence building approach which uses colour coding, symbols and signs. It aims to:

- develop understanding of *wh-* questions;
- increase sentence complexity;
- develop children's vocabulary;
- increase range and complexity of verbs (children with delayed or disordered spoken language skills often overuse simple verbs such as *do, go* or *get*);
- improve children's written language skills.

This pack provides a detailed approach to developing sentence structure, focusing on key components of a sentence before looking at the sentence as part of a wider narrative. Each component of a sentence is allocated a colour, a symbol and a Makaton sign.

This resource pack is designed for therapists, teachers and other educational personnel who wish to develop the spoken and written language skills of children. Our local Colourful Semantics approach and related resources have been developed in conjunction with education staff.

Most of the resources in this pack have been developed to be used with children from age four up to eight and can be used with individuals, small groups and whole classes. Ready-made session plans are provided, which have been designed by speech and language therapists and teachers. They are a suggestion only and can be easily differentiated for different ages and abilities. Additional resources within the pack include vocabulary pictures, cue cards, sentence planners and example worksheets. The resources can be used to apply Colourful Semantics principles to spoken and written language activities across the curriculum, to generalise children's skills.

We are grateful to the author of the published Easylearn resources *Write About the Picture*, *Sequencing Pictures* and *More Sequencing Pictures* for permission to use their images throughout this pack, including in the sentence building resources and example picture description and picture sequences worksheets. These are resources which are useful tools to complement the Colourful Semantics approach, using images that are clear, interesting and motivating for children to write about. Examples of differentiated picture description and sequencing worksheets are included in this pack in Appendix 7 and support children at a variety of writing ability levels to transfer their spoken language skills to early sentence and story writing. Easylearn resources are available to purchase from www.tes.com.

The Colourful Semantics colour coding system

The Colourful Semantics approach allocates a colour to each key component in a sentence. However, the colour coding system used alongside the approach may differ from area to area.

This Colourful Semantics Resource Pack provides materials that are fully adaptable for different colour coding systems used alongside the Colourful Semantics approach.

Black and white resources are provided which can be adapted for any colour system that may be being used. Additionally, a set of colour online resources is available which will support those using the current colourful semantics colours developed by Alison Bryan, currently in popular use in many areas of the UK and internationally. Finally, resources are also provided online for a further, adapted colour coding system. Developed and used locally in NHS Forth Valley, Scotland, these colours have been successfully used to align with colours used in published narrative resources, such as those developed by Black Sheep Press, which are often used in local education settings alongside Colourful Semantics.

The colours used for each sentence component in the two colour coding systems detailed above are outlined in the table below.

Question	Current Colourful Semantics Colours	NHS Forth Valley Colours
Who	Orange	Orange
Doing (verb)	Yellow	Yellow
What	Green	Blue
Where	Blue	Red
When	Brown	Green
Why	Purple	Brown
To Who	Pink	Pink
How	Black	Purple

Chapter 1
Using Colourful Semantics with individual children

Colourful Semantics is helpful in supporting children with specific difficulties, including those who are on the Speech and Language Therapy caseload, such as children with Developmental Language Disorders, language delay or Hearing Loss.

Sentence components can be introduced individually, to help build up children's understanding of each before being used in sentences. Sentence components can be combined into sentences at each stage of sentence building, from the 'who' plus 'doing' stage onwards.

1. 'Doing' (verbs)

As the verb is the key to the meaning of a sentence, it is important to introduce this first in Colourful Semantics sessions. Many children who have spoken language difficulties have poor verb knowledge and may require a number of sessions to improve their knowledge and storage of verbs. There are many different types of activities that can be used but it is essential that the verb is linked with the correct colour, cue card and sign (yellow in both colour coding systems included within this pack). When introducing the verb, begin by using the word 'doing' but link the word 'verb' as appropriate.

Suggested 'doing' activities
- Encourage the child to identify 'doing' words in stories and books. Children can be given cards to hold up when they hear a 'doing' word being read aloud.
- Using 'doing' pictures, take turns with the child to act out the 'doing' word.
- Make lotto, pairs or snap games using the 'doing' pictures provided.
- Depending on the child's literacy abilities, they can be provided with simple sentences and can be asked to underline the 'doing' word in the correct colour.

2. 'Who'

Once you feel that the child has knowledge of a variety of verbs and is secure in linking them to the correct colour, cue card and sign, 'who' can be introduced. Again it is important to spend time on activities which will help the child link the 'who' to its colour, cue card and sign.

Suggested 'who' activities
- Encourage the child to identify the 'who' in stories and books. Children can be given cards to hold up when they hear a 'who' being read aloud.
- 'Who am I' game – using the 'who' pictures provided, take turns with the child to give clues about the pictures.

Once the child has a good grasp of the meaning of 'who', they can begin activities using the 'who' and the 'doing' together.

Suggested 'who' and 'doing' activities

- Sorting game – the child matches the 'who' and 'doing' pictures to their corresponding cue card.
- Detective game – the child is given cue cards. The adult will then say an example of a 'doing' or 'who' word, such as 'jumping' or 'farmer', and the child has to hold up the correct cue card. This activity can be transferred to the gym hall, where the children can run to corresponding stations.
- Silly sentences – the child is encouraged to choose a 'who' and a 'doing' from their respective piles to make a sentence, by placing them under their corresponding cue card and saying the sentence.
- Use a 'Draw a Line' or 'Cut and Stick' worksheet from this pack with a 'who' and 'doing' word.

At this stage, you can begin to support the child to build sentences using picture supports. Some sample resources can be found in Appendix 3. Appendix 1 also contains cue card sentence template and box templates which support this sentence building. An example of how to carry out a sentence building activity is provided below.

- The child is given a main picture to describe using a sentence and is then given various cues to support the structuring of the sentence.
- A cue card sentence template with question words is used to prompt the child. The cue card sentence template used can be differentiated to support the stage the child is at. The child is given individual pictures (with or without the accompanying written word) that match the components of the sentence.
- The child can then use the blank box template underneath the cue card sentence template to place the pictures in the correct order.
- Alternatively, the child could be given a selection of pictures for each sentence component and then asked to choose the appropriate picture from the selection to make the sentence,
  o e.g. in the example below, for 'who' the child is asked to choose between symbols for 'the boy', 'the baby' and 'the princess'; for 'doing' the child chooses between 'is driving', 'is swinging' and 'is climbing'.
- The child is then supported to say the sentence.
- The child is then asked to identify each component, e.g. 'Who is swinging?', 'What is the boy doing?' or 'Tell me "who" is in the sentence'.

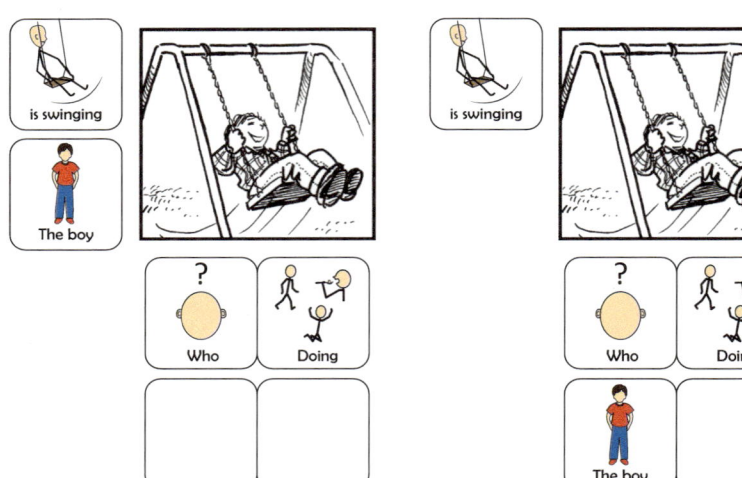
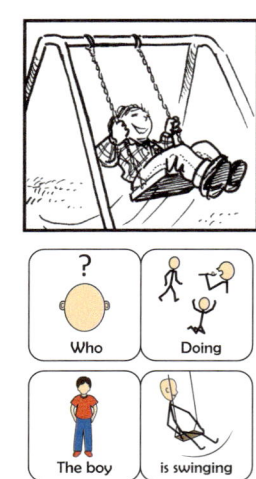

3. 'What'

Next introduce 'what'. Many children have already begun verbally adding 'what' to their sentences so it can usually be introduced quite quickly. A small amount of time should be spent introducing 'what' pictures and linking them to the colour, cue card and sign.

Many of the activities already mentioned can be used to introduce 'what'.

Suggested additional activities

- Fill in the missing word, e.g. The girl is brushing _____. Depending on the child's literacy skills, this may also be done as a written task.
- Encourage the child to provide a simple piece of news including a 'who', 'doing' and 'what'. The child can then draw and/or write their sentence.

4. Where

When carrying out sentence building activities, it is essential to include the step 'who' 'doing' 'where'. This requires omitting the 'what' initially, then reintroducing this once the child is familiar with 'where'. This is important because certain 'doing' words do not need a 'what' and would not make sense if this sentence component were included. Such verbs include 'crawl', 'jump' and 'run'.

Following the above step, reintroduce 'what' as required, to combine 'who' 'doing' 'what' and 'where' into sentences.

All previously suggested activities can be used to consolidate the child's understanding of 'where' using the 'where' pictures.

5. To who

Few verbs contain 'to who' as an essential component. However, when using certain verbs, e.g. give, show, pass, it is important to teach the 'to who' element of the sentence.

The 'who' pictures provided can be used for this stage, but should be linked with the **'to who'** colour, cue card and sign.

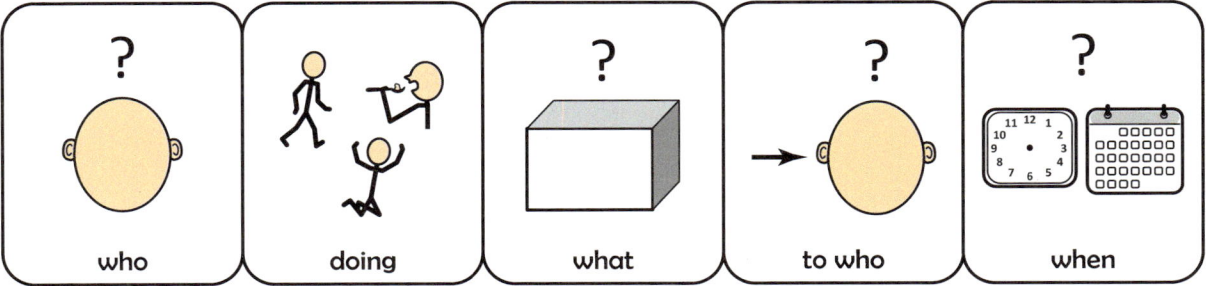

- Silly sentences can be made using 'to who' after 'what', e.g. **the girl is giving the cake *to the dinosaur***. However, omit 'where' until 'to who' is consolidated before adding this in, e.g. **the girl is giving the cake to the dinosaur *in the forest***.
- Many of the previously suggested activities can be used at this stage, including 'Cut and Stick' worksheets provided in this pack.

6. When

'When' would usually be taught after the 'who' 'doing' 'what' 'where' stage, again linking this to the colour, cue card and sign. It should be explained to the children that the 'when' does not have a fixed position in a sentence and can be placed at the beginning or end.

Time concepts can often be difficult for children with language disorder to learn and retain. Additional time may need to be spent teaching the child about days of the week, months of the year and concepts like 'today', 'tomorrow' and 'yesterday'. The introduction of 'when' is a good opportunity to introduce past, present and future verb tenses and highlight the different forms verbs can take dependent on 'when' something happened.

7. Why and how

'Why' should be taught first and linked to the cue card, colour and sign. At this stage the child is being encouraged to expand beyond a simple sentence.

- 'Why' can be introduced using a simple 'who doing what' sentence, e.g. 'the man is drinking the juice *because he is thirsty*'. Children will often require lots of examples before being able to generate their own 'why'.
- This can be a difficult stage to teach if the child relies heavily on visual material. Why/because cards can be a useful resource to help children learn this concept.
- Sentence length can be increased by adding 'where', 'when' or even 'to who' if appropriate.

'How', meaning the way an action is carried out, can be introduced in a similar way, linking it to its cue card, colour and sign. Use a simple 'who doing what' sentence, e.g. 'the man is painting the fence', and support the child to generate how he might do this, e.g. '*with paint and a brush*'.

Adjectives (what like)

The Colourful Semantics approach enables you to easily integrate teaching of adjectives, supporting children to increase the complexity of their sentences. Once children are confident in building who, doing, what sentences, they can be encouraged to use adjectives to add description. Examples of adjectives which relate to 'who', 'what', 'where' or 'when' can be provided by the teacher or speech and language therapist before supporting the children to generate their own. Adjectives can be visually represented in the sentence in the form of a cloud, which can be placed within or above the sentence component that it describes, e.g.

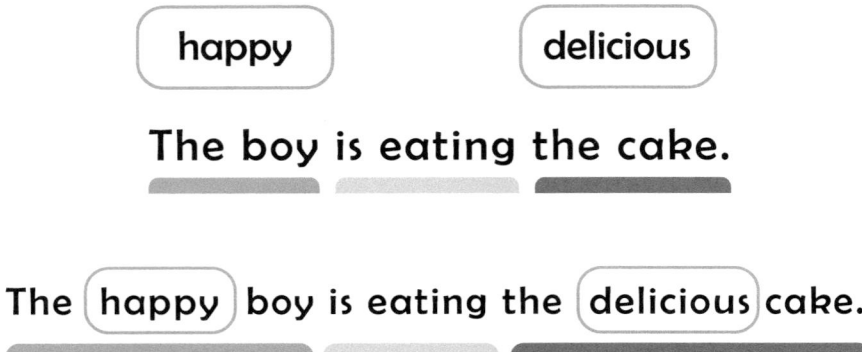

Chapter 2

Colourful Semantics for classes and groups

Introduction

There is a solid evidence base from researchers and practitioners of the key importance of spoken language and its link to learning. The link between spoken and subsequent success in written language is clear. Colourful Semantics has been developed to support children's spoken language but is easily adapted to support development of written language skills.

The session plans in this pack have been developed to be used with children from approximately age four to eight years but can be adapted to be used with older children. The session plans focus on both spoken and written language skills and can be used with whole classes and small groups. Our education partners have been very influential in the design of our whole class and group lesson plans. These session plans are a guide only and can be easily adapted to different ages and abilities. They are designed for sentences up to the 'why' stage, but can easily be adapted and extended to include teaching of 'how' and 'to who' depending on the learners' abilities.

The session plans in this pack are provided in black and white. However, you should use resources in colour as directed, according to the colour coding system you are using.

Colourful Semantics session plans – ages 4–6 years

Session 1

Aims	Description and strategies	Differentiation	Resources
• To be familiar with the cue card colour, name and Makaton sign for 'who?' and 'doing?' • To independently match the cue card colour and name with the Makaton sign.	**Whole class** Introduce large cue cards to class for 'who' and 'doing', demonstrating the Makaton signs for each. Explain that 'who' refers to a person/animal/character and 'doing' refers to an action you can do. Get the whole class to join in copying the signs and saying the words. **Small group** Children work in groups of four to practise the signs together. Adults move around groups and check children know the signs that match each cue card. Select children to show to the class.	**Step up** Ask children to generate 'who' and 'doing' vocabulary by asking about a class story. **Step down** Reinforce the 'who' and 'doing' vocabulary by playing guessing games with the children, e.g. 'Who swims in a pond?', 'Who puts out fires?' etc.	Large coloured cue cards for 'who' and 'doing'.
• To be familiar with the 'doing' cue card. • To be able to name 'doing' words (verbs). • To act out a 'doing' word for others to guess.	**Whole class** Review the 'doing' card. Ask the class to show you the Makaton sign for 'doing'. Show class a coloured verb vocabulary card. Model acting this out with another adult guessing the 'doing' word. **Pairs** Give a child in each pair a verb vocabulary picture card. When directed by the adult, they can look at it and mime it for their partner to guess. Get feedback from children: Could they guess? Did anyone have a tricky one? Ask them out to the front and help them model it. Invite the child to choose someone else doing still, quiet sitting to take a guess. Now the other partner gets a go. Adult(s) move around the pairs to ensure children are talking about the verbs and can think of actions for their given word.	**Step up** Give more challenging action word pictures to more able children. Ask them if they can use the 'doing' word from their picture in a sentence. **Step down** Consider grouping less able children together and giving adult support with modelling of action words.	Large coloured 'doing', 'what', 'where' and 'when' cue card. Small coloured verb ('doing') vocabulary cards.

- To know the order that words come in a sentence.
- To know how to make a silly sentence.
- To be able to identify parts of a sentence.
- To be able to colour code written vocabulary.

Whole class

Put the cue cards in the correct order for the children on the board, getting the children to name and sign 'who' and 'doing' as you go along.

Model a silly sentence containing a 'who' and 'doing' word using the A5 vocabulary cards. Get the class to say it together.

Model another but this time ask the children to tell you where the words go. Then have all the children say it together.

Worksheet – whole class

Model an example of a 'Draw a Line' worksheet with a 'who' and 'doing' on the board first.

Worksheet – individual

Children then make their own silly sentence by completing a 'Draw a Line' worksheet with 'who' and 'doing'. Individually, children choose their favourite silly sentence by joining a 'who' and 'doing' word. They then write out their sentence, underlining each sentence component in the correct colour. They can then draw a picture of it.

Whole class or pairs

Share your favourite silly sentence with the class or your partner.

Step up

More able children can write the sentence on the board.

Step down

Less able children will need individual or small group reinforcement of the colour, Makaton sign and word type.

Large coloured cue cards for 'who' and 'doing'.

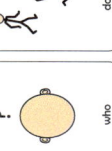
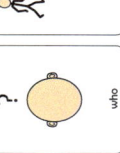

A5 coloured vocabulary cards for 'who' and 'doing'.

(N.B. Use only the 'doing' words on pages 118–119 for this activity, since these do not require a 'what' in order for the sentences made to make sense).

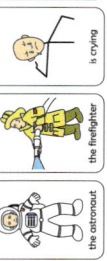
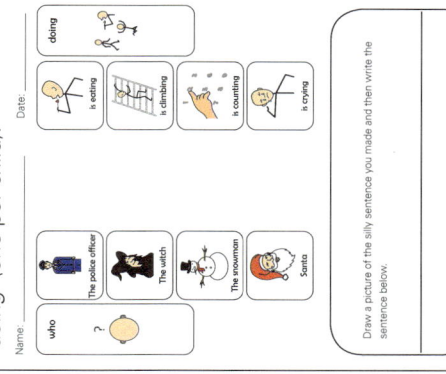

Silly sentences 'Draw a Line' worksheet with a 'who' and 'doing' (one per child).

Writing pencils.

Coloured pencils or pens to match the 'who' and 'doing' colours.

Colourful Semantics session plans – ages 4–6 years

Session 2

Aims	Description and strategies	Differentiation	Resources
• To revise the cue card colour, name and sign for 'who?' and 'doing?' • To be familiar with the cue card colour, name and sign for 'what'.	**Whole class** Ask the children to help you put the cue cards in the correct order and stick on the board. As you go along, get them to name the cue card, say its colour and sign the word. Explain today there's a new card: 'what'. Introduce with the Makaton sign. Can anyone think of a 'what' word? It may be necessary to clarify the difference between the question being asked and the answer to the question (i.e. the vocabulary you want the children to generate).	**Step up** More able children could generate a word to go with each cue card. **Step down** Ensure less able children are joining in with the Makaton sign and saying the word on each cue card.	Large coloured cue cards for 'who', 'doing' and 'what'.
• To be familiar with the 'doing' card. • To be able to name 'doing' words (verbs). • To act out a 'doing' word for others to guess.	**Whole class** Review the 'doing' card. Ask the class to show you the Makaton sign for 'doing'. Show the class a coloured verb vocabulary picture card. Model acting this out with another adult guessing the 'doing' word. **Pairs** Give a child in each pair a verb vocabulary picture card. When directed by the adult, they can look at it and mime it for their partner to guess. Get feedback from children: Could they guess? Did anyone have a tricky one? Ask them out to the front and help them model it. Invite the child to choose someone else doing still, quiet sitting to take a guess. Now other partner gets a go. Adult(s) move around the pairs to ensure children are talking about the verbs and can think of actions for their given word.	**Step up** Give more challenging action word pictures to more able children. Ask them if they can use the 'doing' word in a sentence. **Step down** Consider grouping less able children together and giving adult support with modelling of action words.	Large coloured cue card for 'doing'. Small coloured verb ('doing') vocabulary cards.

Objectives	Activity	Step up / Step down	Materials
• To be able to identify parts of a sentence. • To use the given vocabulary to make a silly sentence.	**Small group** Give each group a 'who', 'doing' or 'what' word on a coloured A5 vocabulary card. Give groups one or two minutes to discuss and agree on the type of word they have been given. **Whole class** When the time is up, ask class what word is first in the sentence ('who'). Ask a group that thinks they have the 'who' to come out to the front with their card. Repeat for 'doing' and 'what'. Once you have completed the sentence say it as a class, write the sentence on the board and colour code it by underlining the written words.	**Step up** More able children can write up the silly sentence on the board as the cards are brought up to the front, or have a turn at being the teacher and asking the 'wh' question to other children. **Step down** Less able children can colour code the written words on board. Reinforce the word type by asking e.g. 'who is in your sentence?'	Large coloured cue cards for 'who', 'doing' and 'what'. A5 coloured vocabulary cards for 'who', 'doing' and 'what'.
• To be able to sort vocabulary into 'who', 'doing' and 'what'. • To be able to make silly sentences with a 'who', 'doing' and 'what'.	**Pairs** Model the use of a story planner grid and small vocabulary cards to make silly sentences. Give each pair a selection of 'who', 'doing' and 'what' cards (two of each kind) and a story planner grid. Adult moves around the pairs and asks the children to say their sentences out loud. Model for the children how to use 'little words' in their sentences, e.g. 'the' and 'is'. Children in each pair then say one silly sentence they have made out loud to the class.		Coloured story planner grids with 'who', 'doing' and 'what'. Small coloured vocabulary cards for 'who', 'doing' and 'what'.

Session 2 follow-up activity

Aims	Description and strategies	Differentiation	Resources
• To know how to make a silly sentence. • To be able to write and colour code a sentence.	**Worksheet – whole class** Model an example of a 'Draw a Line' worksheet with a 'who', 'doing' and 'what' on the board first. **Worksheet – individual** Children complete a 'Draw a Line' worksheet with a 'who', 'doing' and 'what', writing out their sentence, underlining each sentence component in the correct colour and drawing a picture of it underneath.	**Step down** Use a 'who' and 'doing' worksheet for less able children.	Silly sentences 'Draw a Line' worksheet with a 'who', 'doing' and 'what'. Writing pencils. Coloured pencils to match the 'who', 'doing' and 'what' colours.

Colourful Semantics session plans – ages 4–6 years

Session 3

Aims	Description and strategies	Differentiation	Resources
• To revise the cue card colour, name and Makaton sign for 'who' and 'doing'. • To be familiar with the cue card, sign and colour for 'where'.	**Whole class** Briefly recap the 'who' and 'doing' cue cards, reinforcing the colour, name and Makaton sign. Introduce 'where' cue card. Explain today there's a new card – introduce with Makaton sign and emphasise what colour 'where' is. Explain that not all 'doing' words need a 'what' so we are missing that out today. Can anyone think of a 'where' word? Have some 'where' questions prepared as a quiz. May need to clarify the difference between the question word on the cue card and the answers (i.e. the vocabulary you want the children to generate).	**Step up** More able children could generate vocabulary to go with each card. More able children generate own clues/think of own 'where' word to describe. **Step down** Ensure less able children are joining in with the sign and saying the word. Could have visual prompts for 'where' and adult supports them to generate clues.	Large coloured cue cards for 'who', 'doing' and 'where'. Prepared questions for a 'where' quiz.
• To identify vocabulary as 'who', 'doing' or 'where'. • To use given vocabulary to make silly sentences with a 'who', 'doing' and 'where'.	**Groups** Give each group an A5 vocabulary card with either a 'who', 'doing' or 'where' word on it. Give each group two minutes to discuss and agree on the type of word they have been given. When the time is up ask what word is first in the sentence ('who'). Ask a group that thinks they have a 'who' word to come out to the front with their card. Repeat for 'doing' and 'where' and for a few sentences. (Note: use the 'doing' words on pages 118 and 119 for this task, as these do not require a 'what' word for the sentence to make sense.) Once you have completed the sentences, say them as a class and colour code the written sentences on the board by underlining.	**Step up** More able children can be asked to use the word on their card in a sentence. If class are more able writers, can get them to write their ideas on the board. **Step down** Prompt less able children by asking specific questions to help them name the words.	Large coloured cue cards for 'who', 'doing' and 'where'. A5 coloured vocabulary cards for 'who', 'doing' and 'where'.

Session 3 follow-up activity

Aims	Description and strategies	Differentiation	Resources
• To be able to make a silly sentence with a 'who', 'doing' and 'where'. • To be able to write and colour code a sentence with a 'who', 'doing' and 'where'. • To understand the difference between the 'wh' question and the 'wh' answers to the 'wh' questions.	**Worksheet – whole class** Model an example of a 'Draw a Line' worksheet with a 'who' 'doing' and 'where' on the board first. **Worksheet – individual** Children then complete a 'Draw a Line' worksheet with a 'who', 'doing' and 'where', writing out their sentence, underlining each sentence component in the correct colour and drawing a picture of it underneath. **Pairs** In pairs, children take turns to be the teacher and ask their partner a 'wh' question about their sentence and their partner has to answer. This can also be done as a whole class activity.	**Step up** More able children can be asked to up-level their sentences with adjectives. **Step down** Less able children could be supported by adults to identify the vocabulary in the pictures first and, if necessary, colour code them as a reminder for when they come to build the sentence. Could use a 'who', 'doing' worksheet instead. Adult can write sentence and the child can underline the vocabulary.	Large coloured cue cards for 'who', 'doing' and 'where'. Silly sentences 'Draw a Line' worksheet with a 'who', 'doing' and 'where' (one per child). Writing pencils. Coloured pencils to match the 'who', 'doing' and 'where' colours.

Colourful Semantics session plans – ages 4–6 years

Session 4

Aims	Description and strategies	Differentiation	Resources
• To revise the cue card colour, name and Makaton sign for 'who', 'doing', 'what' and 'where'.	**Whole class** Revise the 'who', 'doing', 'what' and 'where' cards and their meaning. As you go along, ask children to name, say the colour and sign. Remind children of recent sessions on 'who', 'doing' and 'what', and 'who', 'doing' and 'where'. Explain that now we are going to make longer silly sentences that put all these words together. Put the cue cards in the correct order on the board. Alternatively, give each cue card to one child, on a piece of string to wear as a necklace. Support the children wearing the necklaces to arrange themselves into the right order for a sentence.	**Step up** More able children could generate vocabulary to go with each cue card. **Step down** Ensure less able children are joining in with the sign and saying the name of the cue cards.	Large coloured cue cards for 'who', 'doing', 'what' and 'where'.
• To identify vocabulary as 'who', 'doing', 'what' or 'where'. • To use given vocabulary to make a silly sentence with a 'who', 'doing', 'what' and 'where'.	**Groups** Give a coloured vocabulary card to each group/table. Give each group two minutes to discuss and agree on the type of word they have been given. When the time is up ask what word is first in the sentence ('who'). Ask which group(s) think they have a 'who'. One person from a group with 'who' comes out to the front with their card and/or gives their card to the person wearing the 'who' necklace. Repeat for 'doing', 'what' and 'where' and for a few sentences. Once you have completed the sentences, say them as a class and colour code written sentences on the board by underlining.	**Step up** If class are more able writers, can get them to write their ideas on the board. **Step down** Less able children can be prompted by asking specific questions to support them to name the word pictured on the vocabulary card.	Large coloured cue cards for 'who', 'doing', 'what' and 'where' (enough for all tables). A5 coloured vocabulary cards for 'who', 'doing', 'what' and 'where'.

Session 4 follow-up activity

Aims	Description and strategies	Differentiation	Resources
• To know how to make a silly sentence with 'who', 'doing', 'what' and 'where' words in the correct order. • To be able to write and colour code a sentence.	**Worksheet – Whole class** Model an example of a 'Cut and Stick' worksheet with a 'who', 'doing', 'what' and 'where' word for the whole class/on the board first. **Worksheet – Individual** Children then complete a 'Cut and Stick' worksheet with a 'who', 'doing', 'what' and 'where'. Children then write out their sentence, underlining each sentence component in the correct colour and drawing a picture of it on the back.	**Step down** Use a 'who', 'doing' and 'what' worksheet for less able children.	Silly sentences 'Cut and Stick' worksheet with a 'who', 'doing', 'what' and 'where'. Writing pencils. Coloured pencils to match the 'who', 'doing', 'what' and 'where' colours.

- To use a 'who', 'doing', 'what' and 'where' word in a sentence that is more personal.

This is an activity that can be done during the week, e.g. at news time, where the children's news can be structured using the colourful semantics prompts.

Whole class

Ask children to tell what they were doing at the weekend, using a 'who', 'doing', 'what' and 'where' word.

Step up

More able children could write down their ideas independently or could add a describing word to one of the parts of their sentence.

Step down

Less able children could generate a 'who', 'doing', 'what' and 'where' sentence using a colourful semantics story planner grid to plan.

Large coloured cue cards for 'who', 'doing', 'what' and 'where'.

Coloured story planner grids with a 'who', 'doing', 'what' and 'where'.

Colourful Semantics session plans — ages 4–6 years

Session 5

Aims	Description and strategies	Differentiation	Resources
• To be able to recall cue card colours, names and Makaton signs for 'who', 'doing', 'what' and 'where' from previous session. • To put 'who', 'doing', 'what' and 'where' words in the correct order for a sentence.	**Whole class** Ask children to help you organise the cue cards in the correct sequence, stick on board at front or give cue cards to children on silly sentence necklaces. As you go along get them to name, say the colour and do the sign for each cue card. Ask children to generate vocabulary for each cue card.	**Step down** Ensure that less able children are joining in with the sign and saying the words, colours and signs for the cue cards. Prompt less able children with clues, e.g. 'where' can you find a sheep, horse and pig?	Large coloured cue cards for 'who', 'doing', 'what' and 'where'.
• To identify vocabulary as 'who', 'doing', 'what' or 'where' words, without colour clues. • To sequence and use given vocabulary to make a silly sentence with a 'who', 'doing', 'what' and 'where'.	**Whole class** Explain that you are challenging the children to think about what kind of words they have been given by using only white vocabulary cards with no colour clues. **Groups** Give each group a white vocabulary card. Give two minutes for groups to discuss and agree on the type of word they have been given – a 'who', 'doing', 'what' or 'where' word. When the time is up ask what word is first in the sentence ('who'). Ask someone from the group that thinks they have the 'who' to come out to the front with their card/give it to the person with the 'who' necklace on. Once you have completed the sentence say it as a class, write it on the board and colour code it by underlining.	**Step up** More able children could use the word they were given in a sentence of their own. If class are more able writers, they could write their ideas on the board themselves. **Step down** Prompt less able children by asking specific questions, e.g. 'who' makes your dinner after school?	Large coloured cue cards for 'who', 'doing', 'what' and 'where'. Optional: cue cards above attached to string to wear as a necklace. A5 white vocabulary cards for 'who', 'doing', 'what' and 'where'.

Objective	Activity	Differentiation	Resources
• To describe a picture using a 'who', 'doing', 'what' and 'where' word.	**Whole class** Class come to the floor. Use smart board to show a picture (such as Easylearn *Write About the Picture* or a picture related to a current topic). Remind the children that we cannot always make silly sentences. Sometimes we have to be able to make a real sentence about an idea that might be in our heads for a story or something we want to tell someone, so we are going to practise using a picture. Ask the children to look at the picture and in pairs discuss the 'who', 'doing', 'what' and 'where' ideas in the picture.	**Step up** More able children can add a describing word for the 'who' and/or 'where'. **Step down** Adult to support less able children.	Easylearn *Write About the Picture* or other relevant picture to describe.
• To write about a picture using a 'who', 'doing', 'what' and 'where' word. • To identify written words as 'who', 'doing', 'what' or 'where'.	**Individual** Children go back to their table and write about the picture discussed above, using a 'who', 'doing', 'what' and 'where' word, and colour code it by underlining.	**Step up** Give more able children worksheets with individual vocabulary mixed up to reorder, or allow them to generate their own vocabulary. **Step down** Give less able children worksheets with vocabulary already in the correct order. Less able children could write just the 'who', 'doing' and 'what'.	Worksheet containing the picture discussed above (differentiated for different abilities). Worksheet: Autumn Leaves Name: _____ Date: _____ Write a sentence about the autumn leaves picture, using the question words below for ideas. Colour the question words the correct colours first to help you. After writing your sentence, underline the 'who', 'doing', 'what' and 'where' words in the correct colour. who doing what where

Aims	Description and strategies	Differentiation	Resources
			Name: _____ Date: _____ Write a sentence about the autumn leaves picture. Colour the question words and small pictures in the correct colours first to help you. After writing your sentence, underline the 'who', 'doing', 'what' and 'where' words in the correct colour. Worksheet: Autumn Leaves

Session 5 follow-up activity

Aims	Description and strategies	Differentiation	Resources
• To generate spoken and written sentences with 'who', 'doing', 'what' and 'where' words based on a picture.	**Whole class** Introduce the picture to the class. Children work with a partner and share with each other what is happening in the picture. Display the picture and the colourful semantics story planner grid on the smart board, helping the class generate vocabulary related to it, i.e. ask them to tell you the 'who', then 'doing', then 'what' and 'where'.		Picture to discuss, e.g. *Write About the Picture*. Coloured story planner grid with 'who', 'doing', 'what' and 'where' on large piece of paper or smart board.

Colourful Semantics session plans – ages 4–6 years

Session 6

Aims	Description and strategies	Differentiation	Resources
• To generate vocabulary for 'who', 'doing', 'what' and 'where'.	**Whole class** Put 'who', 'doing', 'what', 'where' cue cards in the middle of a circle. Children take it in turns to throw the beanbag onto one of the cue cards and then generate a related word.	**Step up** More able children could be asked to make a sentence using the word they thought of. **Step down** Support less able children to generate words using questions and gestures.	Large coloured cue cards for 'who', 'doing', 'what' and 'where'. Bean bag.
• To be familiar with cue card colour, name and Makaton sign for 'when'.	**Whole class** Introduce the 'when' cue card. Discuss the colour and demonstrate Makaton sign. Talk about the position of 'when' in the sentence – it can go at the start or the end of the other cue cards.	**Step down** Support less able children to identify a 'when' word by giving them a choice of two, e.g. 'When would you see fireworks? At Halloween or on Bonfire Night?'	As above plus coloured 'when' cue card.
• To be familiar with 'when' vocabulary.	**Whole class** Help the children generate 'when' words. Have a selection of 'when' vocabulary on the board; ask 'when' questions and the children choose the correct answer from the choices. **Pairs** Optional: Hand out some 'when' cards so the children can describe their word to a partner.	**Step up** Ask more able children to come out and choose a card and give clues. Other children to guess 'when' it is they are describing. **Step down** Provide additional support for less able children to describe their 'when', e.g. giving choices (is it Easter or Christmas?), sentence completion (you get a cake with candles when it's your ...?).	Selection of A5 coloured 'when' vocabulary.

21

Session 6 follow-up activity

Aims	Description and strategies	Differentiation	Resources
• To be able to sort words into 'who', 'doing', 'what', 'where' and 'when'.	**Whole class** Have the large coloured cue cards in order on the board and put A5 vocabulary pictures for each into piles. Children take it in turns to come up to the front of the class and pick a picture from each pile and put the word under the correct colour of cue card. Once all the parts of the sentence have a picture, children say the sentence together. Link to verb tenses by explaining to the class that when we use the 'when' words it often changes the 'doing' words. Give some examples, using mixture of past/present/future tenses. Sometimes stop in the middle of the sentence and ask children next to each other to discuss a silly or sensible ending to the sentence.	**Step up** More able children could be asked to use describing words in their sentence. **Step down** For less able children, do not ask them to use 'when' in their sentence.	Large coloured cue cards for 'who', 'doing', 'what', 'where' and 'when'. Selection of A5 coloured vocabulary cards.
• To be able to make a silly sentence with a 'who', 'doing', 'what', 'where' and 'when'. • To be able to write and colour code a sentence with a 'who', 'doing', 'what', 'where' and 'when'. • To understand the difference between the 'wh' question and answers given (vocabulary).	**Worksheet – whole class** Model an example of a 'Draw a Line' worksheet with a 'who', 'doing', 'what', 'where' and 'when' on the board first. **Worksheet – individual** Children then complete a 'Draw a Line' worksheet with a 'who', 'doing', 'what', 'where' and 'when'. Ask them to write out their sentence, underlining each sentence component in the correct colour and drawing a picture of it on the back. **Pairs** In pairs, children take turns to be the teacher and ask their partner a 'wh' question about their sentence and their partner has to answer. This can also be done as a whole class activity.	**Step up** More able children can up-level their sentences with describing words. **Step down** Less able children can be supported by adults to identify the vocabulary in the pictures first and colour code them as a reminder for when they come to build the sentence. Adult can write sentence and child can underline the vocabulary.	Large coloured cue cards for 'who', 'doing', 'what', 'where' and 'when'. Silly sentences 'Draw a Line' worksheet with a 'who', 'doing', 'what', 'where' and 'when' (one per child).

Writing pencils.

Coloured pencils to match the 'who', 'doing', 'what', 'where' and 'when' colours.

Colourful Semantics session plans – ages 4–6 years

Session 7

Aims	Description and strategies	Differentiation	Resources
• To generate words related to 'who', 'doing', 'what', 'where' and 'when'.	**Whole class** Ask children to help you organise the cue cards in the correct sequence and stick them on the board. As you go along get them to name, say the colour and use the Makaton sign for each cue card. Ask children to generate vocabulary for each cue card.	**Step up** More able children can be asked to make a sentence about the word they have chosen. **Step down** Support less able children to generate vocabulary by giving verbal and gesture clues.	Large coloured cue cards for 'who', 'doing', 'what', 'where' and 'when'.
• To describe a picture using a 'who', 'doing', 'what', 'where' and 'when' word.	**Whole class** Show a stimulus picture and have individual vocabulary pictures/symbols on the board to go with the different parts of the sentence. Ask children to organise the symbols into the right order on a story planner to describe the picture. Children to read out sentence as a class. Children to ask each other questions about the picture.	**Step up** More able children could be encouraged to use describing words for e.g. the 'who' or 'where'. **Step down** Provide prompts for less able children.	Picture to describe, e.g. Easylearn *Write About the Picture* 'The Airport'. Symbols, such as Boardmaker PCS symbols, to represent parts of the sentence.

- To write about a picture using a 'who', 'doing', 'what', 'where' and 'when' word.

Individual
Children to complete a worksheet at a level appropriately differentiated for them, e.g. 'Cut and Stick', written worksheet.

Step up
Give more able children written worksheets with mixed up vocabulary, or ask them to generate their own vocabulary about the picture for their sentences.

Step down
Use written worksheets with vocabulary already in the correct order for less able children.

Coloured sentence planner on board with 'who', 'doing', 'what', 'where' and 'when'.

Picture description worksheet, differentiated for different ability levels but with same content.

Worksheet: The Airport

Name: _____ Date: _____

Write a sentence about the airport picture. Colour the question words and small pictures in the correct colours first to help you. After writing the sentence, underline the 'who', 'doing', 'what', 'where' and 'when' words in the correct colour.

Session 7 follow-up activity

Aims	Description and strategies	Differentiation	Resources
			Worksheet: The Airport Name: _____ Date: _____ Write a sentence about the airport picture. Colour the question words and small pictures in the correct colour first to help you. Then work out which order the words in the sentence should come in. After writing your sentence, underline the 'who', 'doing', 'what', 'where' and 'when' words in the correct colour. when · who · when · what · where watched · the family · at the airport · Yesterday · aeroplanes doing

Colourful Semantics session plans – ages 4–6 years

Session 8

Aims	Description and strategies	Differentiation	Resources
• To recall the colours, names and Makaton signs for all cue cards – 'who', 'doing', 'what', 'where' and 'when'. • To generate vocabulary for 'who', 'doing', 'what', 'where' and 'when'.	**Whole class** Choose a cue card – get children to demonstrate the Makaton sign for the cue card and name the card. Select children to take a turn to think of a word for a particular cue card, e.g. 'can you think of a "who" word?' Select children by getting them to listen and stand up if they match the criteria that you call, e.g. 'if you're a girl with a pink ribbon in your hair, think of a "who" word', 'if you're a boy with Velcro on your shoes, think of a "where" word', etc.	**Step up** Ask more able children to make a sentence with the word they have given. **Step down** Prompt less able children to generate vocabulary by offering gestural or descriptive clues.	Large coloured cue cards for 'who', 'doing', 'what', 'where' and 'when'.
• To generate spoken sentences with 'who', 'doing', 'what', 'where' and 'when' words related to a two-part picture sequence.	**Whole class** Introduce the idea of writing about more than one picture. Explain that this means we can tell a story. Look at a two-part picture sequence as a class first. **Pairs** Pairs of children work together and tell each other what they think is happening in the story. Use a story planner grid (hard copy or on the smart board), helping the class to generate vocabulary related to the story, i.e. point to the first picture and ask them to say what is the 'who', then 'doing', then 'what', 'where' and 'when'. Explain that the sentence about the first picture should include all the sentence components. However, we don't need them all for the second sentence. Discuss that we could make two sentences or we could use 'joining words' to make one longer sentence about the story.	**Step up** Encourage more able children to use describing words, e.g. for the 'who' or 'where'. **Step down** Prompt less able children to generate words by giving clues or a choice of two possible words.	Two-part picture sequences, e.g. Easylearn Sequencing Pictures/ More Sequencing Pictures or Black Sheep Press 2 Part sequences. Story planner grid with a 'who', 'doing', 'what', 'where' and 'when'.

Session 8 follow-up activity

Aims	Description and strategies	Differentiation	Resources
• To write about a two-part picture sequence using 'who', 'doing', 'what', 'where' and 'when' words.	**Individual** Children go back to their tables to complete a worksheet about the two-part picture sequence discussed above.	**Step up** More able children write their own sentences and add describing words. **Step down** Support less able children to plan the sentences together first. Provide symbols to sort for children who find it difficult to write or generate vocabulary. Write the sentence for them if needed, for them to copy or overwrite. Get them to colour code/underline the sentence parts.	Two-part picture sequence worksheets, differentiated according to different children's ability levels. Worksheet: The picnic Worksheet: The picnic

Colourful Semantics session plans – ages 4–6 years

Session 9

Aims	Description and strategies	Differentiation	Resources
• To recap cue card names, colours and signs for 'who', 'doing', 'what', 'where' and 'when'. • To correctly sequence cue cards to make a sentence.	**Whole class** Ask children to help you organise the cue cards in the correct sequence and stick them on the board at front. As you go along get them to name the cue card and say its colour and sign. Ask children to generate vocabulary for each cue card.	**Step up** You can ask more able children to make a sentence using the word they generated. **Step down** Prompt less able children to generate vocabulary by giving clues.	Large coloured cue cards for 'who', 'doing', 'what', 'where' and 'when'.
• To generate spoken sentences with 'who', 'doing', 'what', 'where' and 'when' words related to a two-part sequence picture.	**Whole class** Look at sequence on the smart board as a class first. Use symbols to represent different sentence components that make up the story. Support the children to organise the symbols on the board to generate two sentences about the sequence. Choose children to ask the class 'wh' questions about the sequence.	**Step up** Encourage more able children to ask their peers questions about the story. **Step down** Prompt less able children to generate vocabulary by giving clues.	Two-part picture sequences, e.g. Easylearn *Sequencing Pictures/ More Sequencing Pictures* or Black Sheep Press 2 Part sequences. Symbols, such as Boardmaker PCS, to go with the picture sequence.

Session 9 follow-up activity

Aims	Description and strategies	Differentiation	Resources
• To generate written sentences with *'who'*, *'doing'*, *'what'*, *'where'* and *'when'* words related to a two-part sequence picture.	**Individual** Children go back to their tables to complete a worksheet about the two-part picture sequence discussed above.	**Step up** Use written worksheets with mixed up vocabulary or without given vocabulary for more able children. **Step down** Use worksheets with vocabulary that is already in the correct order or give symbols to 'Cut and Stick' for less able children.	Two-part picture sequence worksheets, differentiated according to different children's ability levels.
• Celebration task.	Support the children to reflect on what they have learned and why it has been useful. Give certificates to all children.		

Colourful Semantics session plans – ages 5–8 years

Session 1

Aims	Description and strategies	Differentiation	Resources
• To be familiar with cue card colour, name and Makaton sign for 'who', 'doing' and 'what'.	**Whole class** Introduce large cue cards to class for 'who', 'doing' and 'what' with Makaton signs for each. Explain that 'who' refers to a person/animal/character, 'doing' refers to an action you can do and 'what' refers to an object/thing. Get whole class to join in copying the signs and saying the words. **Small group** Children work in groups of four to practise the signs together. Adults to move around groups and check children know the signs that match each cue card. Select children to show to the class.	**Step up** Ask children to generate 'who', 'doing' and 'what' vocabulary by asking about a class story. **Step down** Reinforce the 'who', 'doing' and 'what' vocabulary by playing guessing games with the children, e.g. 'Who swims in a pond?', 'Who puts out fires?' etc.	Large coloured cue cards for 'who', 'doing' and 'what'.
• To be familiar with the 'doing' card. • To be able to name 'doing' words (verbs). • To act out a 'doing' word for others to guess.	**Whole class** Review the 'doing' card. Ask the class to show you the Makaton sign for 'doing'. Show the class a coloured verb vocabulary picture card. Model acting this out with another adult guessing the 'doing' word. **Pairs** Give a child in each pair a verb vocabulary picture card. When directed by the adult, they can look at it and mime it for their partner to guess. Get feedback from children: Could they guess? Did anyone have a tricky one? Ask them out to the front and help them model it. Invite the child to choose someone else doing still, quiet sitting to take a guess. Now other partner gets a go. Adult(s) move around the pairs to ensure children are talking about the verbs and can think of actions for their given word.	**Step up** Give more challenging action word pictures to more able children. Ask them if they can use the 'doing' word in a sentence. **Step down** Consider grouping less able children together and giving adult support with modelling of action words.	Large coloured verb ('doing') cue card. Small coloured verb ('doing') vocabulary cards.

Session 1 follow-up activity

Aims	Description and strategies	Differentiation	Resources
• To know the order that words come in a sentence. • To know how to make a silly sentence. • To be able to identify parts of a sentence. • To be able to colour code written vocabulary.	**Whole class** Put the cue cards in the correct order for the children, getting the children to name and sign *who*, *doing* and *what* as you go along. Model a silly sentence containing a *who*, *doing* and *what* word using the A5 vocabulary cards. Get the class to say it together. Model another but this time ask the children to tell you where the words go. Then have all the children say it together. **Worksheet – whole class** Model an example of a 'Draw a Line' worksheet with a *who*, *doing* and *what* on the board first. **Worksheet – individual** Children then make their own silly sentence by completing a 'Draw a Line' worksheet with *who*, *doing* and *what*. Individually, children choose their favourite silly sentence by joining *who*, *doing* and *what* words. They then write out their sentence, underlining each sentence component in the correct colour. They can then draw a picture of it. **Whole class or pairs** Share your favourite silly sentence with the class or your partner.	**Step up** More able children can write the sentence on the board. **Step down** Less able children will need individual or small group reinforcement of the colour, Makaton sign and word type.	Large coloured cue cards for *'who'*, *'doing'* and *'what'*. A5 coloured vocabulary cards for *'who'*, *'doing'* and *'what'*. Silly sentences 'Draw a Line' worksheet with a *'who'*, *'doing'* and *'what'* (one per child).

Colourful Semantics session plans – ages 5–8 years

Session 2

Aims	Description and strategies	Differentiation	Resources
• To revise cue card colour, name and Makaton sign for *'who'* and *'doing'*. • To be familiar with the cue card, sign and colour for *'where'*.	**Whole class** Briefly recap the 'who' and 'doing' cue cards, reinforcing the colour, name and Makaton sign. Introduce 'where' cue card. Explain today there's a new card – introduce with Makaton sign and emphasise what colour *'where'* is. Explain that not all *'doing'* words need a *'what'* so we are missing that out today. Can anyone think of a *'where'* word? Have some *'where'* questions prepared as a quiz. May need to clarify the difference between the question word on the cue card and the answers (i.e. the vocabulary you want the children to generate).	**Step up** More able children could generate vocabulary to go with each card. More able children generate own clues/think of own *'where'* word to describe. **Step down** Ensure less able children are joining in with the sign and saying the word. Could have visual prompts for *'where'* and adult supports them to generate clues.	Large coloured cue cards for *'who'*, *'doing'* and *'where'*. Prepared questions for a *'where'* quiz.
• To identify vocabulary as *'who'*, *'doing'* or *'where'*. • To be able to use given vocabulary to make silly sentences with a *'who'*, *'doing'* and *'where'*.	**Groups** Give each group an A5 vocabulary card with either a *'who'*, *'doing'* or *'where'* word on it. Give each group two minutes to discuss and agree on the type of word they have been given. When the time is up ask what word is first in the sentence (*'who'*). Ask someone from a group that thinks they have a *'who'* word to come out to the front with their card. Repeat for *'doing'* and *'where'* and for a few sentences. (Note: use the *'doing'* words on pages 118 and 119 for this task, as these do not require a *'what'* word for the sentence to make sense.) Once you have completed the sentences, say them as a class and colour code the written sentences on the board by underlining.	**Step up** More able children can be asked to use the word on their card in a sentence. If class are more able writers, can get them to write their ideas on the board. **Step down** Prompt less able children by asking specific questions to help them name the words.	Large coloured cue cards for *'who'*, *'doing'* and *'where'*. A5 coloured vocabulary cards for *'who'*, *'doing'* and *'where'*.

Session 2 follow-up activity

Aims	Description and strategies	Differentiation	Resources
• To be able to make a silly sentence with a 'who', 'doing' and 'where'. • To be able to write and colour code a sentence with a 'who', 'doing' and 'where'. • To understand the difference between the 'wh' question and the vocabulary, i.e. the answers to the 'wh' questions.	**Worksheet – whole class** Model an example of a 'Draw a Line' worksheet with a 'who', 'doing' and 'where' on the board first. **Worksheet – individual** Children then complete a 'Draw a Line' worksheet with a 'who', 'doing' and 'where', writing out their sentence, underlining each sentence component in the correct colour and drawing a picture of it. **Pairs** In pairs, children take turns to be the teacher and ask their partner a 'wh' question about their sentence and their partner has to answer. This can also be done as a whole class activity.	**Step up** More able children can be asked to up-level their sentences with adjectives. **Step down** Less able children could be supported by adults to identify the vocabulary in the pictures first and, if necessary, colour code them as a reminder for when they come to build the sentence. Could use a worksheet with just 'who' and 'doing' instead. Adult can write sentence and the child can underline the vocabulary.	Large coloured cue cards for 'who', 'doing' and 'where'. Silly sentences 'Draw a Line' worksheet with a 'who', 'doing' and 'where' (one per child). Writing pencils. Coloured pencils to match the 'who', 'doing' and 'where' colours.

Colourful Semantics session plans – ages 5–8 years

Session 3

Aims	Description and strategies	Differentiation	Resources
• To revise the cue card colour, name and Makaton sign for *'who'*, *'doing'*, *'what'* and *'where'*.	**Whole class** Revise the *'who'*, *'doing'*, *'what'* and *'where'* cards and their meaning. As you go along, ask children to name, say the colour and sign. Remind children of recent sessions on *'who'*, *'doing'* and *'what'*, and *'who'*, *'doing'* and *'where'*. Explain that now we are going to make longer silly sentences that put all these words together. Put the cue cards in the correct order on the board. Alternatively, give each cue card to one child, on a piece of string to wear as a necklace. Support the children wearing the necklaces to arrange themselves into the right order for a sentence.	**Step up** More able children could generate vocabulary to go with each cue card. **Step down** Ensure less able children are joining in with the sign and saying the name of the cue cards.	Large coloured cue cards for *'who'*, *'doing'*, *'what'* and *'where'*.
• To be able to generate vocabulary for *'who'*, *'doing'*, *'what'* and *'where'*.	**Small groups** Split the class into groups. Each group is given a different cue card. Set the timer for 2–3 minutes. On 'go', the children pass the card around the table so that each child has the opportunity to generate vocabulary for that cue card. Swap cards after 2–3 minutes and repeat until each group has had a turn for each 'wh' cue card. Adult(s) move around groups supporting children to generate vocabulary.	**Step up** More able children could use the word they have generated in a sentence. If class are more able writers, can get them to write their ideas on a large piece of paper. **Step down** Prompt less able children by asking specific questions to support them to name words.	Large coloured cue cards for *'who'*, *'doing'*, *'what'* and *'where'*. Timer. Optional: large piece of paper.
• To identify vocabulary as *'who'*, *'doing'*, *'what'* or *'where'*. • To use given vocabulary to make a silly sentence with a *'who'*, *'doing'*, *'what'* and *'where'*.	**Groups** Give each group a *'who'*, *'doing'*, *'what'* or *'where'* vocabulary card. Give each group one or two minutes to discuss and agree on the type of word they have been given.	**Step up** More able children can write up the silly sentence on the board as the cards are brought up to the front. Get the children to have a turn at being the teacher and asking the 'wh' question to other children.	Large coloured cue cards for *'who'*, *'doing'*, *'what'* and *'where'* (enough for all tables). Optional: attach cue cards to string for chosen children to wear as 'necklaces'.

Session 3 follow-up activity

Aims	Description and strategies	Differentiation	Resources
	Whole class When the time is up ask what word is first in the sentence ('*who*'). Ask which group(s) think they have a '*who*'. One person from a group with '*who*' comes out to the front with their card and/or gives their card to the person wearing the '*who*' necklace. Repeat for '*doing*', '*what*' and '*where*' and for a few sentences. Once you have completed the sentences, say them as a class and colour code written sentences on the board by underlining.	**Step down** Less able children can colour code the written words on board. Reinforce the word type by asking a question, e.g. '*who* is in your sentence?' Prompt less able children by asking specific questions to support them to name the word pictured on the vocabulary card.	A5 vocabulary cards for '*who*', '*doing*', '*what*' and '*where*'. Use coloured cards or white cards, depending on ability level of group. is washing the firefighter is zipping the astronaut the elephant the cereal in the kitchen in the haunted house Timer.

• To be able to identify vocabulary as *'who'*, *'doing'*, *'what'* or *'where'* words. • To be able to make silly sentences with *'who'*, *'doing'*, *'what'* and *'where'* words.	**Pairs** Model the use of a story planner grid and small vocabulary cards to make silly sentences. Give each pair a selection of *'who'*, *'doing'*, *'what'* and *'where'* cards (eight cards in total) in an envelope and a story planner grid. Practise making up 'silly' sentences in their grids. Adult move around the pairs and ask the children to say their sentences out loud. Choose children to say a silly sentence they have made out loud to the class.	**Step up** Get more able children to have a turn at being the teacher and asking the 'wh' questions to other children. 	Coloured story planner grid with *'who'*, *'doing'*, *'what'* and *'where'*. Envelopes with small, coloured vocabulary cards for *'who'*, *'doing'*, *'what'* and *'where'* – two of each card per pair.

During the week you can get the children to complete a *'who'*, *'doing'*, *'what'*, *'where'* silly sentence worksheet.

Colourful Semantics session plans – ages 5–8 years

Session 4

Aims	Description and strategies	Differentiation	Resources
• To revise the cue card colour, name and Makaton sign for 'who', 'doing', 'what' and 'where'.	**Whole class** Revise the 'who', 'doing', 'what' and 'where' cards and their meaning. As you go along, ask the children about the colour, the name of the cue card, the Makaton sign and where in the sentence the word goes.	**Step up** More able children could generate vocabulary to go with each cue card. **Step down** Ensure less able children are joining in with the sign and saying the name of the cue cards.	Large coloured cue cards for 'who', 'doing', 'what' and 'where'.
• To be able to identify the 'who', 'doing', 'what' and 'where' parts of a sentence. • To be able to use the given vocabulary to make a silly sentence.	**Small group** Split the class into either four or eight groups. Each table gets a different vocabulary card. Give each group two minutes to discuss and agree on the type of word they have been given. When the time is up ask what word is first in the sentence ('who') and ask which group thinks they have a 'who'. That group come out to the front with their card. Repeat for 'doing', 'what' and 'where'. **Whole class** Once you have completed the sentences say them as a class and colour code written sentences on the board.	**Step up** More able children to use the word in a sentence. If class more able writers, can get them to write their ideas on the board. **Step down** Prompt less able children by asking specific questions, e.g. 'where would you see a nurse?'	Large coloured cue cards for 'who', 'doing', 'what' and 'where' (enough for all tables to have one). A5 white vocabulary cards for 'who', 'doing', 'what' and 'where'. Timer.

- To be able to sort vocabulary correctly as 'who', 'doing', 'what' or 'where'.
- To be able to make a silly sentence with a 'who', 'doing', 'what' and 'where' word.
- To understand the difference between the 'wh' question and the 'wh' vocabulary (answer to the 'wh' question).
- To be able to write and colour code a sentence with a 'who', 'doing', 'what' and 'where'.

Worksheet – whole class

Model an example of a 'Cut and Stick' worksheet with a 'who', 'doing', 'what' and 'where' at the front of the class.

Worksheet – individual

Children then complete a 'Cut and Stick' worksheet with a 'who', 'doing', 'what' and 'where'. Children cut, sort and stick their favourite vocabulary to make their own silly sentence. They then write out their sentence, underlining each sentence component in the correct colour and drawing a picture of it on the back.

Pairs

In pairs, children take turns to be the teacher and ask their partner a 'wh' question about their sentence and their partner has to answer. This can also be done as a whole class activity.

Step up

More able children can up-level their sentences with adjectives/wow words.

Step down

For less able children, the adult can support to identify the pictures first and if necessary colour code them as a reminder for when children come to build the sentence.

Could simplify using a 'who', 'doing', 'what' worksheet instead.

Adult could write sentence and child can underline the vocabulary.

Silly sentences 'Cut and Stick' worksheet with 'who', 'doing', 'what' and 'where'.

Coloured pencils.

Scissors.

Glue.

Writing pencil.

Colourful Semantics session plans – ages 5–8 years

Session 5

Aims	Description and strategies	Differentiation	Resources
• To be familiar with colour, name and Makaton sign for *'when'*. • To be able to identify *'when'* words from clues.	**Whole class** Recap *'who'*, *'doing'*, *'what'*, *'where'* cue cards. Introduce the *'when'* cue card, referring to its colour and demonstrating its Makaton sign. Discuss that *'when'* refers to time. CT to discuss some *'when'* words from the classroom by referring to timetable/days of the week/seasons, etc. **Small group** Each group is given a *'when'* picture to discuss – *'when'* is it? Give two minutes to discuss. Feedback on *'when'* words from group task to put on board. Adults can give clues for the children to guess the *'when'* word, e.g. *'when'* do we get a cake with candles?' Give points to the team the answer came from. Whichever team reaches e.g. five points first wins. Talk about how *'when'* can go at the beginning or end of the sentence and demonstrate this.	**Step up** Ask more able children to be the teacher and give the clues. Ask the children about *'when'* the current class text is set. **Step down** Give each individual group clues until they are able to guess the word so that they have more time to think.	Large coloured cue cards for *'who'*, *'doing'*, *'what'*, *'where'* and *'when'*. A5 coloured *'when'* vocabulary cards. Timer. A5 coloured vocabulary cards for *'who'*, *'doing'*, *'what'*, *'where'* and *'when'*, to demonstrate the position of *'when'*.

- To be able to make silly sentences with 'who', 'doing', 'what', 'where' and 'when' words.

Pairs

Give each pair 10 cards (two for each cue card), which they should put in order to construct two 'silly' sentences on their story planner grid.

Adult to move around the pairs and ask the children to say their sentences out loud. Pairs choose their favourite sentence to feed back to class.

Step up

More able children can use plain white cards– not colour coded and/or write a sentence about what happens next.

Step down

Less able children can have all cards colour coded and adult support to name the vocabulary.

Coloured story planner grid with a 'who', 'doing', 'what', 'where' and 'when'.

Small coloured vocabulary cards for 'who', 'doing', 'what', 'where' and 'when', in envelopes, or white cards for more able children.

Session 5 follow-up activity

Aims	Description and strategies	Differentiation	Resources
• To be able to make a silly sentence with a 'who', 'doing', 'what', 'where' and 'when' word. • To be able to write and colour code a sentence with a 'who', 'doing', 'what', 'where' and 'when'.	**Worksheet – whole class** Model an example of a 'Draw a Line' worksheet with a 'who', 'doing', 'what', 'where' and 'when' at the front of the class. **Worksheet – Individual** Children then complete a 'Draw a Line' worksheet with a 'who', 'doing', 'what', 'where' and 'when'. Children draw lines between their favourite vocabulary to make their own silly sentence. They then write out their sentence, underlining each sentence component in the correct colour and drawing a picture of it underneath. **Pairs** In pairs, children take turns to be the teacher and ask their partner a 'wh' question about their sentence and their partner has to answer. This can also be done as a whole class activity.	**Step up** More able children can up-level their sentences with wow words. **Step down** For less able children, the adult can support to identify the pictures first and if necessary colour code them as a reminder for when they come to build the sentence. Could use a 'who', 'doing', 'what', 'where' worksheet instead. Adult could write sentence and child can underline the vocabulary.	Silly sentences 'Draw a Line' worksheet with 'who', 'doing', 'what', 'where' and 'when'. Writing pencil. Coloured pencils.

Colourful Semantics session plans – ages 5–8 years

Session 6

Aims	Description and strategies	Differentiation	Resources
• To revise cue card colour, name and Makaton sign for 'who', 'doing', 'what', 'where' and 'when'. • To be able to generate vocabulary for 'when'.	**Whole class** Recap 'who', 'doing', 'what', 'where' and 'when' cue cards. Discuss cue card colours, revise Makaton signs and names of cards. Remind children of new 'when' card from last session and that it refers to a time. Ask the children to identify where in the sentence each cue card comes as they are put up. Children are asked to discuss 'when' with a partner and generate vocabulary for it. Ask for feedback from pairs on the words they identified.	**Step up** Ask more able child to be the teacher and give the clues. Ask the children about 'when' the current class text is set. **Step down** Give each individual group clues until they are able to guess the word so that they have more time to think.	Large coloured cue cards for 'who', 'doing', 'what', 'where' and 'when'. Timer.
• To be able to identify 'who', 'doing', 'what', 'where' and 'when' words. • To be able to use 'who', 'doing', 'what', 'where' and 'when' vocabulary to make a silly sentence.	**Small group** Split the class into five or ten groups. Each group gets a different vocabulary card. Give each group two minutes to discuss and agree on the type of word they have been given. When the time is up ask what word is first in the sentence ('who') and ask which group thinks they have a 'who'. That group come out to the front with their card. Repeat for 'doing', 'what', 'where' and 'when'. **Small group** Once you have completed the sentences say them as a class and colour code written sentences on the board.	**Step up** More able children to use the word in a sentence. If class more able writers, can get them to write their ideas on the board. **Step down** Prompt less able children by asking specific questions to help them name words and identify the kind of word.	Large coloured cue cards for 'who', 'doing', 'what', 'where' and 'when'. A5 white vocabulary cards for 'who', 'doing', 'what', 'where' and 'when'.

Aims	Description and strategies	Differentiation	Resources
• To be able to make spoken sentences with 'who', 'doing', 'what', 'where' and 'when'.	**Pairs** Give each pair ten small vocabulary cards (two for each cue card) and a story planner grid. They should put the vocabulary cards in order on their grid to construct two 'silly' sentences. Adult to move around the pairs and ask the children to say their sentences out loud. Pairs choose their favourite sentence to feed back to the class.	**Step up** More able children can use plain white cards – not colour coded and/or write a sentence about what happens next. **Step down** Less able children can have all cards colour coded and adult support to name the vocabulary.	Coloured story planner grids with a 'who', 'doing', 'what', 'where' and 'when'. Small coloured vocabulary cards for 'who', 'doing', 'what', 'where' and 'when', in envelopes, or white cards for more able children.

- To be able to describe a picture using a 'who', 'doing', 'what', 'where' and 'when' word.

Whole class

Class come to the floor. Use smart board to show a picture (such as Easylearn Write About the Picture). Explain that we cannot always make silly sentences. Sometimes we have to be able to make a real sentence about an idea that might be in our heads for a story or something we want to tell someone so we are going to practise using a picture.

Ask the children to look at the picture and in pairs discuss the 'who', 'doing', 'what', 'where' and 'when' in the picture.

Large cue cards for 'who', 'doing', 'what', 'where' and 'when'.

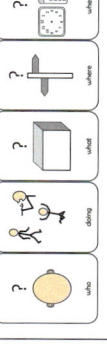

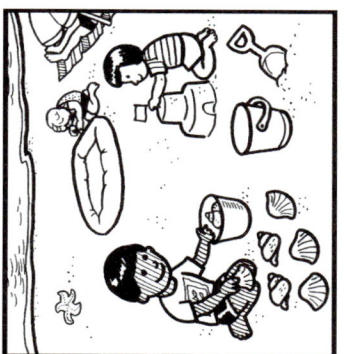

Picture to describe, containing a 'who', 'doing', 'what', 'where' and 'when', e.g. Easylearn *Write About the Picture* – 'The Beach'.

Step up

More able children to up-level their sentence using a wow word.

Step down

Less able children to make a sentence using a 'who', 'doing' and 'what' or 'who', 'doing', 'what' and 'where'.

Colourful Semantics session plans – ages 5–8 years

Session 7

Aims	Description and strategies	Differentiation	Resources
• To be able to generate vocabulary for 'who', 'doing', 'what', 'where' and 'when'. • To be able to generate a sentence with a 'who', 'doing', 'what', 'where' and 'when'.	Recap cue cards. **Groups** Have children at tables. Give each table a coloured cue card (either a 'who', 'doing', 'what', 'where' or 'when') and give each child at the table a piece of that colour of paper. They are to think of any word in that group, write or draw the word on the piece of paper and write the word at the top. Remind children they can speak to an adult/a partner to check if unsure.	**Step up** More able children could add in a wow word to describe their chosen word. **Step down** Adult to support less able children with questions/clues.	Large coloured cue cards for 'who', 'doing', 'what', 'where' and 'when' (enough for all tables). Blank squares of card/paper in variety of colours to match the 'who', 'doing', 'what', 'where' and 'when' cue cards (enough for one card per child). Writing pencils. Colouring pencils.
• To be able to construct a sentence with 'who', 'doing', 'what', 'where' and 'when' words in the correct order.	**Whole class** Explain that from the last task there are now enough words to make up silly sentences and it is the children's job to get into groups that would make a sentence. Children to make up groups of five that have a 'who', 'doing', 'what', 'where' and 'when'. Once they have found all members, they sit down in their groups and put their pictures in the correct order to tell a sentence. Each group tells the class the silly sentence they have made. To support children to get into groups, perhaps call them first into groups by word type, e.g. all the people with a 'who' sit together.	**Step up** Encourage more able children to use extra description/wow words. **Step down** Adult to support less able children to generate a word for their sentence component.	Coloured squares of card/paper with hand drawn/written vocabulary from previous activity.

- To be able to describe a picture using a 'who', 'doing', 'what', 'where' and 'when' word.

Whole class

Class come to the floor and do a practice picture together as last session.

Show them a picture, such as one from Easylearn *Write About the Picture* or related to a current class topic.

Children look at picture on board or a hard copy and with a partner discuss the 'who', 'doing', 'what', 'where' and 'when'. Then take ideas from the class and write the ideas on a story planner displayed on the board.

Picture to describe, e.g. Easylearn *Write About the Picture* – 'The Airport' picture.

Coloured story planner grids with a 'who', 'doing', 'what', 'where' and 'when'.

Step up

More able children can add a wow word, e.g. to describe the 'who' or 'where'.

Step down

Adult to support less able children.

Session 7 follow-up activity

Aims	Description and strategies	Differentiation	Resources
• To write about a picture using a 'who', 'doing', 'what', 'where' and 'when' word.	**Individual** Children then complete a picture description worksheet, differentiated to appropriate levels – e.g. with sorted vocabulary, with mixed up vocabulary, or without vocabulary given so that children can generate their own ideas.		Picture description worksheet for the picture described above, differentiated for different ability levels but with same content. Worksheet: The Airport Name: _____ Date: _____ Write a sentence about the airport picture. Colour the question words and small pictures in the correct colour first to help you. After writing the sentence, underline the 'who', 'doing', 'what', 'where' and 'when' words in the correct colour.

Name: _____ Worksheet: The Airport Date: _____

Write a sentence about the airport picture, using the question words below for ideas. Colour the question words the correct colours first to help you. After writing yours sentence, underline the 'who', 'doing', 'what', 'where' and 'when' words in the correct colour.

| when ? | who ? | doing ? | what ? | where ? |

During the week, children can be asked to use a *'who'*, *'doing'*, *'what'*, *'where'* and *'when'* word in a sentence that is more personal, for example when sharing news. Use the Colourful Semantics prompts to help facilitate news time.

Colourful Semantics session plans – ages 5–8 years

Session 8

Aims	Description and strategies	Differentiation	Resources
• To be able to generate vocabulary related to 'who', 'doing', 'what', 'where' and 'when'.	**Whole class** Recap cue cards. Choose a cue card and ask children to name the card, say its colour and show the Makaton sign. Split class into two groups. Each group sits in a circle with cue cards in the centre. Throw a beanbag and generate vocabulary for the cue card the beanbag landed on.	**Step up** Ask more able children to use the word they generated to make a sentence. **Step down** Support less able children by asking specific questions or giving choices to help them generate ideas.	Two copies of large cue cards for 'who', 'doing', 'what', 'where' and 'when'.
• To generate spoken sentences with 'who', 'doing', 'what', 'where' and 'when' words related to a two-part picture sequence.	**Whole class** Introduce the idea of writing about more than one picture. Explain that this means we can tell a story. Look at a two-part picture sequence as a class first. **Pairs** In pairs, children tell each other what they think is happening in the story. Use a story planner grid (hard copy or on the smart board), to write up vocabulary generated related to the story, i.e. point to the first picture and ask them to say what is the 'who', then 'doing', then 'what', 'where' and 'when'. Explain that the sentence about the first picture should include all the sentence components. However, we don't need them all for the second sentence. Discuss that we could make two sentences or we could use 'joining words' to make one longer sentence about the story.	**Step up** Encourage more able children to use describing words, e.g. for the 'who' or 'where'. **Step down** Prompt less able children to generate words by giving clues or a choice of two possible words.	Two-part picture sequences, e.g. Easylearn *Sequencing Pictures/ More Sequencing Pictures* or Black Sheep Press 2 Part sequences. Story planner grid with a 'who', 'doing', 'what', 'where' and 'when'.

- To write about a two-part picture sequence using 'who', 'doing', 'what', 'where' and 'when' words.

Individual

Children go back to their tables to complete a worksheet about the two-part picture sequence discussed above.

Step up

More able children can write their own sentences without vocabulary given, or could add describing words.

They could write about what they think might happen next.

Step down

Support less able children to plan the sentences together first.

Provide symbols to sort for children who find it difficult to write or generate vocabulary.

Write the sentence for them if needed, for them to copy or overwrite. Get them to colour code/underline the sentence parts.

Two-part picture sequence worksheets, differentiated according to different children's ability levels.

Colourful Semantics session plans – ages 5–8 years

Session 9

Aims	Description and strategies	Differentiation	Resources
• To be able to generate spoken sentences with *'who'*, *'doing'*, *'what'*, *'where'* and *'when'* words related to a two-part picture sequence.	**Whole class** Recap all the cue cards, naming them and revisiting the Makaton signs. Ask children to help you put the cards in the correct order. Introduce the two-part picture sequence to the class. Children work with a partner to tell each other what they think is happening in the story. Using a large piece of paper or story planner grid on the smart board, help the class generate vocabulary related to the story, i.e. point to the first picture and ask them to say what is the *'who'*, then *'doing'*, then *'what'*, *'where'* and *'when'*. Discuss the connectives you could use to join two sentences together.	**Step up** More able children could be encouraged to use describing words. **Step down** Could do a small group for less able children where you support them to plan the sentence together first on a planner that they can use. If needed, write the sentence for them to colour code.	Large cue cards for *'who'*, *'doing*, *'what'*, *'where'* and *'when'*. Two-part picture sequences, e.g. Easylearn *Sequencing Pictures/ More Sequencing Pictures* or Black Sheep Press 2 Part sequences. Story planner grid with *'who'*, *'doing'*, *'what'*, *'where'* and *'when'* on large piece of paper or smart board.

- To be able to generate written sentences with *'who'*, *'doing'*, *'what'*, *'where'* and *'when'* words related to a two-part picture sequence.

Individual–worksheet

Children go back to their tables and complete a two-part picture sequence worksheet based on the picture sequence discussed above.

Worksheet: Bedtime   Name: _____   Date: _____

Worksheet: Bedtime   Name: _____   Date: _____

Two-part picture sequence worksheets, differentiated according to different children's ability levels.

Step up

Give more able children a worksheet with mixed up vocabulary to sort, allow them to generate their own vocabulary or use the ideas generated by class on the story planner above.

Step down

Use worksheets with vocabulary that is already in the correct order or give symbols to 'Cut and Stick'.

Colourful Semantics session plans – ages 5–8 years

Session 10

Aims	Description and strategies	Differentiation	Resources
• To be familiar with colour, name and Makaton sign for 'why' cue card.	**Whole class** Introduce the 'why' cue card, referring to its colour and demonstrating its Makaton sign. Discuss that 'why' refers to a reason for something happening. Say that we can use connective words such as 'because', 'so' or 'to' to give an answer to a 'why' question. Talk about where the 'why' comes in the sentence, using the opportunity to review and discuss all the other cue cards.	**Step up** More able children could make a whole sentence using a 'why'. **Step down** Give less able children choices of answers to 'why'.	Large cue card for 'why'. Large cue cards for 'who', 'doing', 'what', 'where', 'when' and 'why'.
• To be able to generate vocabulary for 'who', 'doing', 'what', 'where', 'when' and 'why'. • To be able to make a sentence about a picture including a 'who', 'doing', 'what', 'where', 'when' and 'why'.	**Whole class** Use pre-prepared question and answer to support children to answer 'why' questions, e.g. published 'why ... because' cards. Select some pictures, such as from the Easylearn *Write About the Picture* resource. In pairs, ask children to talk about the 'who', 'doing', 'what', 'where' and 'when' from the pictures. Afterwards, can they end the sentence by giving a 'why'? Challenge the children to see how many different ideas they can think of.	**Step up** More able children could use 'why' to ask a question to a peer. **Step down** Ask less able children to recall the ideas they heard shared by a peer.	Why-because pictures, e.g. Black Sheep Press *Why ... because* resource. Selection of pictures to describe, e.g. Easylearn *Write About the Picture*.

• To be able to write about a picture, including a 'who', 'doing', 'what', 'where', 'when' and 'why'.	**Individual** Children then complete a picture description worksheet, related to one of the pictures discussed above and differentiated to appropriate levels, e.g.: – with vocabulary provided, to 'Cut and Stick' – with sorted vocabulary – with mixed up vocabulary – without given vocabulary so children can generate their own ideas.

Step up

More able children could add describing words to their sentence, be given a worksheet with mixed up vocabulary or be asked to generate their own ideas.

Step down

Less able children could write a sentence but miss out the 'why' or have it scribed for them.

'Who', 'doing', 'what', 'where', 'when' and 'why' picture description worksheet, differentiated according to different children's ability levels.

Worksheet: Firefighters

Name: _____ Date: _____

Write a sentence about the firefighters picture. Colour the question words and small pictures in the correct colours first to help you. After writing the sentence, underline the 'when', 'who', 'doing', 'what', 'where' and 'why' words in the correct colour.

Worksheet: Firefighters

Name: _____ Date: _____

Write a sentence about the firefighters picture, using the question words below for ideas. Colour the question words the correct colours first to help you. After writing your sentence, underline the 'when', 'who', 'doing', 'what', 'where' and 'why' words in the correct colour.

Colourful Semantics session plans – ages 5–8 years

Session 11

Aims	Description and strategies	Differentiation	Resources
• To be familiar with the colour, name and Makaton sign for all the cue cards. • To be familiar with the meaning and use of 'why'.	**Whole class** Recap all the 'wh' cue cards, focusing especially on the 'why' card, referring to its colour and demonstrating its Makaton sign. Recap that 'why' refers to a reason for something happening and usually starts with a connective like 'because', 'so' or 'to'. Talk about where the 'why' comes in the sentence, using the opportunity to discuss all the other cue cards.	**Step up** More able children could generate a sentence using a 'why'. **Step down** Give less able children choices of answers to 'why'.	Large cue cards for 'who', 'doing', 'what', 'where', 'when' and 'why'.
• To generate spoken and written sentences with 'who', 'doing', 'what', 'where', 'when' and 'why' based on a two- or three-part sequence picture.	Introduce the sequence pictures to the class. Children work with a partner to tell each other what they think is happening in the story and 'why' it might be happening. Use a story planner grid on the smart board to help the class generate vocabulary related to the story, i.e. point to the first picture and ask them to say what is the 'who', 'doing', 'what', 'where', 'when' and 'why'. Time permitting, children could write two or three sentences using a class story planner, or do a worksheet related to the sequence discussed (or could do this at a later point).	**Step up** More able children to think of more than one 'why'. **Step down** Less able children can just think of a 'who', 'doing', 'what', 'where' and 'when'. Give worksheet with pre-prepared vocabulary to those who need it.	Two- or three-part picture sequences, e.g. Easylearn *Sequencing Pictures/More Sequencing Pictures* or Black Sheep Press 2 Part Sequences/3 Part Sequences.

• Celebration task	Support the children to reflect on what they have learned and why it has been useful. Give certificates to all children.	Story planner grid with 'who', 'doing', 'what', 'where', 'when' and 'why' on large piece of paper or smart board. Optional: two- or three-part sequence worksheets, differentiated for different ability levels.

Colourful Semantics small group session plans
Session 1

Aims	Description and strategies	Resources
• To be familiar with cue card colour, name and sign for '*who*', '*doing*' and '*what*'.	Show the children the '*who*' cue card and ask what colour is it. Show them the Makaton sign for '*who*' and ask them to copy it. Remember to ask the children to say '*who*' at the same time as signing it. Repeat the above with the '*doing*' and '*what*' cue cards.	Large coloured cue cards for '*who*', '*doing*' and '*what*'.
• To be able to generate vocabulary for '*who*', '*doing*' and '*what*'.	Put the large '*who*' cue card up on the board and ask the children to generate examples of '*who*' words. Put '*doing*' up on the board and ask the children to generate some '*doing*' words (i.e. verbs). Prompt them with relevant questions: 'What do you do at playtime?' 'What do you like to do at home?' Repeat again for '*what*' words. Write the words up on a piece of A3 paper for the children – the words can be used at a later date to make up silly sentences. Ask questions to give extra prompts, e.g. '*who* lives in your house?' or '*who* is your friend?'	Pens to match the '*who*', '*doing*' and '*what*' colours. A3 piece of paper. Blu Tack.
• To develop verb vocabulary.	Remind the children about the correct colour for '*doing*' words and revisit the Makaton sign. Use the small verb cards and play 'guess the "*doing*" word' with the children. Demonstrate looking at a verb picture yourself and acting out the picture. Ask the children to guess what you are '*doing*'. If the children say '*brushing* her hair', emphasise which word is the '*doing*' word in the sentence. Give the children a turn at acting out two verbs each for the rest of the children to guess.	Small coloured '*doing*' (verb) cards (approximately 20).
• To create silly sentences containing a '*who*', '*doing*' and '*what*'.	This can be done on the table or on the board. Put up the three cue cards for '*who*', '*doing*' and '*what*'. Arrange piles of coloured vocabulary cards for '*who*', '*doing*' and '*what*'. Each child gets a turn at picking a picture from each pile and putting them below the correct cue card. Support the child to say the sentence. Once they have said it ask them to tell you the '*who*' in the sentence, the '*doing*' and then the '*what*'. Remember to use the Makaton signs to reinforce meaning.	Cue cards for '*who*', '*doing*' and '*what*'. Small piles of coloured vocabulary cards for '*who*', '*doing*' and '*what*' for making sentences.

Colourful Semantics small group session plans
Session 2

Aims	Description and strategies	Resources
• To consolidate familiarity with cue card colour, name and sign for '*who*', '*doing*' and '*what*'.	Show the children the '*who*' cue card and ask the group what colour it is. Show them the Makaton sign for '*who*' and ask them to copy it. Remind the children to say '*who*' at the same time as signing it. Repeat for '*doing*' and '*what*'.	Large coloured cue cards for '*who*', '*doing*' and '*what*'.
• To create silly sentence containing a '*who*', '*doing*' and '*what*'.	This can be done on the table or on the board. Put up the three cue cards for '*who*', '*doing*' and '*what*'. Arrange piles of coloured vocabulary cards for '*who*', '*doing*' and '*what*' above the cue cards. Each child gets a turn at picking a picture from each pile and putting them below the correct cue card. Support the child to say the sentence. Once they have said it ask them to tell you the '*who*' in the sentence, the '*doing*' and then the '*what*'. Remember to use the Makaton signs to reinforce meaning.	Cue cards for '*who*', '*doing*' and '*what*'. Small piles of coloured vocabulary cards for '*who*', '*doing*' and '*what*' for making sentences.
• To write a sentence containing '*who*', '*doing*' and '*what*'.	Carry out a '*who*', '*doing*', '*what*' silly sentence worksheet. Children colour in the '*who*', '*doing*' and '*what*' boxes in the correct colours. Children make simple sentences by drawing a line from a '*who*' to a '*doing*' to a '*what*'. For example, 'The firefighter is peeling the beetle'. The child chooses their favourite sentence, draws a quick picture of it, then writes the sentence below. Children colour code their written sentence by underlining each element in the correct colour to match '*who*', '*doing*' and '*what*', i.e. '*The firefighter*' would be underlined in the correct colour for '*who*', '*is peeling*' would be underlined in the correct colour for '*doing*' and '*the beetle*' would be underlined in the correct colour for '*what*'. Remember to reinforce with the children the importance of including the little function words, e.g. the 'the' within the '*who*' element or the 'is' within the '*doing*' element.	Silly sentences 'Draw a Line' worksheet with a '*who*', '*doing*' and '*what*' (one per child). Coloured pens/pencils.

Aims	Description and strategies	Resources
• To be familiar with cue card colour, name and sign for '*where*'. • To generate vocabulary for '*where*'.	Introduce the '*where*' cue card, its colour and Makaton sign. Support the children to generate '*where*' words. You can ask them questions to help them think of words such as '*where* did you go at the weekend?' Make a 'poster' with '*where*' words written in the correct colour.	Large coloured cue card for '*where*'. ? where A3 piece of paper for poster. Blu Tack.

Colourful Semantics small group session plans
Session 3

Aims	Description and strategies	Resources
• To be familiar with cue card colour, name and sign for '*who*', '*doing*' and '*where*'.	Show the children the '*who*' and ask the group what colour it is. Show them the Makaton sign for '*who*' and ask them to repeat it. Remember to get the children to say '*who*' at the same time as signing it. Repeat for the '*doing*' and '*where*' cue cards. Explain to the children that sometimes '*doing*' words do not need to be followed by a '*what*' word so today we are going to practise sentences just with '*who*', '*doing*' and '*where*'.	Large coloured cue cards for '*who*', '*doing*' and '*where*'.
• To make silly sentences containing '*who*', '*doing*' and '*where*'.	Model a silly sentence as a whole group first. Each child gets a coloured card and has to say what kind of word it is then all children work together to make up silly sentences. For this task, ensure you use only the '*doing*' vocabulary from pages 118–119, which do not require a '*what*' word after them.	Large coloured cue cards for '*who*', '*doing*' and '*where*'. Coloured vocabulary cards for '*who*', '*doing*' and '*where*'.
• To write a silly sentence containing a '*who*', '*doing*' and '*where*'.	Carry out a silly sentence 'Draw a Line' worksheet with a '*who*', '*doing*' and '*where*' with the children. Children colour in the '*who*', '*doing*' and '*where*' *boxes* at the top of the worksheet in the correct colours. The children make simple sentences by drawing a line from a '*who*' to a '*doing*' to a '*where*', for example '*The angel is swimming at the beach*'. The child says the sentence they have made, draws a picture of it, then writes the sentence below. Children colour code their written sentence by underlining each element, i.e. '*The angel*' would be underlined in the correct colour for '*who*', '*is swimming*' would be underlined in the correct colour for '*doing*', etc. Remember to include the little function words, e.g. emphasise 'the' within the '*who*' element and 'is' within the '*doing*' element.	Silly sentences 'Draw a Line' worksheet with a '*who*', '*doing*' and '*where*' (one per child). Coloured pens/pencils.

Aims	Description and strategies	Resources
• To be secure with the concept of '*where*'. • To generate and describe '*where*' vocabulary.	Recap the '*where*' card and give some examples. Give the children some clues and they have to guess the '*where*' word. For example, 'This is *where* you go to do exercise, where you wear a costume and where you get wet' (swimming pool). More able children can give some clues about a '*where*' word for others to guess.	Large coloured cue card for '*where*'. ? where

Colourful Semantics small group session plans
Session 4

Aims	Description and strategies	Resources
• To consolidate familiarity with cue card colour, name and sign for '*who*', '*doing*', '*what*' and '*where*'.	Show the children the '*who*' and ask the group what colour it is. Show them the Makaton sign for '*who*' and ask them to repeat it. Remember to get the children to say '*who*' at the same time as signing it. Repeat for all the cue cards.	Large coloured cue cards for '*who*', '*doing*', '*what*' and '*where*'.
• To make silly sentences containing '*who*', '*doing*', '*what*' and '*where*'.	Explain that today we are going to make longer sentences by using all the cue cards we have learned so far. Model a silly sentence as a whole group first. Each child gets a coloured card and has to say what kind of word it is then all children work together to make up silly sentence.	Large coloured cue cards for '*who*', '*doing*', '*what*' and '*where*'. Coloured vocabulary cards for '*who*', '*doing*', '*what*' and '*where*'.
• To write a silly sentence containing a '*who*', '*doing*', '*what*' and '*where*'.	Carry out a silly sentence 'Draw a Line' worksheet with a '*who*', '*doing*', '*what*' and '*where*' with the children. Children colour in the '*who*', '*doing*', '*what*' and '*where*' boxes at the top of the worksheet in the correct colours. The children make simple sentences by drawing a line from a '*who*' to a '*doing*' to a '*what*' to a '*where*', e.g. 'the baby is baking the grapes in church'. The child says the sentence they have made, draws a picture of it, then writes the sentence below. Children colour code their written sentence by underlining each element, i.e. '*The baby*' would be underlined in the correct colour for '*who*', '*is baking*' would be underlined in the correct colour for '*doing*', etc. Remember to include the little function words, e.g. emphasise '*the*' within the '*who*' element and '*is*' within the '*doing*' element.	Silly sentences 'Draw a Line' worksheet with a '*who*', '*doing*', '*what*' and '*where*' (one per child). Coloured pens/pencils.

Colourful Semantics small group session plans
Session 5

Aims	Description and strategies	Resources
• To consolidate familiarity with cue card colour, name and sign for '*who*', '*doing*', '*what*' and '*where*'.	Show the children the '*who*' and ask the group what colour it is. Ask if they can recall the Makaton sign for '*who*' or model this for them. Remember to get the children to say '*who*' at the same time as signing it. Repeat for all cue cards.	Large coloured cue cards for '*who*', '*doing*', '*what*' and '*where*'.
• To be able to name and sort '*who*', '*doing*', '*what*' and '*where*' vocabulary.	Put white '*who*', '*doing*', '*what*' and '*where*' cards in a feely bag. Children take a turn to pick a card from the bag, name it and then match it to the large cue card it belongs to. For example, '*the man*' would be placed on the '*who*' cue card.	Large coloured cue cards for '*who*', '*doing*', '*what*' and '*where*'. White vocabulary cards for each of the above.
• To create and write silly sentences with a '*who*', '*doing*', '*what*' and '*where*'.	Carry out a silly sentence 'Cut and Stick' worksheet with a '*who*', '*doing*', '*what*' and '*where*' with the children. Children cut, sort and stick their favourite vocabulary to make their own silly sentence. They then write out their sentence, underlining each sentence component in the correct colour and drawing a picture of it on the back.	Silly sentences 'Cut and Stick' worksheet with a '*who*', '*doing*', '*what*' and '*where*' (one per child).

Colourful Semantics small group session plans
Session 6

Aims	Description and strategies	Resources
• To be able to name and sort *'who'*, *'doing'*, *'what'* and *'where'* vocabulary.	Put white *'who'*, *'doing'*, *'what'* and *'where'* cards in a feely bag. Children take a turn to pick a card from the bag, name it and then match it to the large cue card it goes with. For example, *'the flower'* would be placed on the *'what'* prompt card.	Large coloured cue cards for *'who'*, *'doing'*, *'what'* and *'where'*. White vocabulary cards for each of the above.
• To be able to create silly sentences containing a *'who'*, *'doing'*, *'what'* and *'where'*.	Put children into pairs. Each pair has a story planner grid with spaces for a *'who'*, *'doing'*, *'what'* and *'where'* word and a range of eight white vocabulary cards: enough to make two silly sentences. Children choose their favourite silly sentence and write the sentence onto the story planner with each element in the correct column.	Story planner grid with a *'who'*, *'doing'*, *'what'* and *'where'*. White vocabulary cards for each of the above (two of each).
• To be familiar with cue card colour, name and sign for *'when'*. • To generate *'when'* vocabulary.	Introduce the *'when'* cue card, show the Makaton sign for it and link it to its colour. Ask the children to copy and say *'when'* with you whilst doing the sign. **'*When*' quiz** Adults can use *'when'* vocabulary cards to give clues for the children to guess the *'when'* word, e.g. *'when* do we get a cake with candles?'* Give points to the team the answer came from. Whichever team reaches e.g. five points first wins.	Large coloured cue card for *'when'*. A5 coloured *'when'* vocabulary cards.

Colourful Semantics small group session plans
Session 7

Aims	Description and strategies	Resources
• To consolidate familiarity with cue card colour, name and sign for '*who*', '*doing*', '*what*', '*where*' and '*when*'.	Show the children the '*who*' and ask the group to say its colour and show the Makaton sign. Repeat for all cue cards. Talk about how the '*when*' word can go at the beginning or end of the sentence and demonstrate this.	Large coloured cue cards for '*who*', '*doing*', '*what*', '*where*' and '*when*'.
• To create and write silly sentences.	Complete a 'Cut and Stick' silly sentence worksheet containing a '*who*', '*doing*', '*what*', '*where*' and '*when*' with the children. Children must work out which words are which sentence element, e.g. '*The witch*' is a '*who*'; '*on their birthday*' is a '*when*'. They then choose their favourite words for each sentence element to create their own sentence. They stick the vocabulary onto the boxes in the correct order then write the sentence out and underline the written words in the correct colour.	Silly sentences 'Cut and Stick' worksheet with a '*who*', '*doing*', '*what*', '*where*' and '*when*' (one per child).
• To consolidate understanding of the meaning of '*when*'. • To identify and describe '*when*' vocabulary.	Guessing game – children come out and choose a card and give clues for other children to guess '*when*' it is. For example: • '*When*' a chocolate egg is given (Easter time). • '*When*' you get a cake with candles (on your birthday). • '*When*' you see Santa (Christmas time).	Selection of coloured vocabulary cards for '*when*'.

Additional suggestions for extension activities:

• Link silly sentence making to themes from current class topic or text.

• Move on to sensible sentences rather than silly sentences.

• Provide written sentences and ask the children to underline the words in the correct colour according to whether it is a '*who*', '*doing*', '*what*', '*where*' or '*when*' word.

• Word generation game – children are in a circle and a large coloured cue card is placed in the centre of the circle. The children take turns to throw a bean bag and when it lands on the card they must think of a word for that question – for example, if '*what*' is in the middle they could say 'pencil'. Repeat for other 'wh' cue cards.

Appendix 1
Cue cards and sentence templates

Provided here are individual cue cards and sentence templates.

Specific sentence templates for individual sentence structures are also available alongside picture prompts in Appendix 3.

Copyright material from NHS Forth Valley (2020), *Colourful Semantics*, Routledge

A5 cue cards

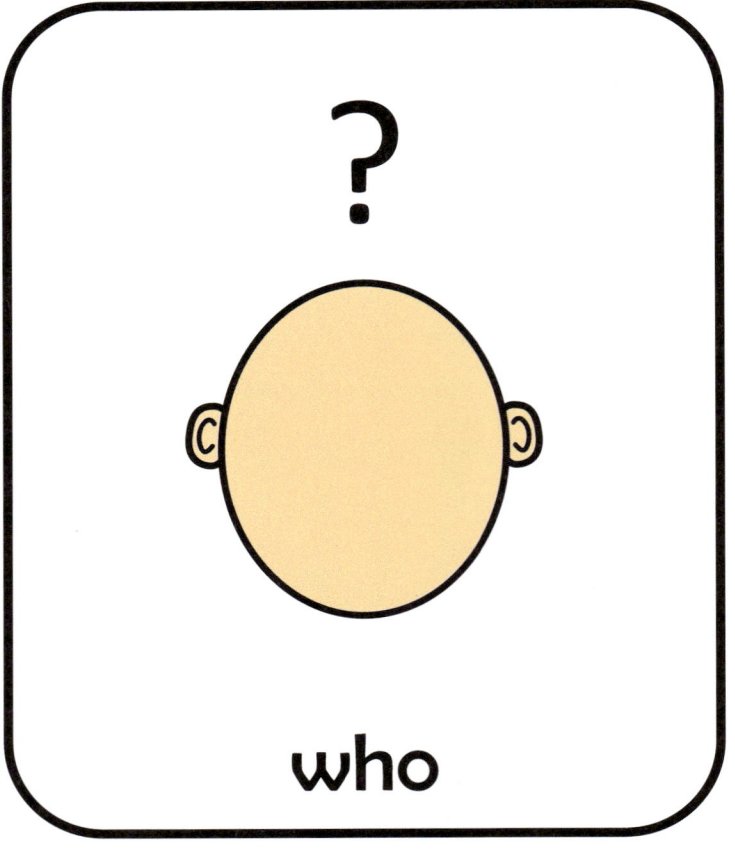

who

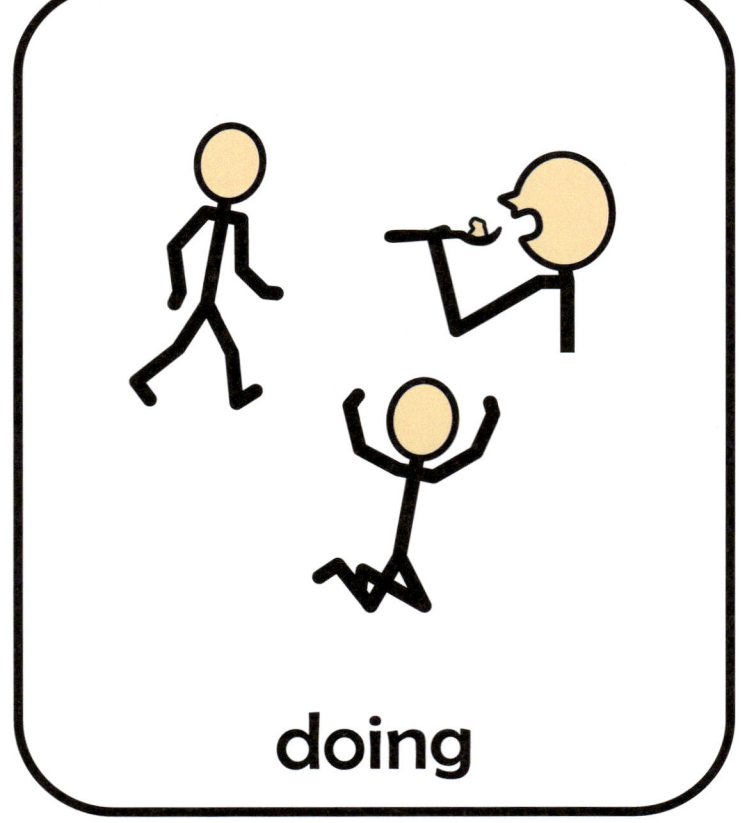

doing

Copyright material from NHS Forth Valley (2020), *Colourful Semantics*, Routledge

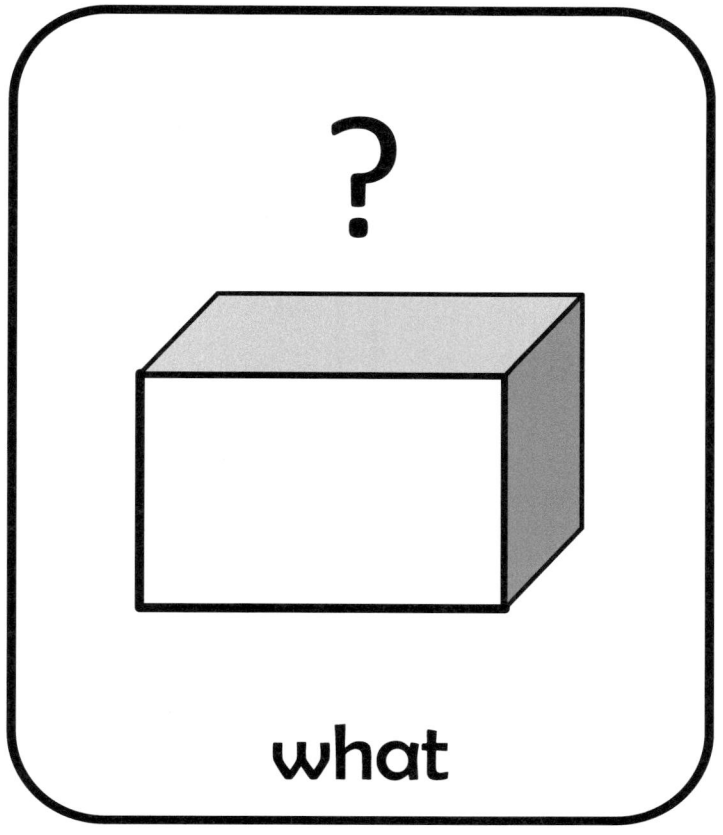

what

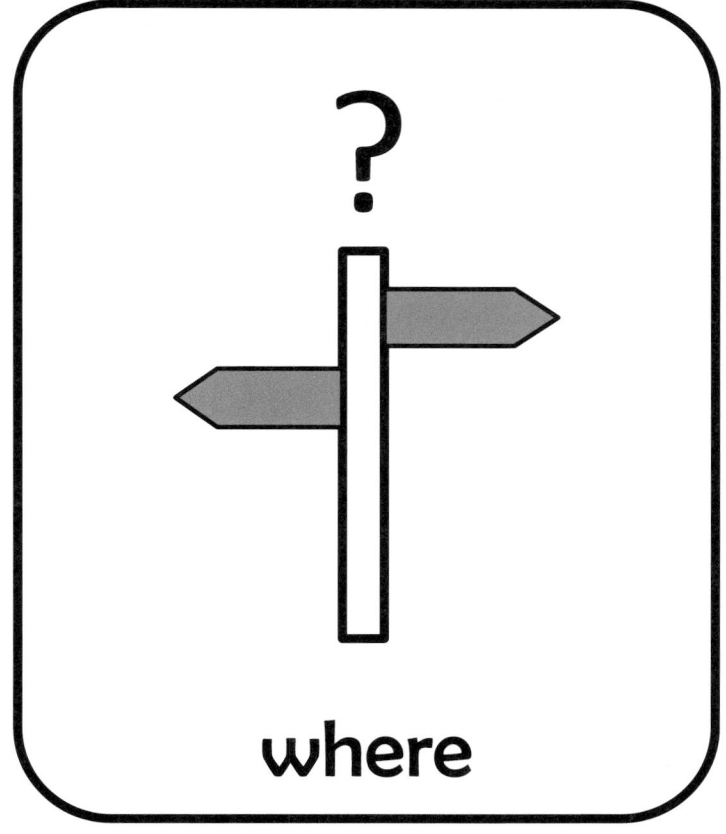

where

Copyright material from NHS Forth Valley (2020), *Colourful Semantics*, Routledge

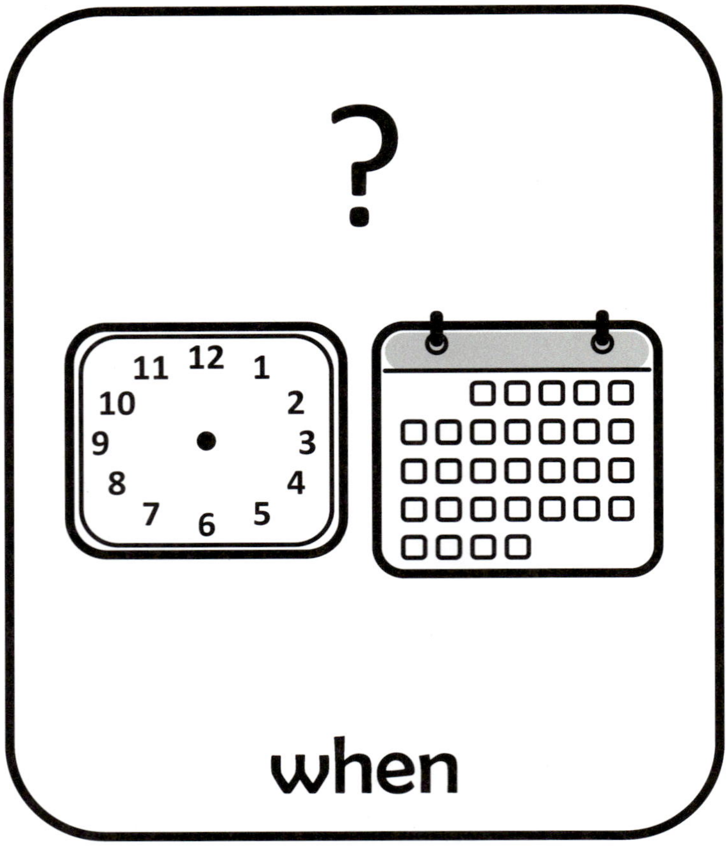

when

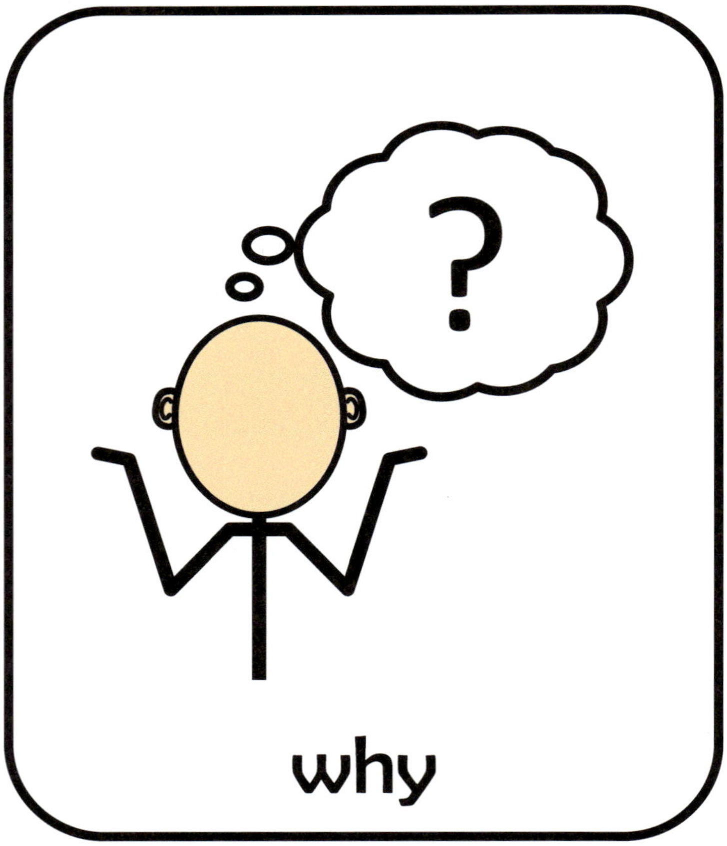

why

Copyright material from NHS Forth Valley (2020), *Colourful Semantics*, Routledge

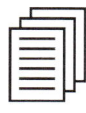

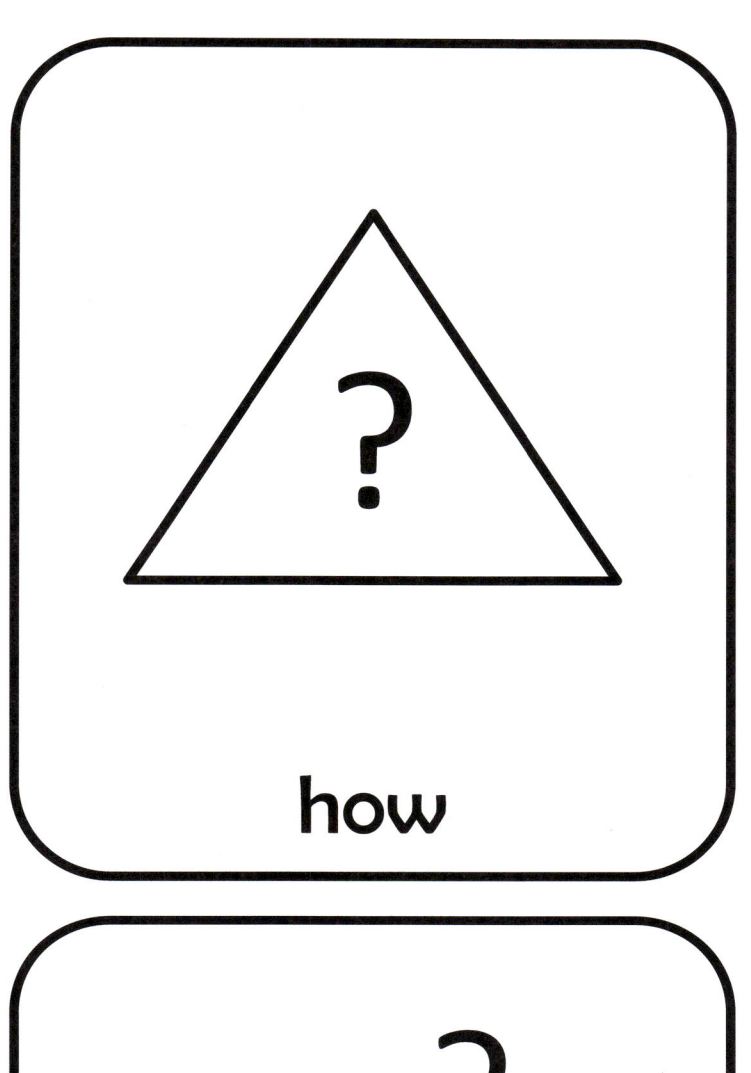

how

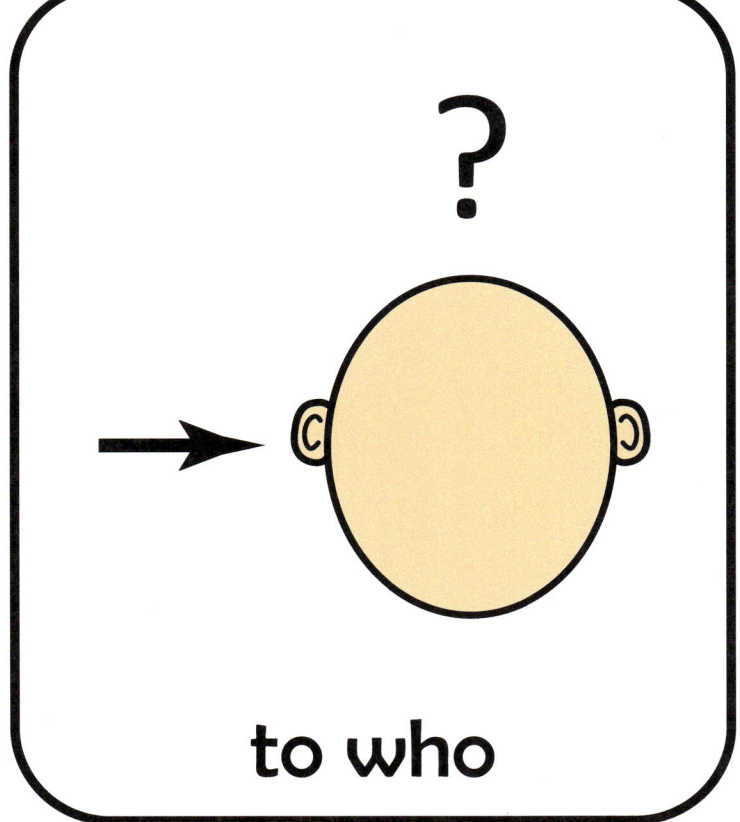

to who

Copyright material from NHS Forth Valley (2020), *Colourful Semantics*, Routledge

A4 cue cards

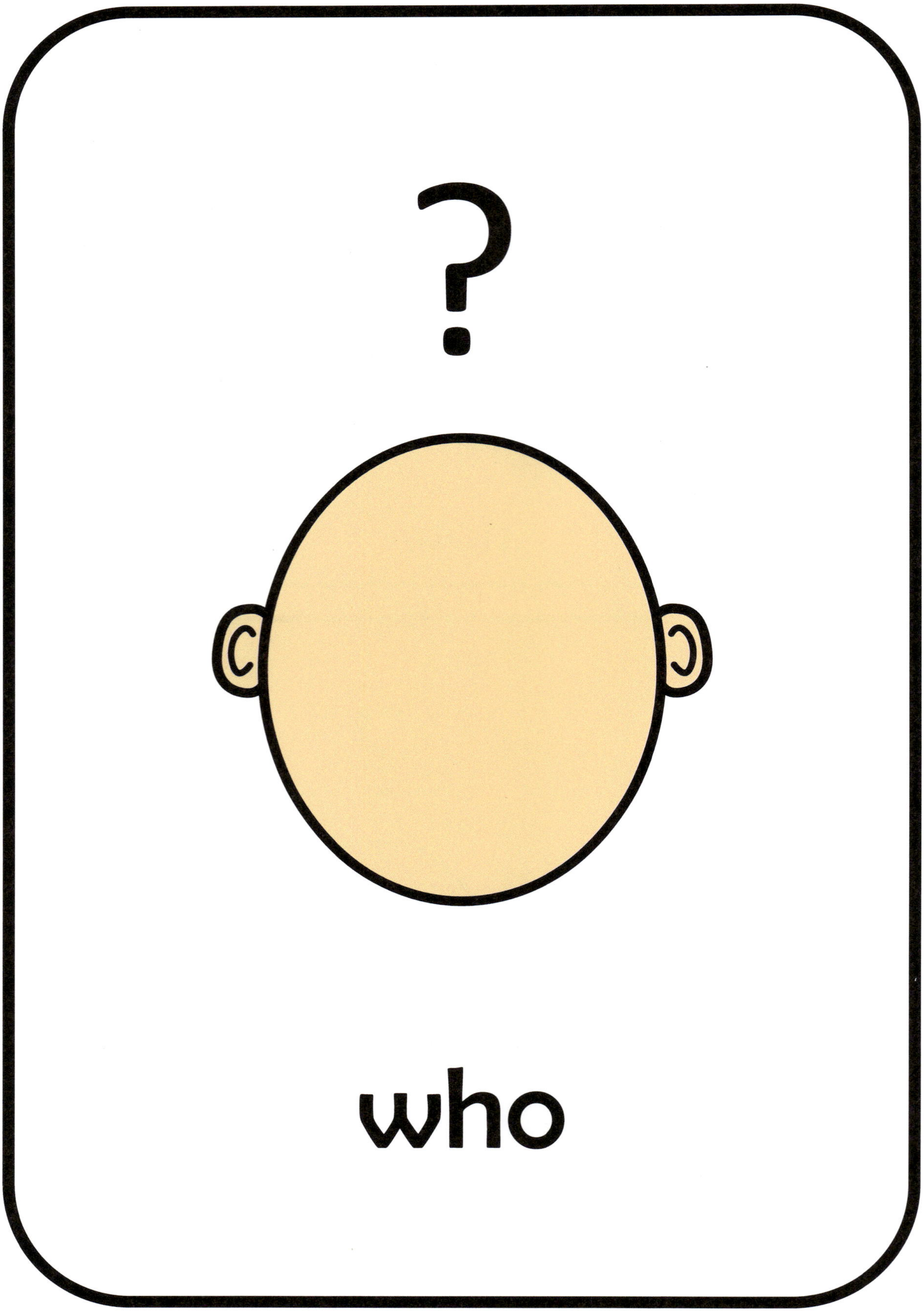

?

who

Copyright material from NHS Forth Valley (2020), *Colourful Semantics*, Routledge

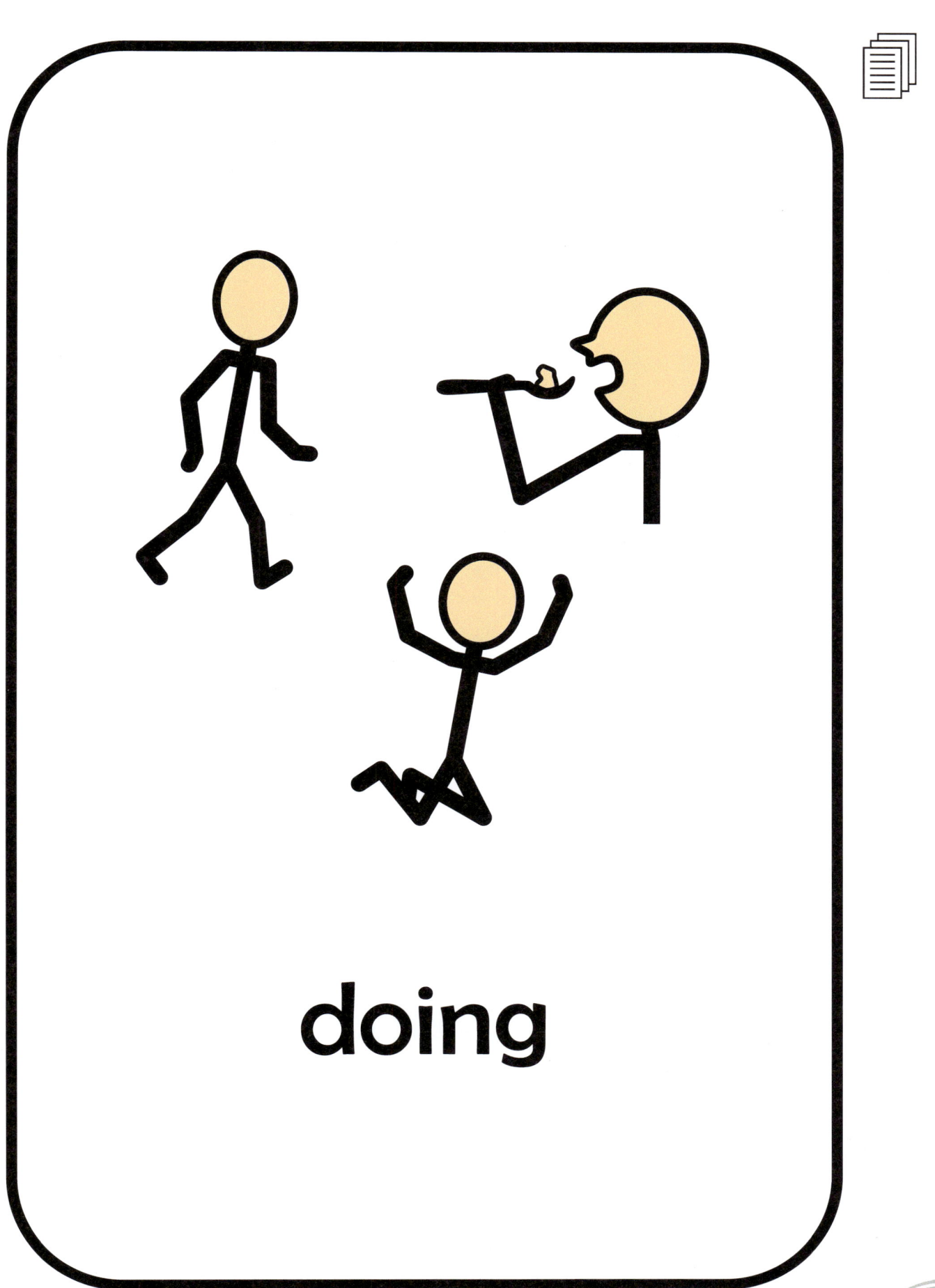

doing

Copyright material from NHS Forth Valley (2020), *Colourful Semantics*, Routledge

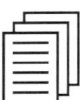

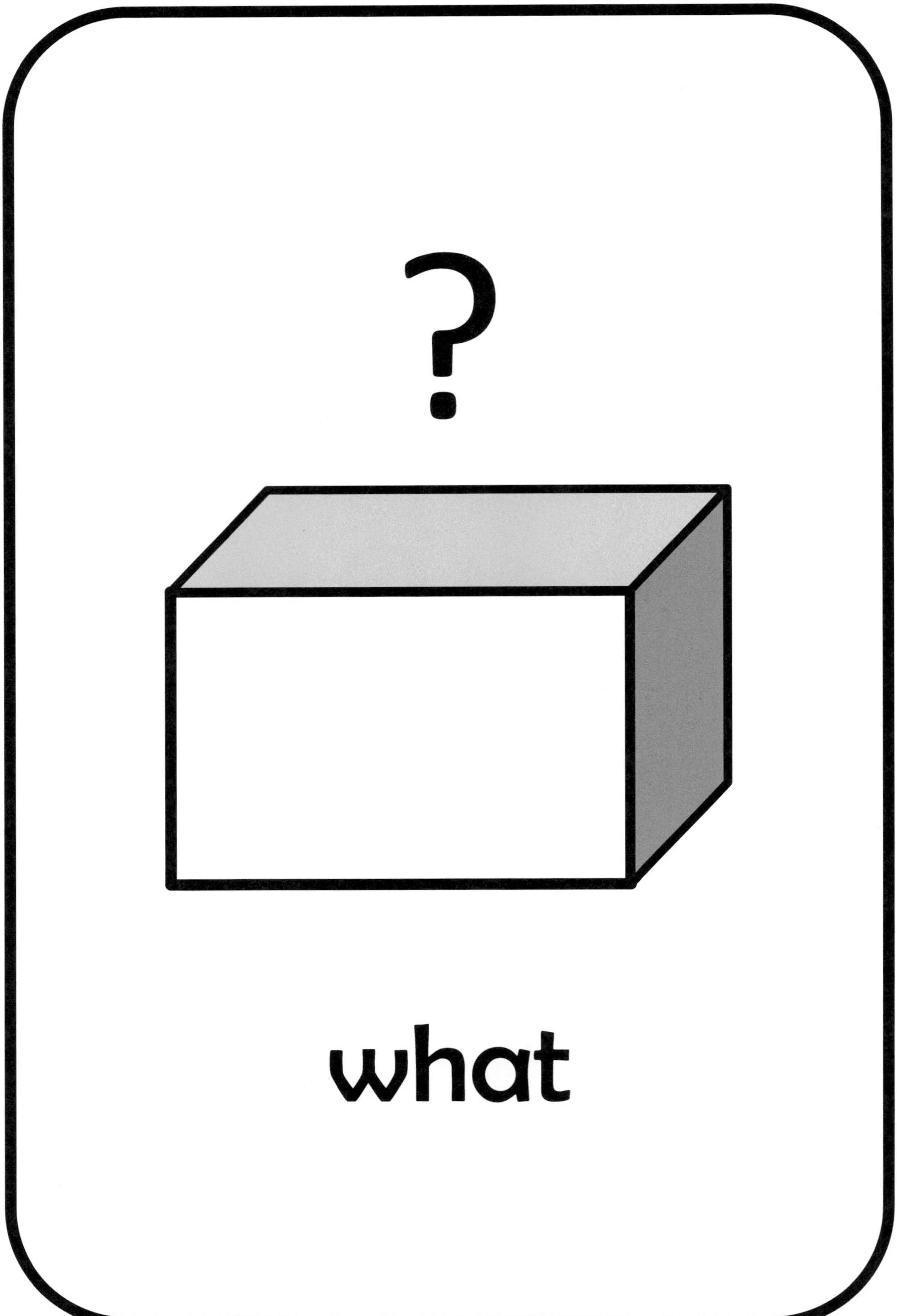

?

what

Copyright material from NHS Forth Valley (2020), *Colourful Semantics*, Routledge

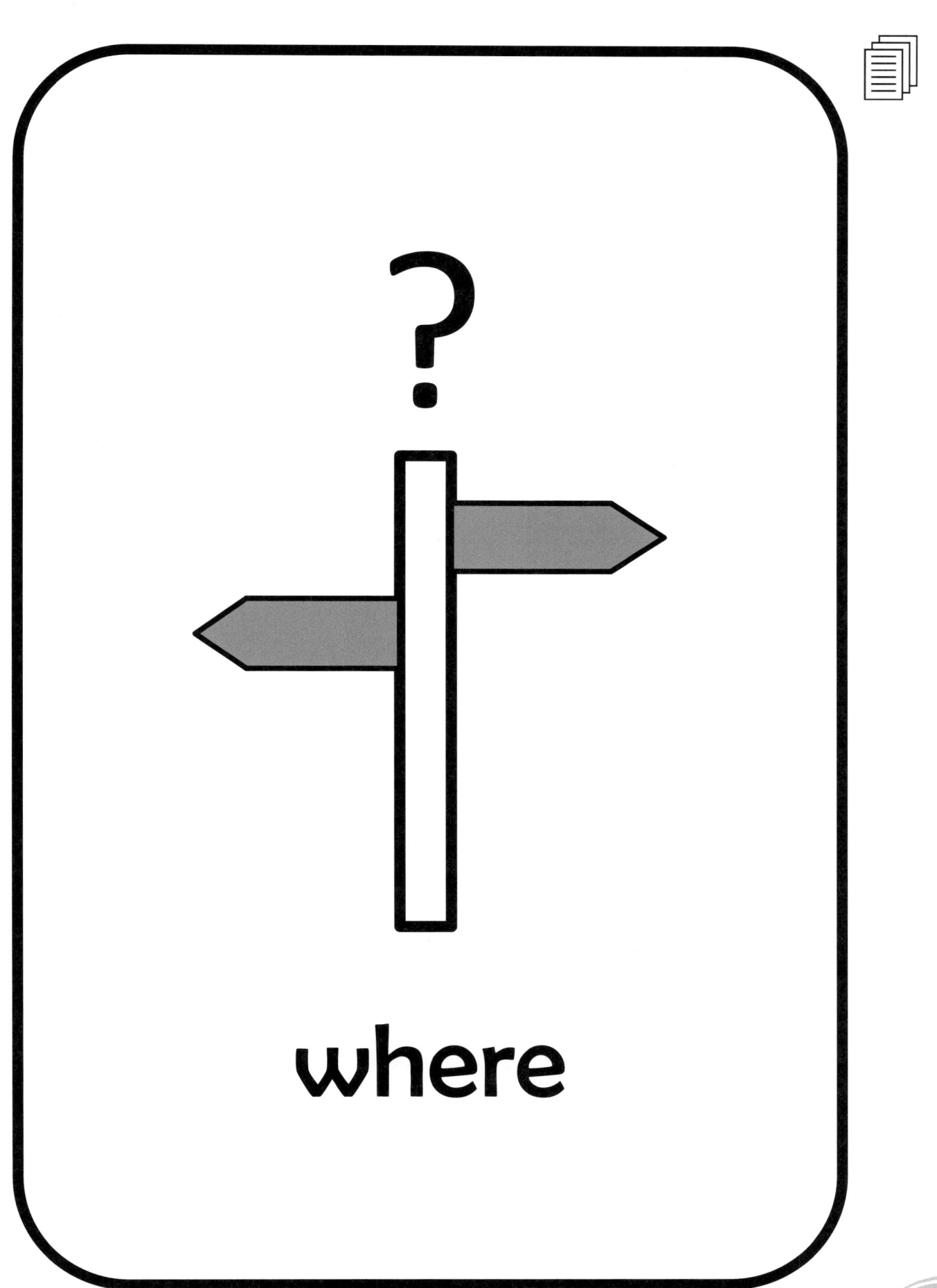

where

Copyright material from NHS Forth Valley (2020), *Colourful Semantics*, Routledge

?

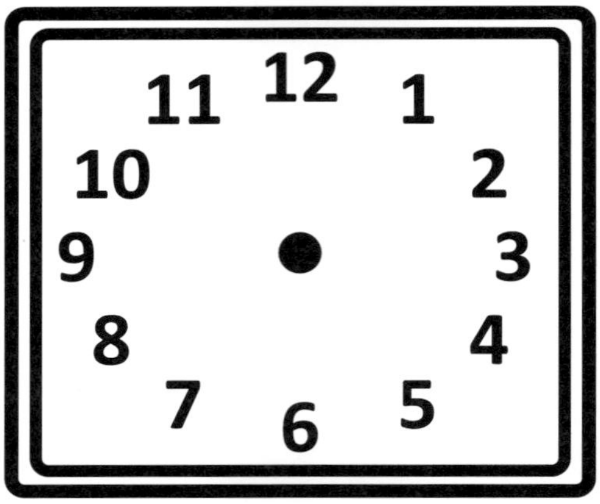

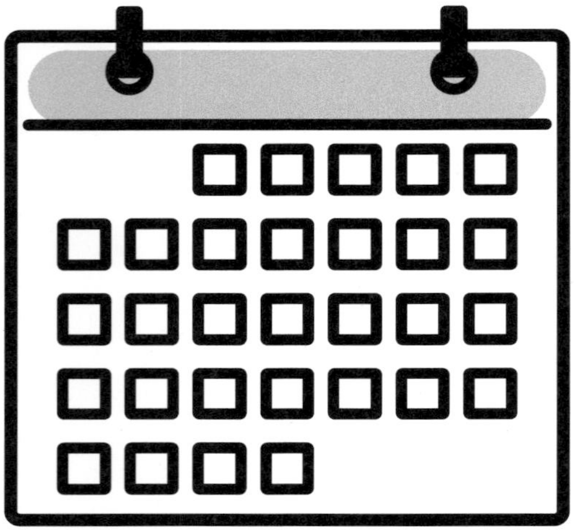

when

Copyright material from NHS Forth Valley (2020), *Colourful Semantics*, Routledge

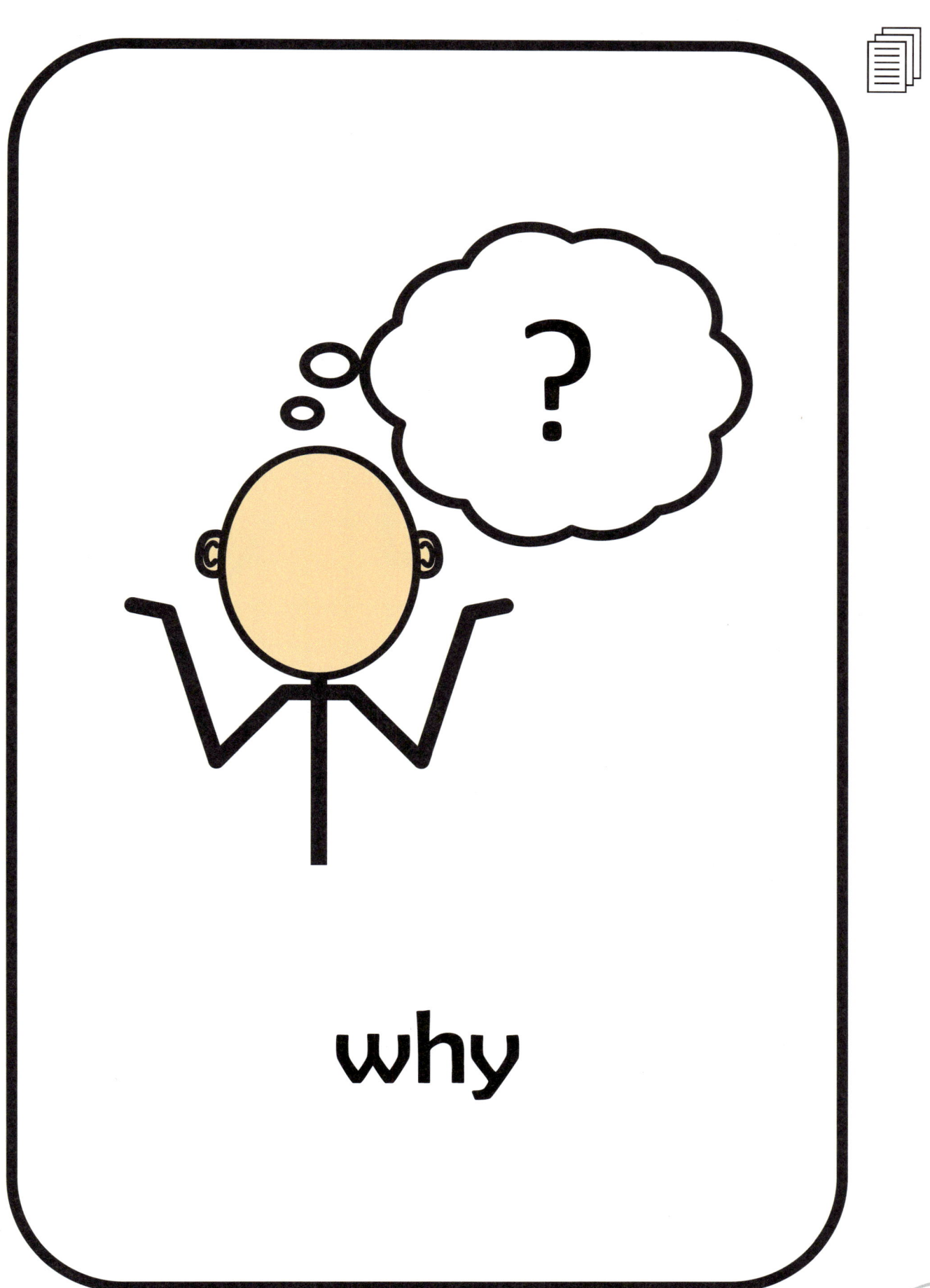

why

Copyright material from NHS Forth Valley (2020), *Colourful Semantics*, Routledge

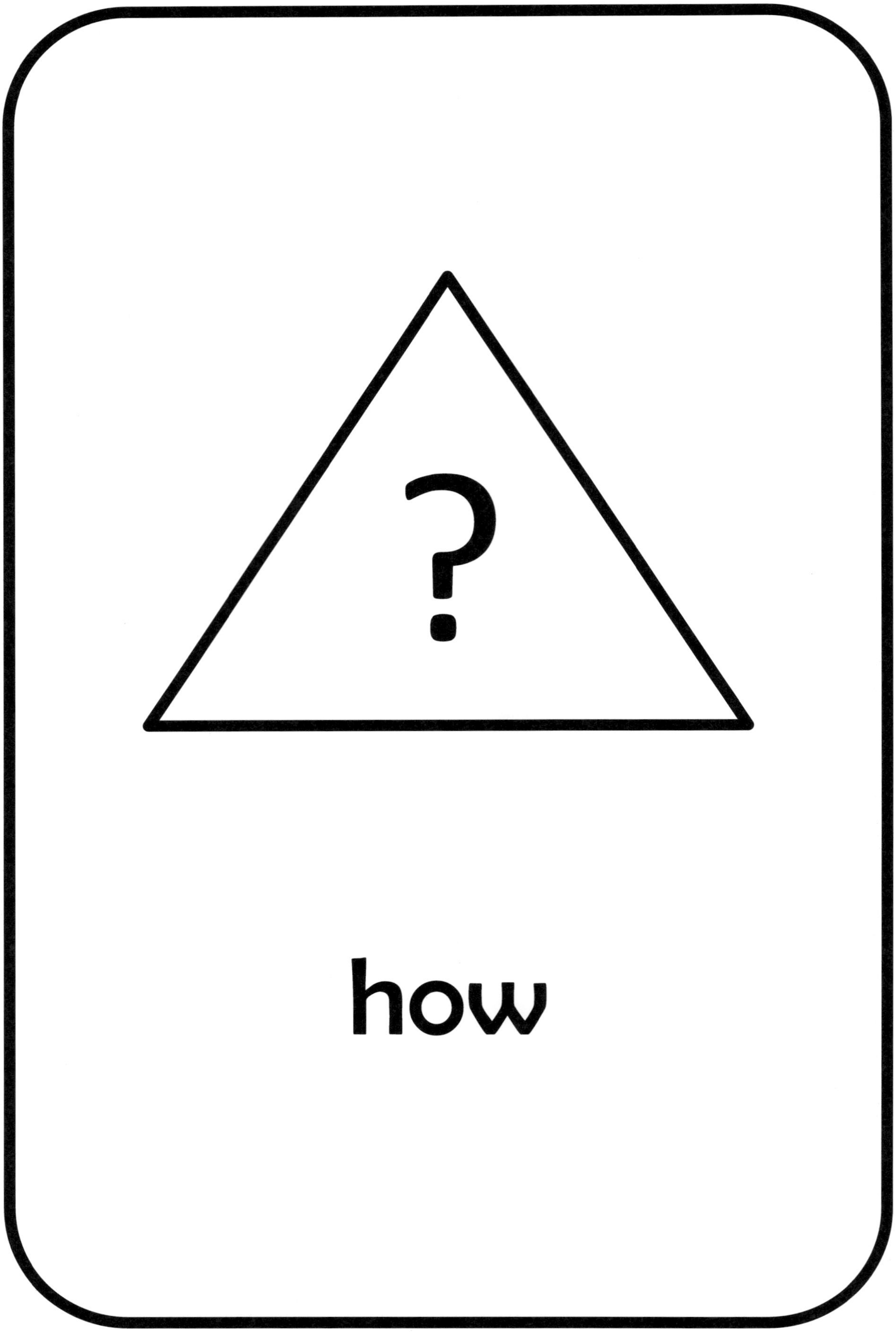

how

Copyright material from NHS Forth Valley (2020), *Colourful Semantics*, Routledge

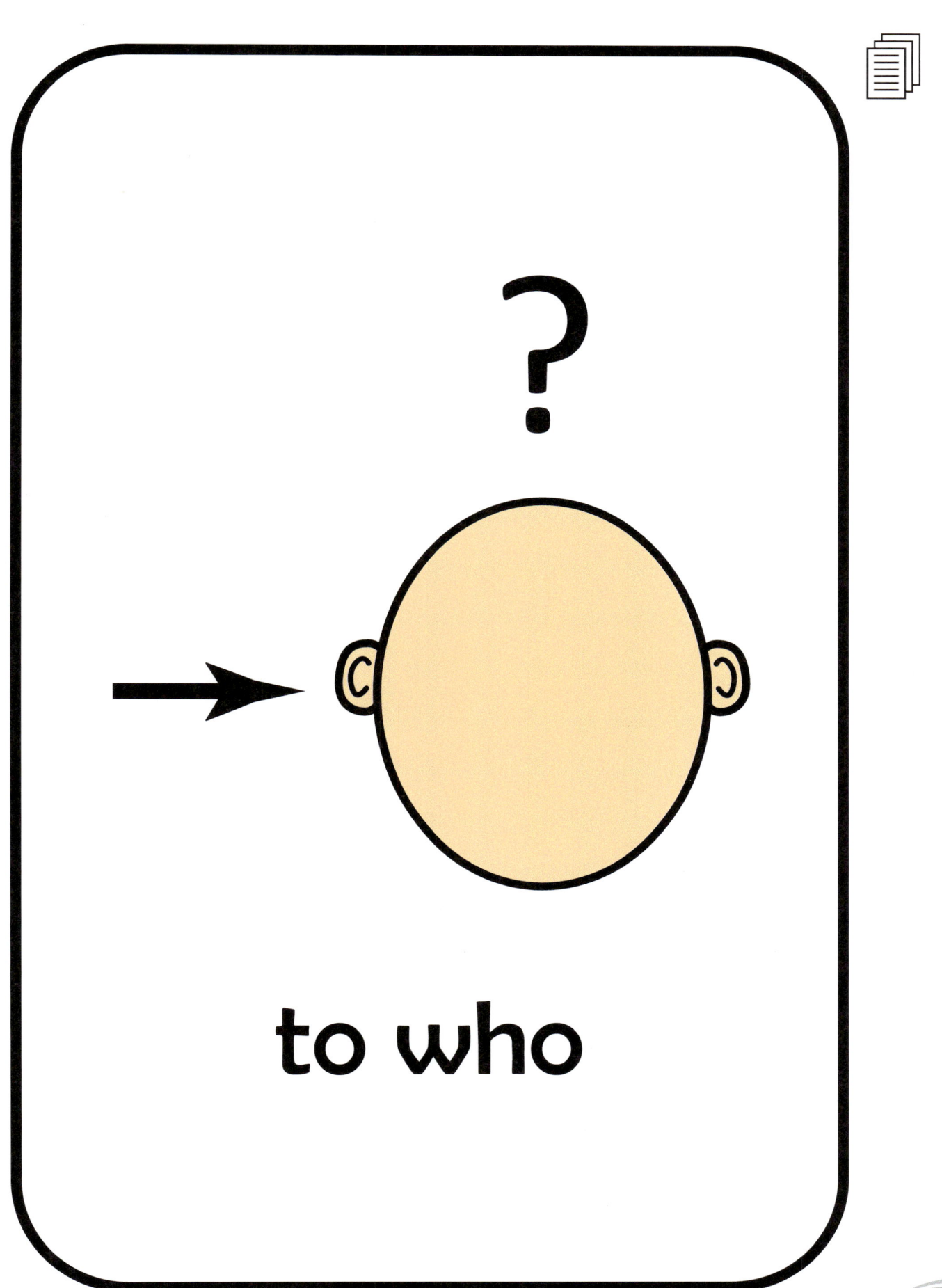

to who

Copyright material from NHS Forth Valley (2020), *Colourful Semantics*, Routledge

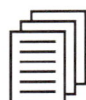

Sentence templates

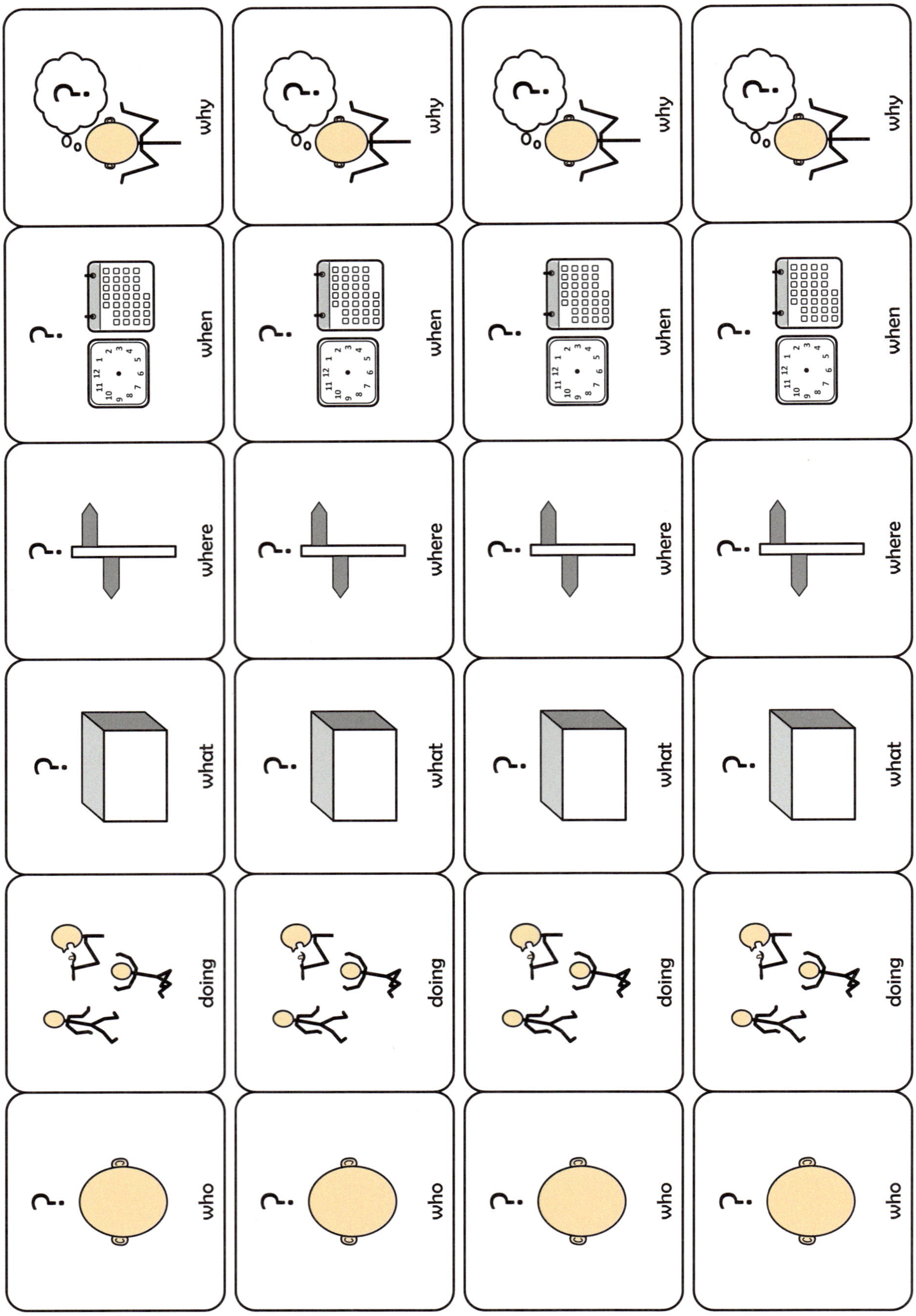

why	why	why	why
when	when	when	when
where	where	where	where
what	what	what	what
doing	doing	doing	doing
who	who	who	who

Copyright material from NHS Forth Valley (2020), *Colourful Semantics*, Routledge

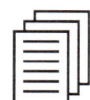

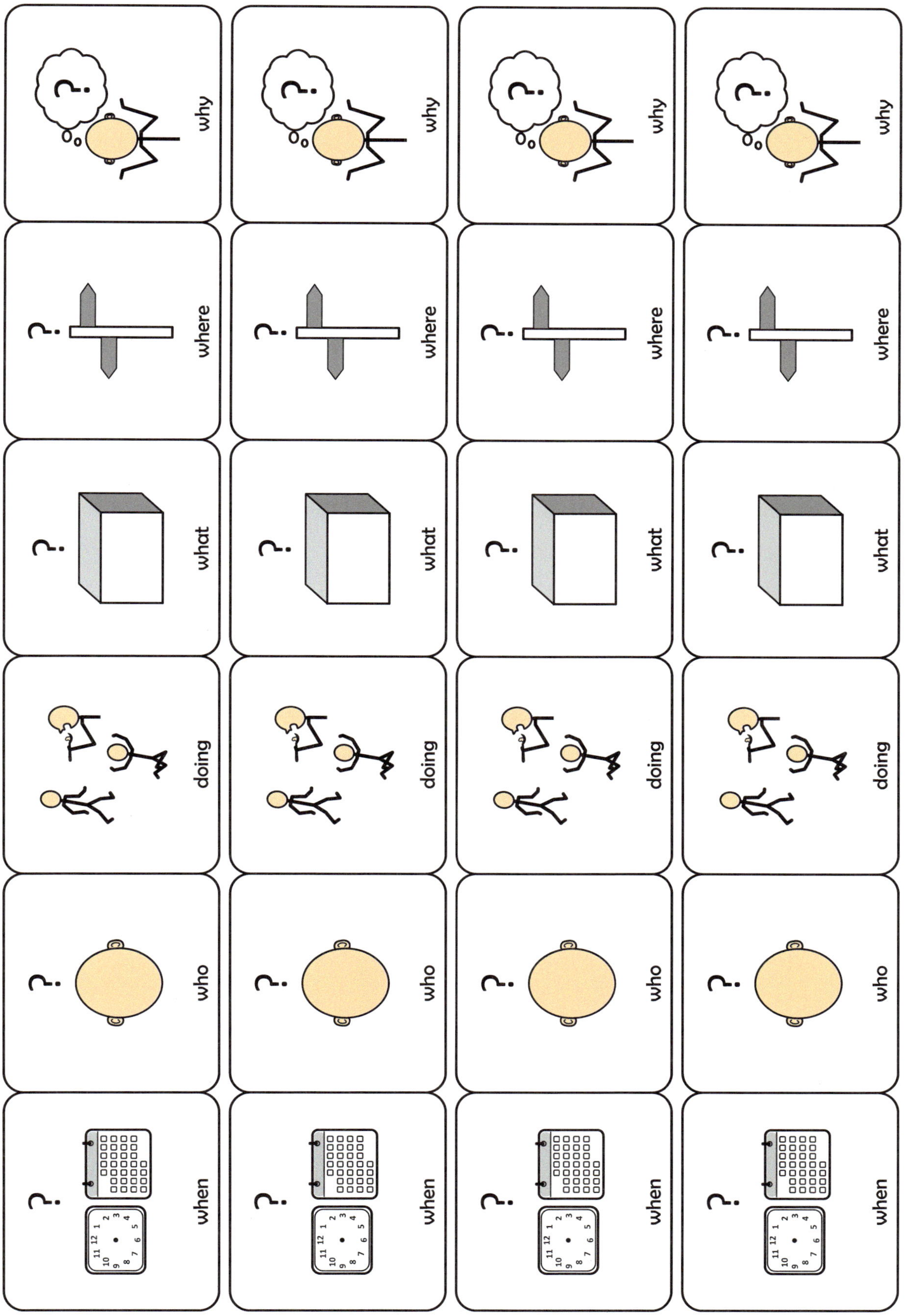

why	why	why	why
where	where	where	where
what	what	what	what
doing	doing	doing	doing
who	who	who	who
when	when	when	when

Copyright material from NHS Forth Valley (2020), *Colourful Semantics*, Routledge

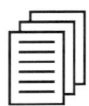

Appendix 2
Story planner grids

This section contains example story planner grids for the most common sentence structures, and which are used to support our Colourful Semantics session plans. However, similar planners could be used to include other sentence components.

Copyright material from NHS Forth Valley (2020), *Colourful Semantics*, Routledge

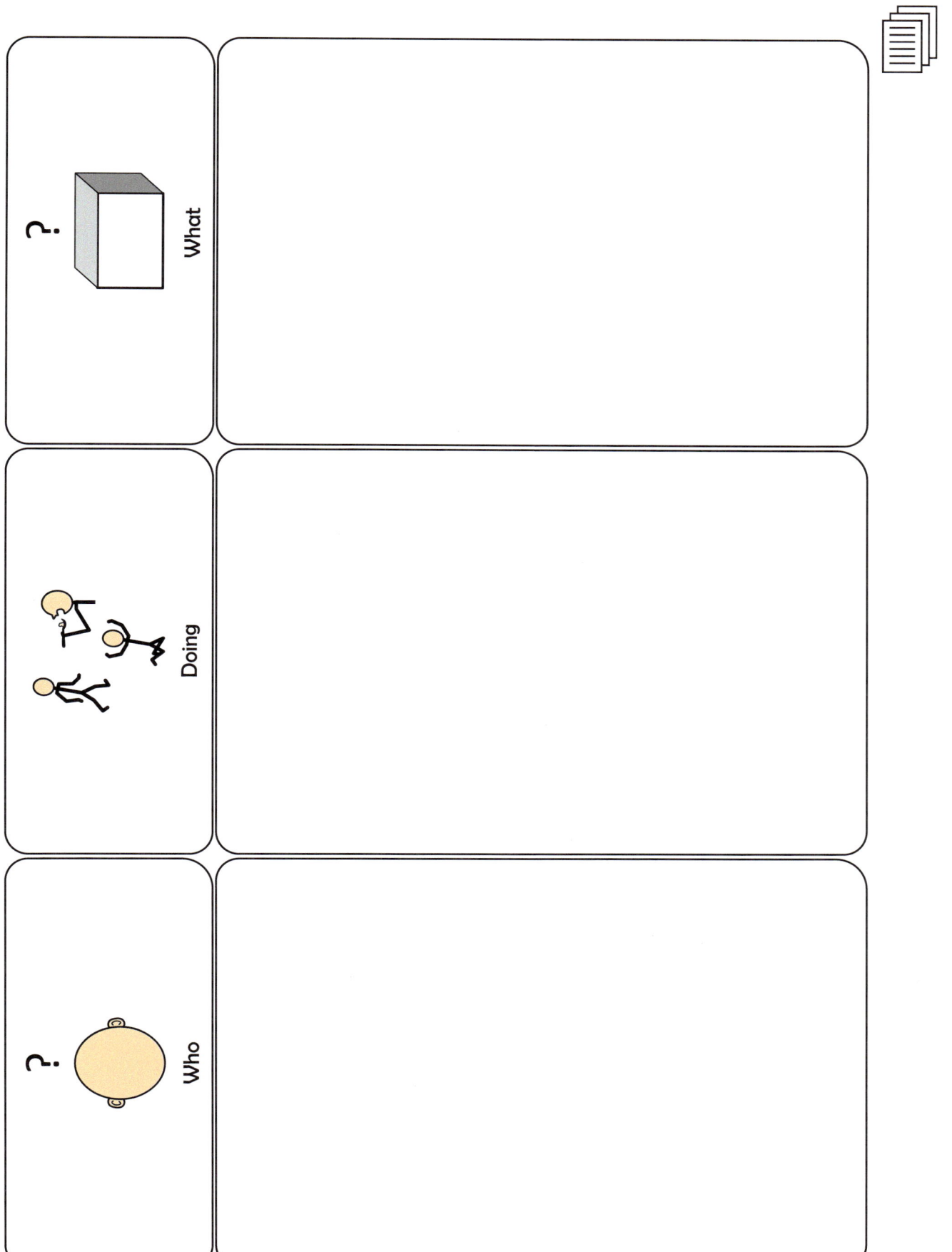

Copyright material from NHS Forth Valley (2020), *Colourful Semantics*, Routledge

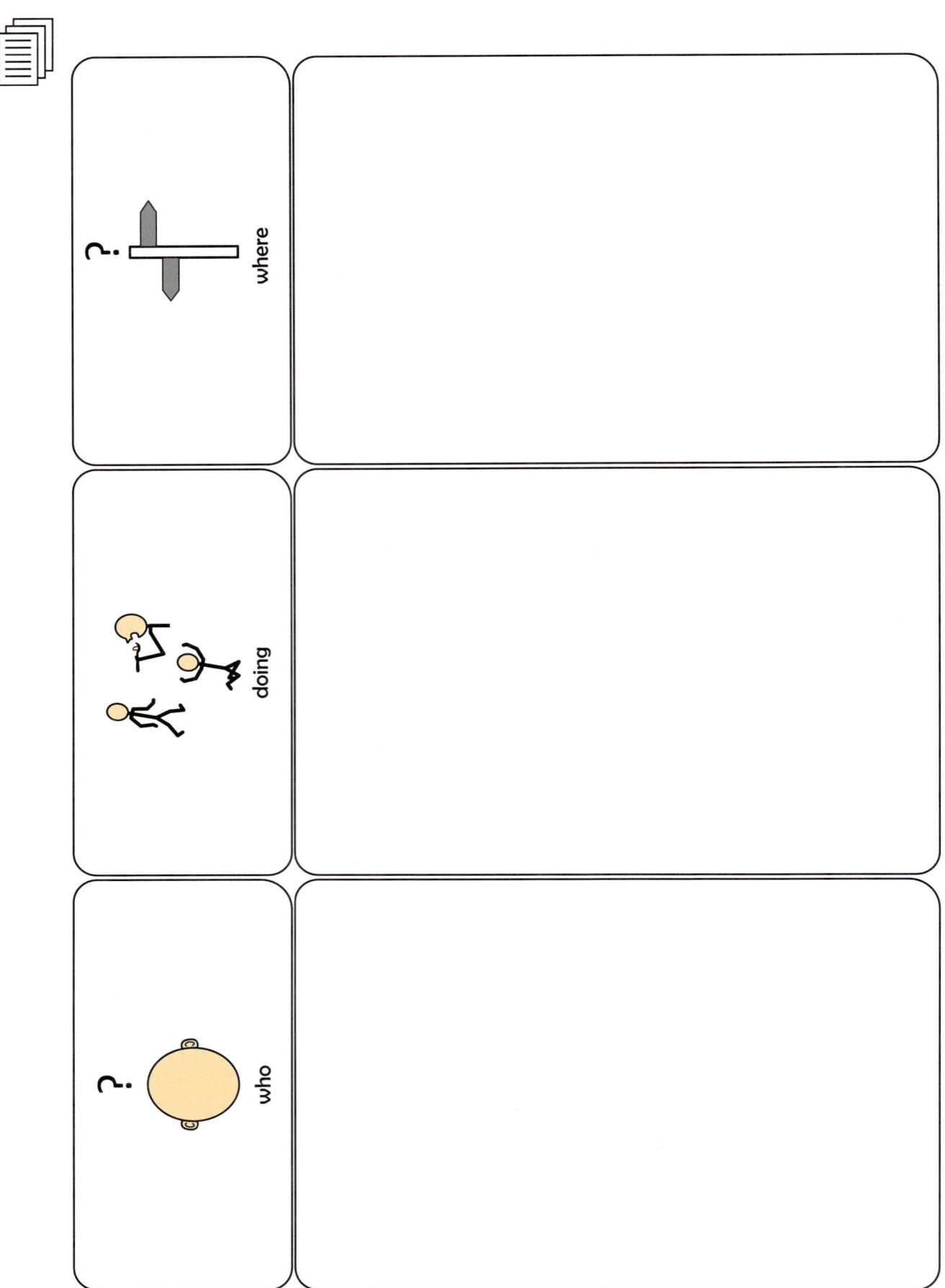

Copyright material from NHS Forth Valley (2020), *Colourful Semantics*, Routledge

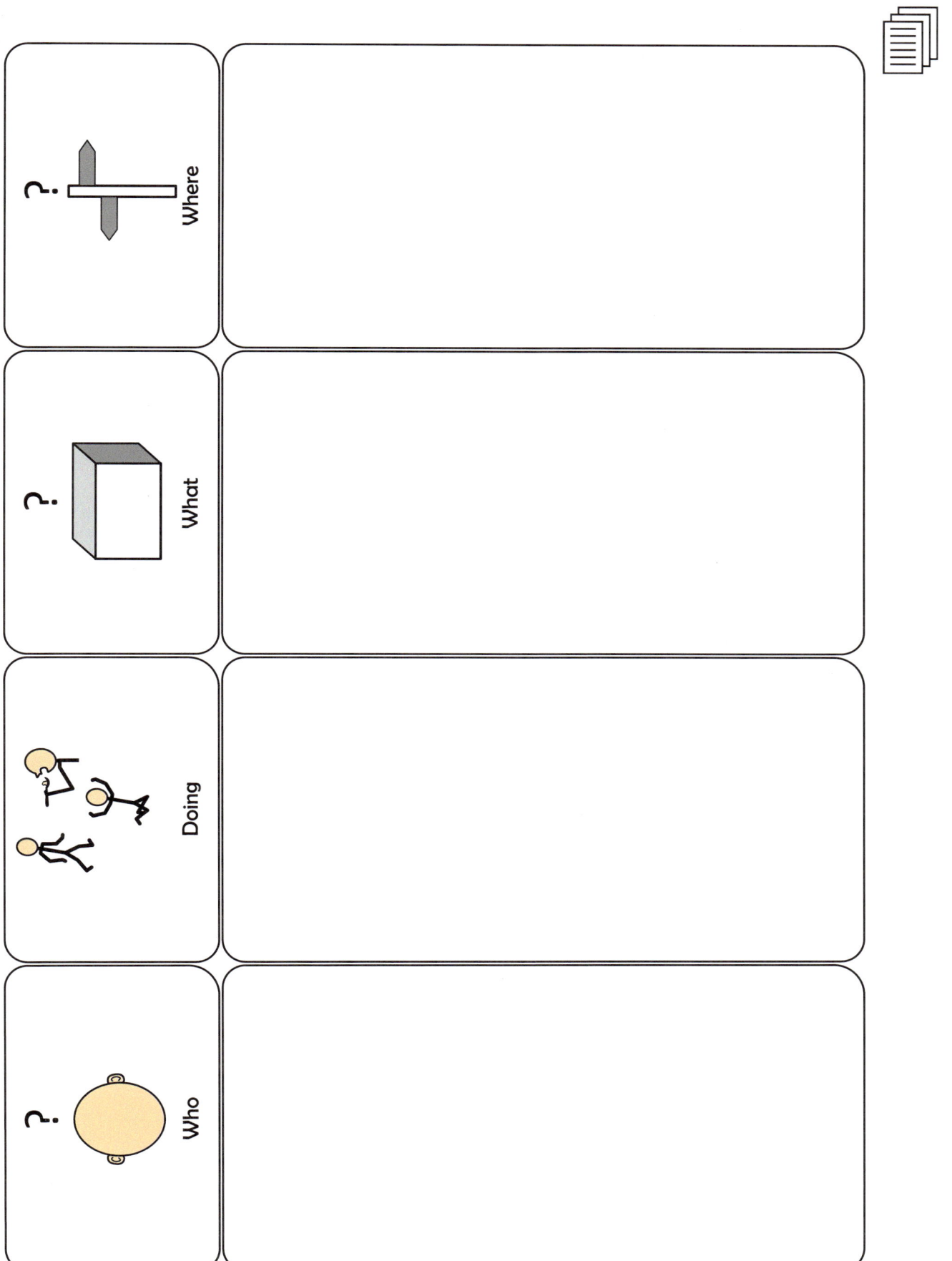

Copyright material from NHS Forth Valley (2020), *Colourful Semantics*, Routledge

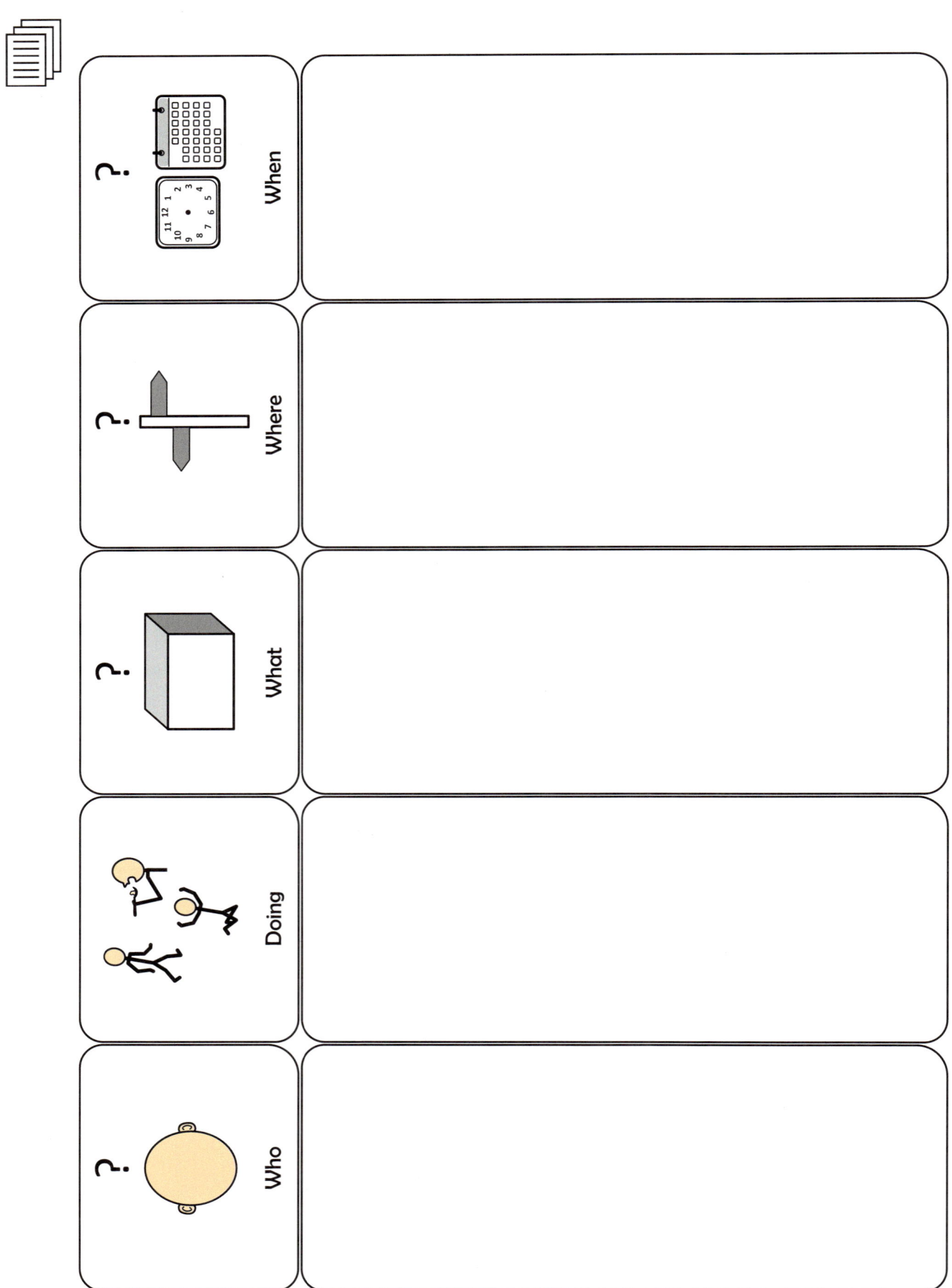

Copyright material from NHS Forth Valley (2020), *Colourful Semantics*, Routledge

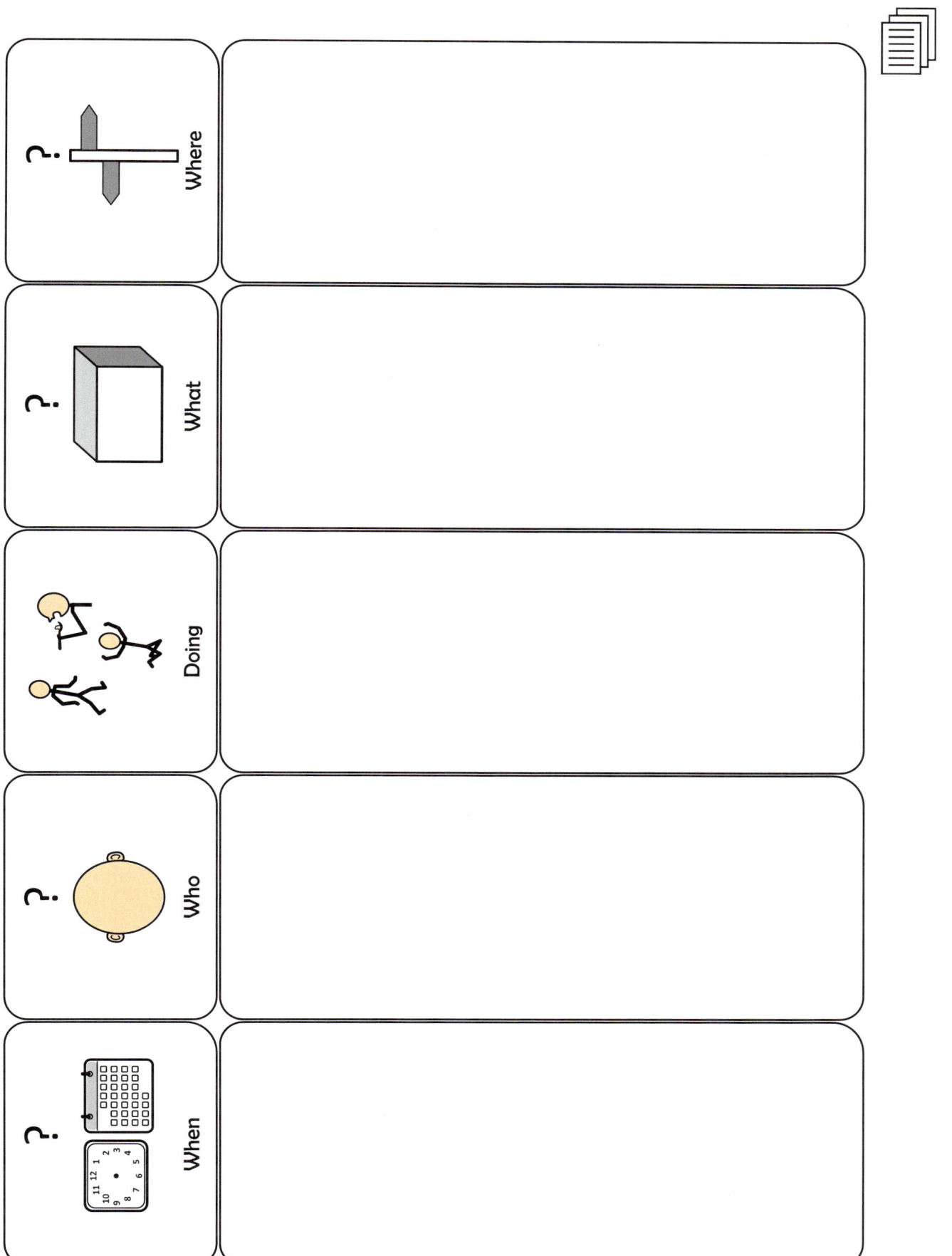

? Where	
? What	
Doing	
? Who	
? When	

Copyright material from NHS Forth Valley (2020), *Colourful Semantics*, Routledge

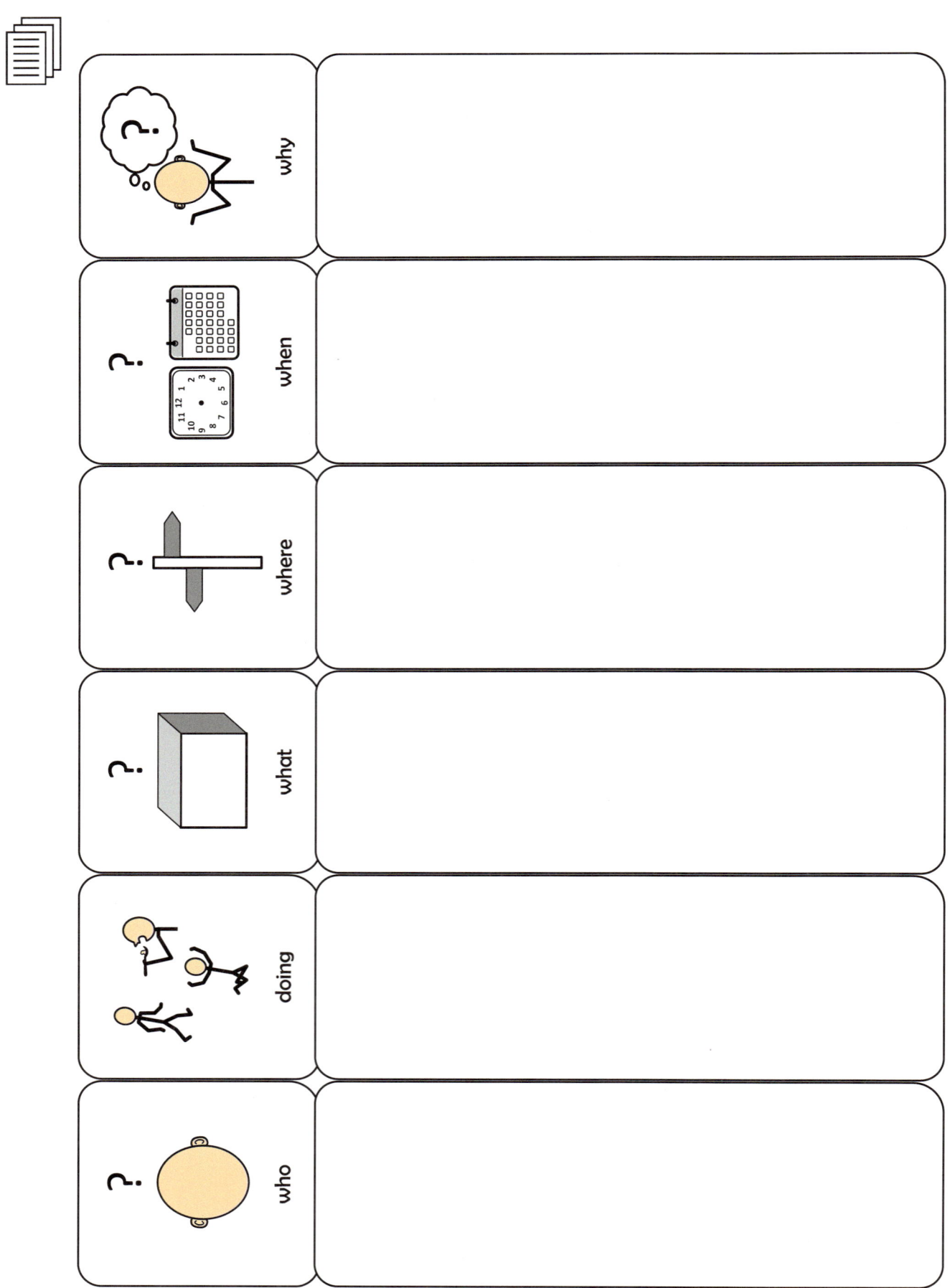

why

when

where

what

doing

who

Copyright material from NHS Forth Valley (2020), *Colourful Semantics*, Routledge

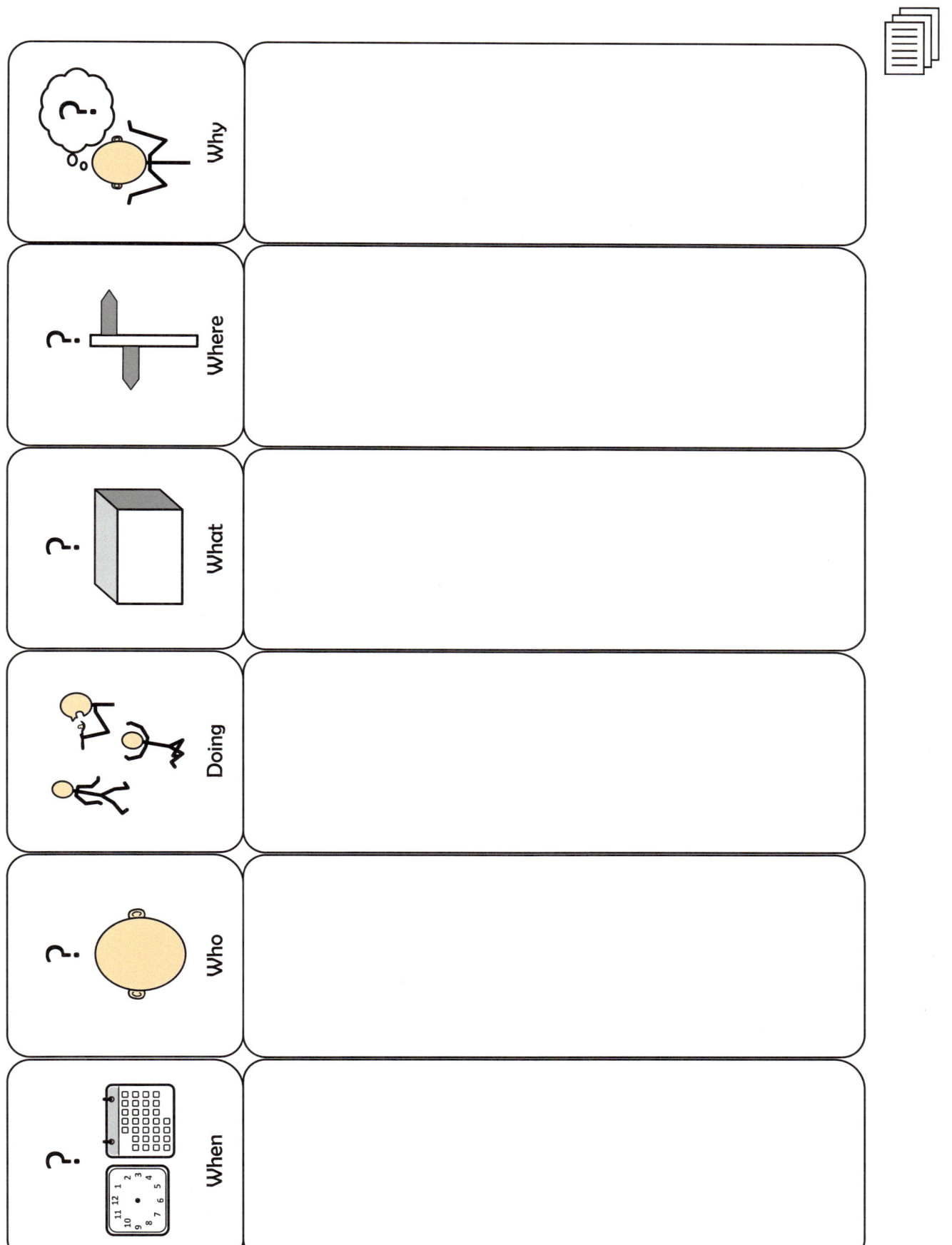

Copyright material from NHS Forth Valley (2020), *Colourful Semantics*, Routledge

Appendix 3
Sentence building resources

These resources and sentence templates may be used to carry out sentence building activities with individuals or small groups, as per the examples demonstrated in Chapter 1. Colour coded sentence templates are also available online.

Copyright material from NHS Forth Valley (2020), *Colourful Semantics*, Routledge

Two-part sentences ('*who*', '*doing*')

Use these alongside the 'Who, Doing' sentence template and blank box template on page 103.

The Swing (*Write About the Picture*, page 6)

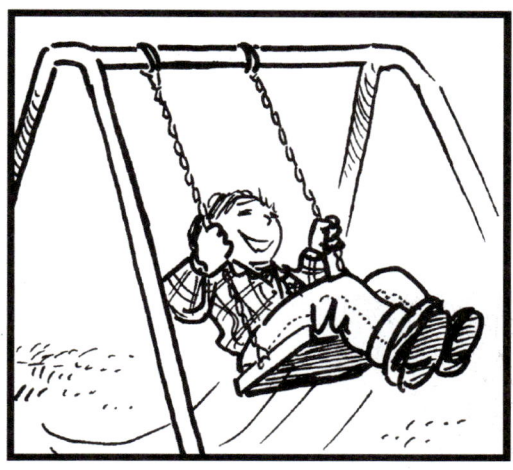
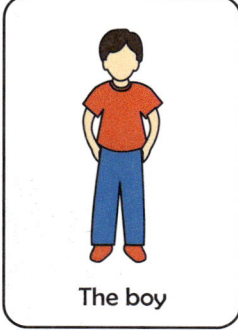
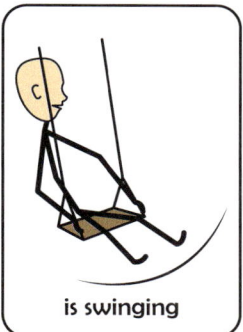

The boy   **is swinging**

The Cat (*Write About the Picture*, page 22)

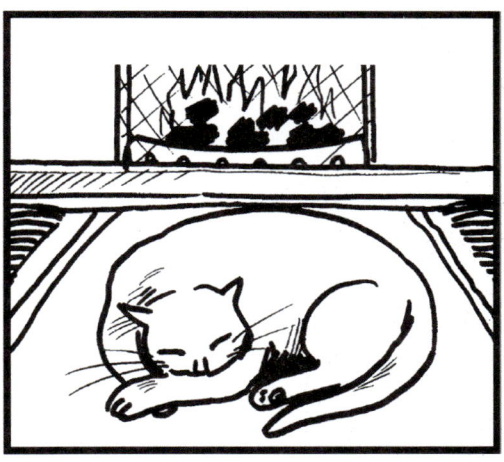
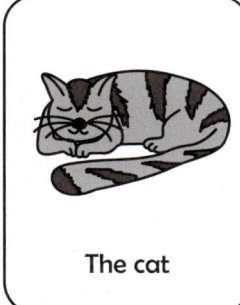
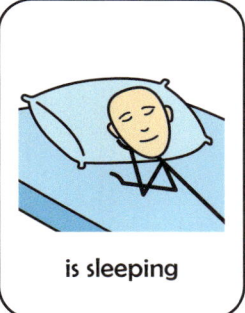

The cat   **is sleeping**

The Baby (*Write About the Picture*, page 17)

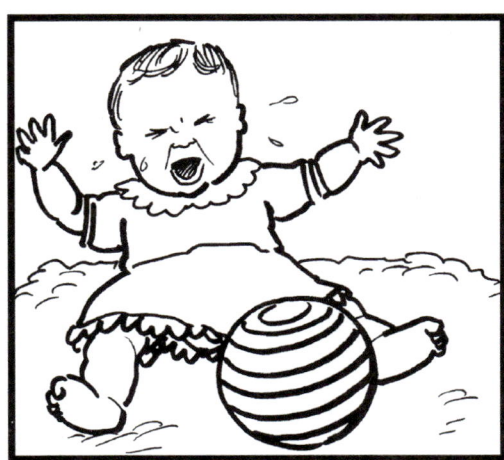
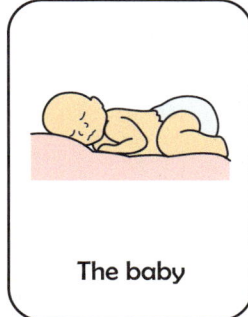
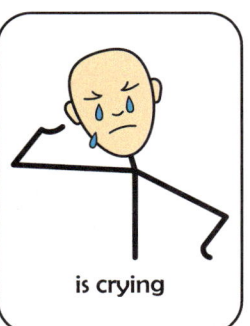

The baby   **is crying**

Copyright material from NHS Forth Valley (2020), *Colourful Semantics*, Routledge

Three-part sentences ('*who*', '*doing*', '*what*')

Use these alongside the 'Who, Doing, What' sentence template and blank box template on page 103.

The Painter (*Write About the Picture*, page 14)

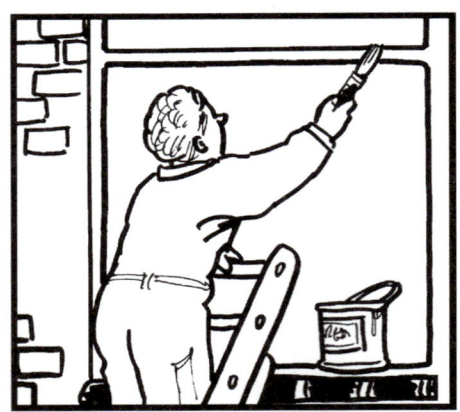

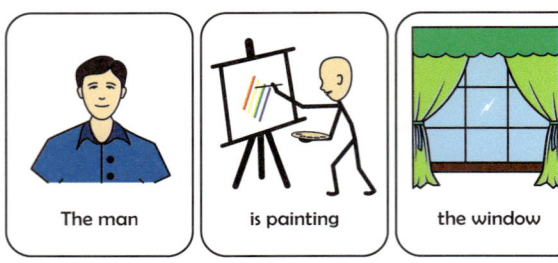

| The man | is painting | the window |

Fruit (*Write About the Picture*, page 18)

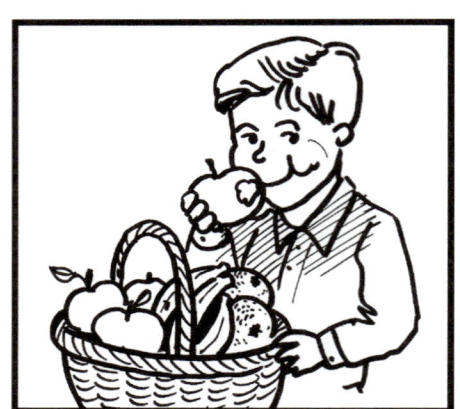

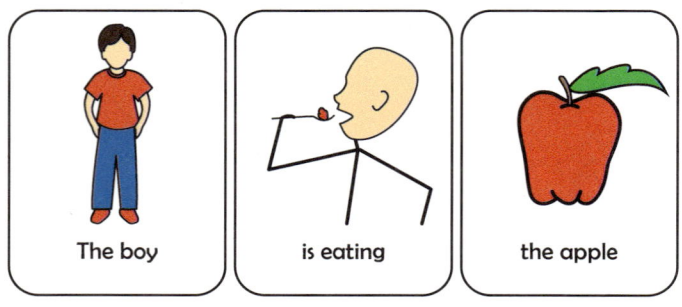

| The boy | is eating | the apple |

Copyright material from NHS Forth Valley (2020), *Colourful Semantics*, Routledge

The Picture (*Write About the Picture*, page 19)

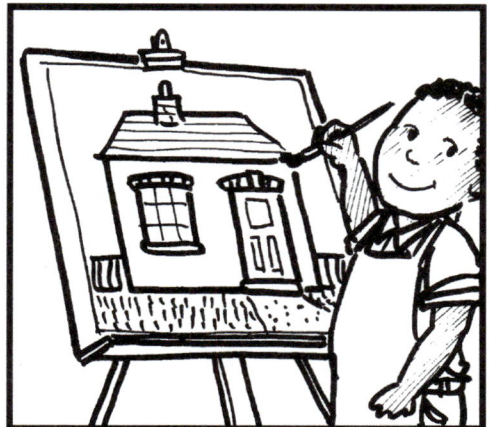

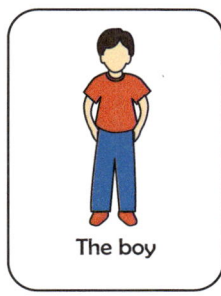
The boy

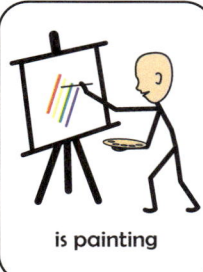
is painting

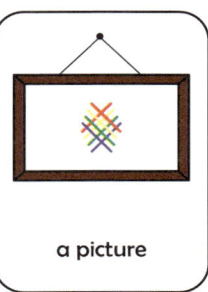
a picture

The Car (*Write About the Picture*, page 16)

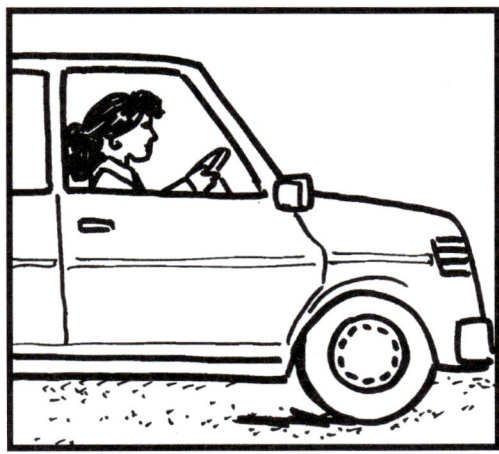

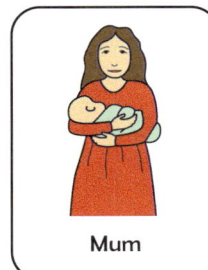
Mum

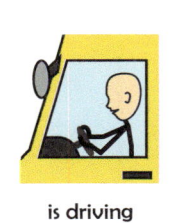
is driving

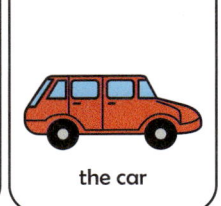
the car

Copyright material from NHS Forth Valley (2020), *Colourful Semantics*, Routledge

Three-part sentences ('*who*', '*doing*', '*where*')

Use these alongside the 'Who, Doing, Where' sentence template and blank box template on page 104.

The Sandpit (*Write About the Picture*, page 14)

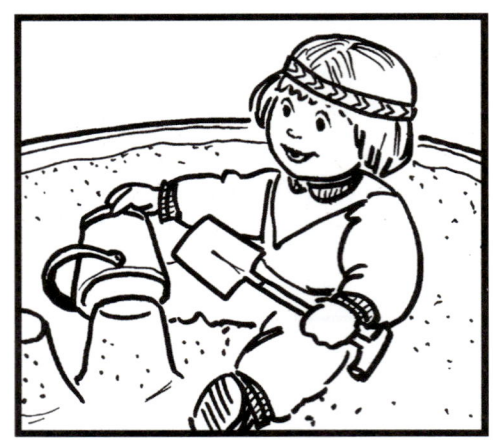

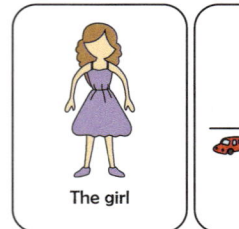
The girl

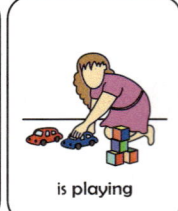
is playing

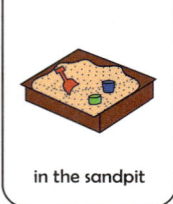
in the sandpit

Bedtime (*Write About the Picture*, page 21)

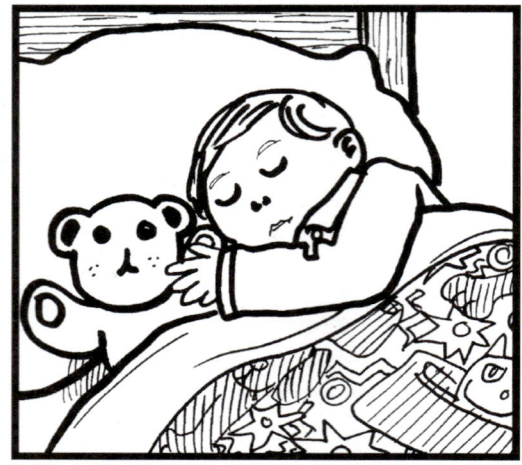

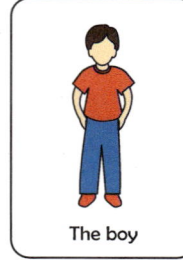
The boy

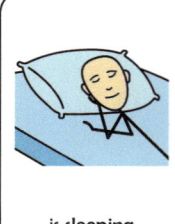
is sleeping

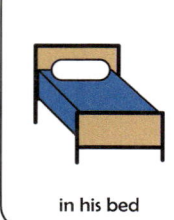
in his bed

Copyright material from NHS Forth Valley (2020), *Colourful Semantics*, Routledge

Bathtime: (*Write About the Picture 2*, page 10)

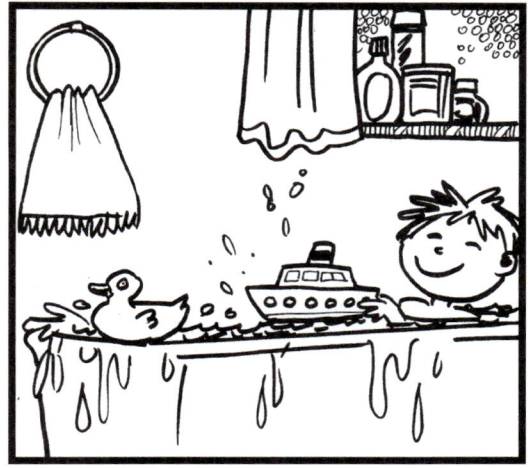

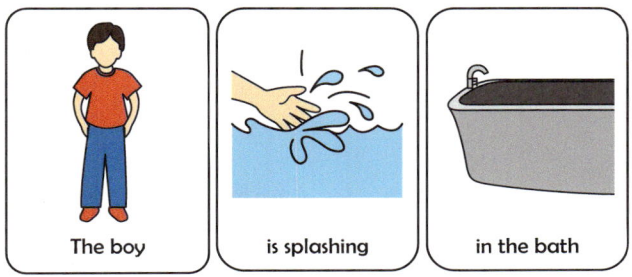

The boy | is splashing | in the bath

Cooking (*Write About the Picture 2*, page 5)

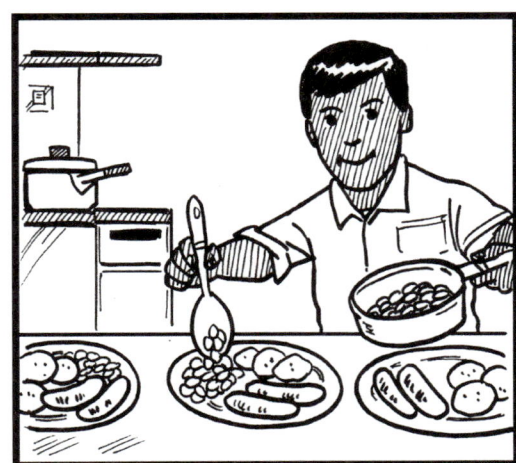

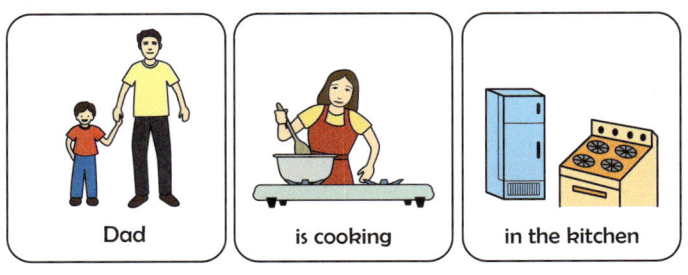

Dad | is cooking | in the kitchen

Copyright material from NHS Forth Valley (2020), *Colourful Semantics*, Routledge

Four-part sentences ('*who*', '*doing*', '*what*', '*where*')

Use these alongside the 'Who, Doing, What, Where' sentence template and blank box template on page 104.

The Farmer (*Write About the Picture*, page 8)

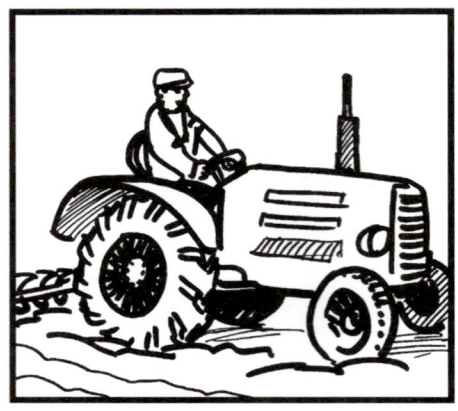

 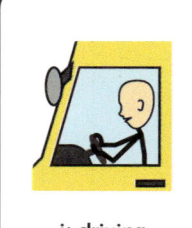 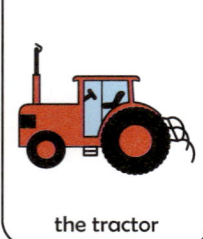 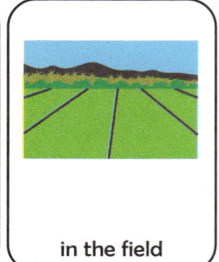

| The farmer | is driving | the tractor | in the field |

Autumn Leaves (*Write About the Picture*, page 9)

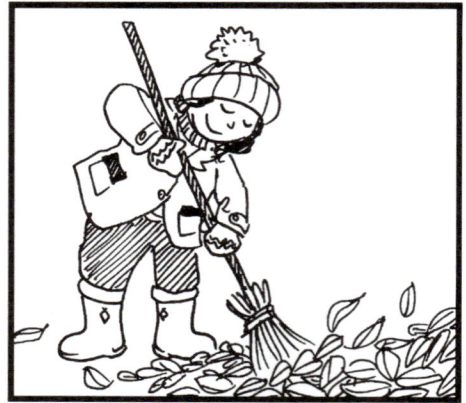

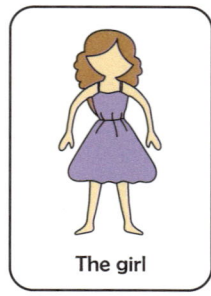 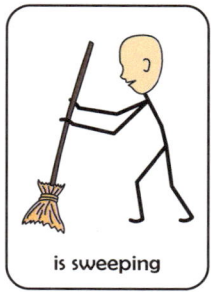 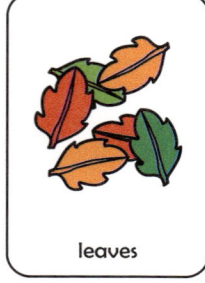 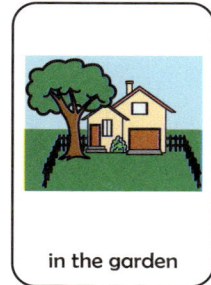

| The girl | is sweeping | leaves | in the garden |

Copyright material from NHS Forth Valley (2020), *Colourful Semantics*, Routledge

Ice cream (*Write About the Picture*, page 15)

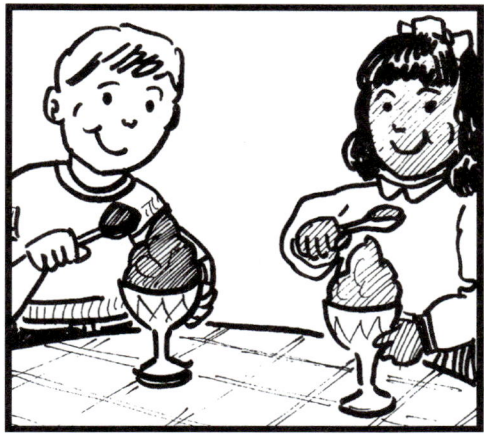

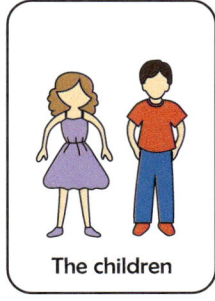

The children

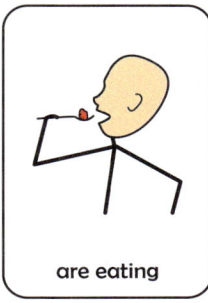

are eating

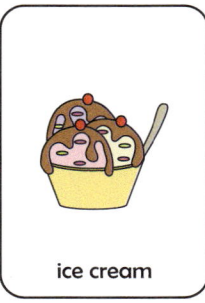

ice cream

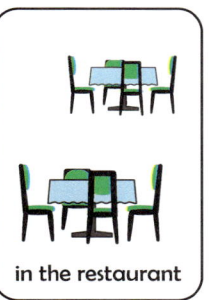

in the restaurant

Dinosaurs (*Write About the Picture 2*, page 25)

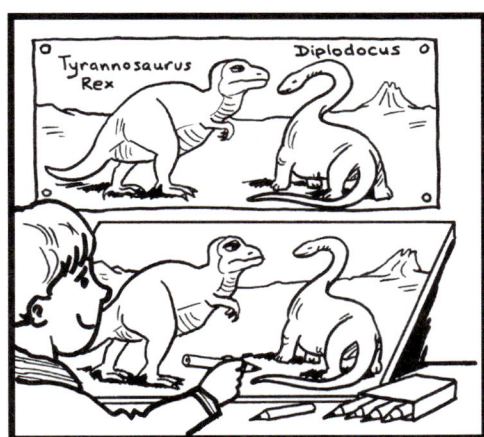

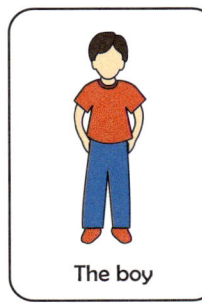

The boy

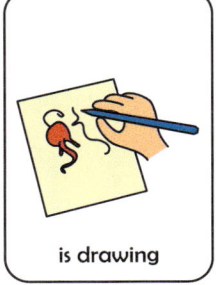

is drawing

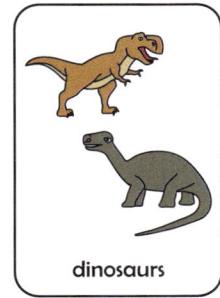

dinosaurs

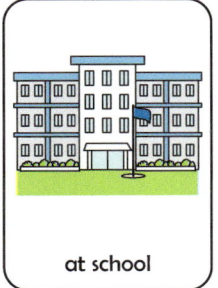

at school

Copyright material from NHS Forth Valley (2020), *Colourful Semantics*, Routledge

Five-part sentences ('*when*', '*who*', '*doing*', '*what*', '*where*')

Use these alongside the 'When, Who, Doing, What, Where' sentence template on page 105.

The Beach (*Write About the Picture 3*, page 1)

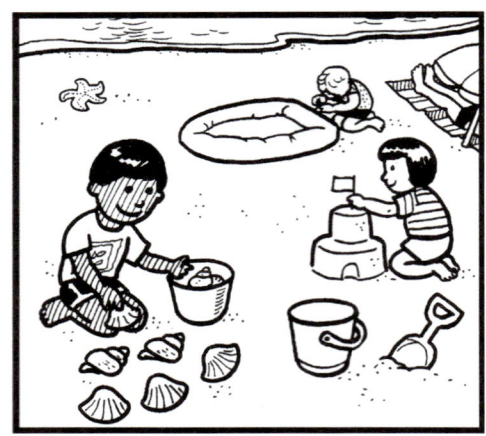

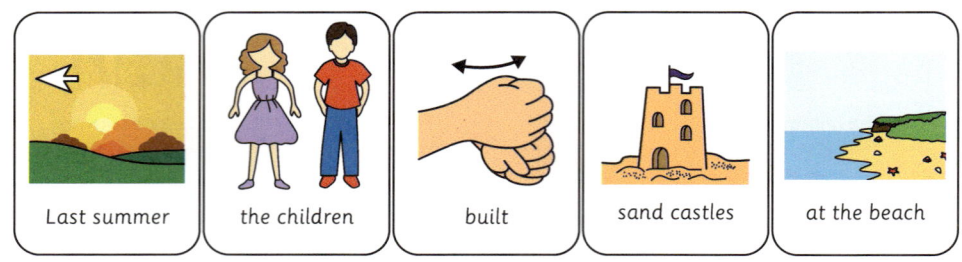

| Last summer | the children | built | sand castles | at the beach |

The Airport (*Write About the Picture 3*, page 6)

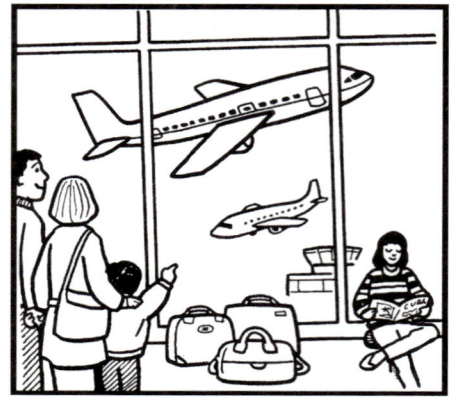

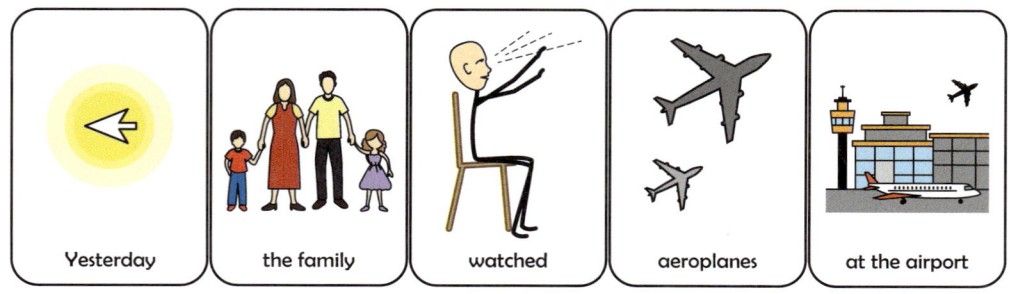

| Yesterday | the family | watched | aeroplanes | at the airport |

Copyright material from NHS Forth Valley (2020), *Colourful Semantics*, Routledge

Playing in the Snow (*Write About the Picture 3*, page 20)

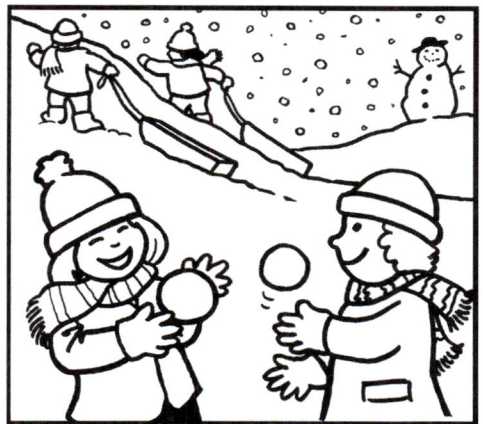

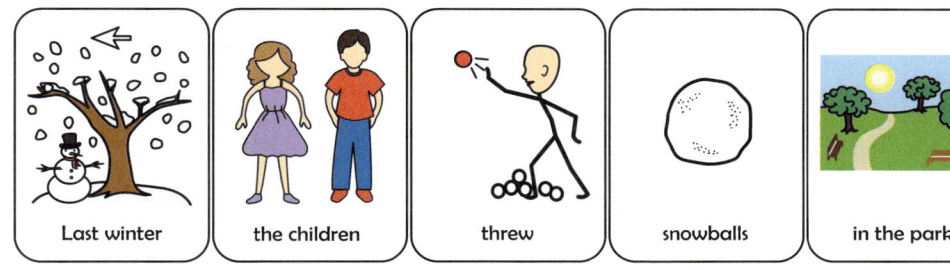

| Last winter | the children | threw | snowballs | in the park |

The Pet Shop (*Write About the Picture 3*, page 14)

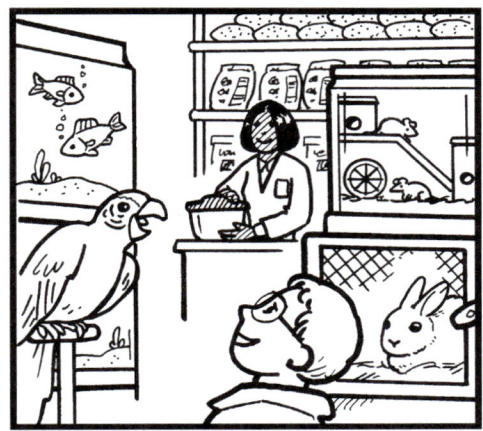

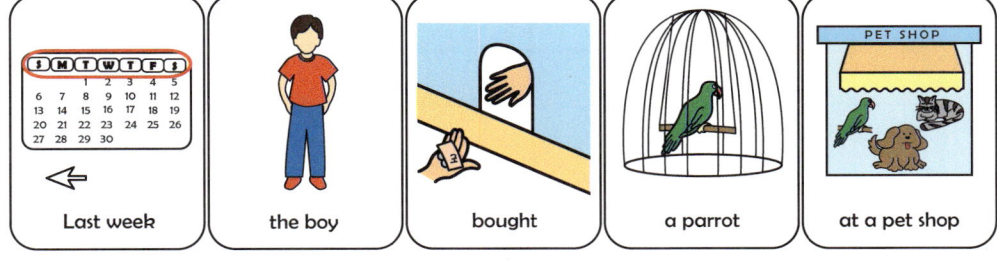

| Last week | the boy | bought | a parrot | at a pet shop |

Copyright material from NHS Forth Valley (2020), *Colourful Semantics*, Routledge

Sentences including 'why'

Making Cakes (*Write About the Picture 3*, page 18)

Use alongside the 'Who, Doing, What, Why' sentence template and blank box template on page 106.

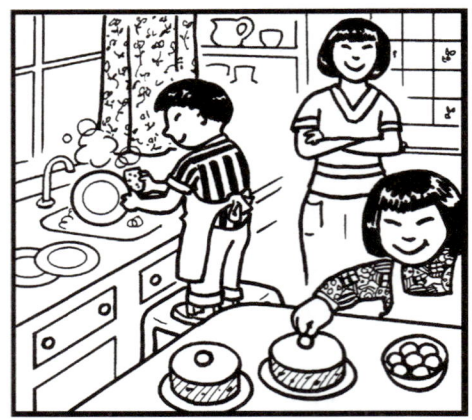

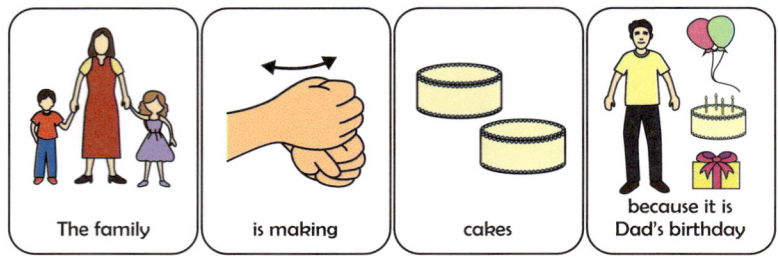

| The family | is making | cakes | because it is Dad's birthday |

Firefighters (*Write About the Picture 3*, page 18 ('who', 'doing', 'what', 'where', 'why'))

Use with the 'Who, Doing, What, Where, Why' sentence template and blank box template on page 106.

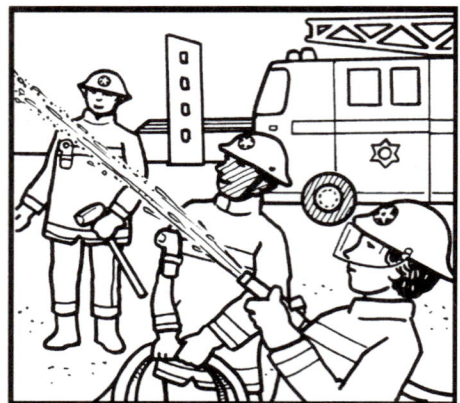

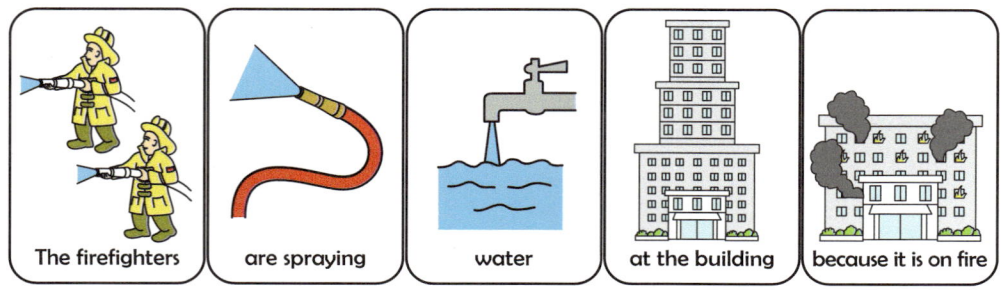

| The firefighters | are spraying | water | at the building | because it is on fire |

Copyright material from NHS Forth Valley (2020), *Colourful Semantics*, Routledge

Sentences including '*to who*'

Plastic Models (*Write About the Picture 5*, page 4 (*'who'*, *'doing'*, *'what'*, *'to who'*))

Use with the 'Who, Doing, What, to Who' sentence template and blank box template on page 107.

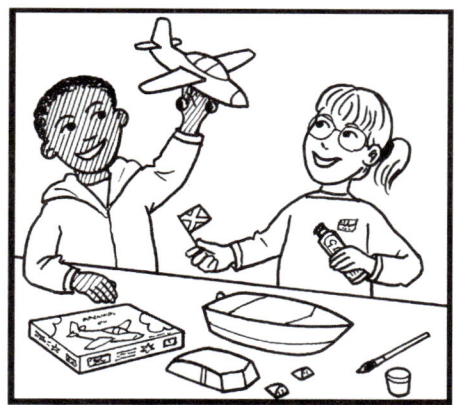

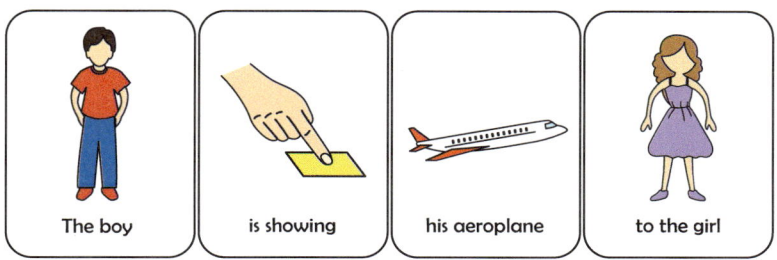

Mother's Day (*Write About the Picture 6*, page 25 (*'when'*, *'who'*, *'doing'*, *'what'*, to *'who'*))

Use with the 'When, Who, Doing, What, to Who' sentence template and blank box template on page 107.

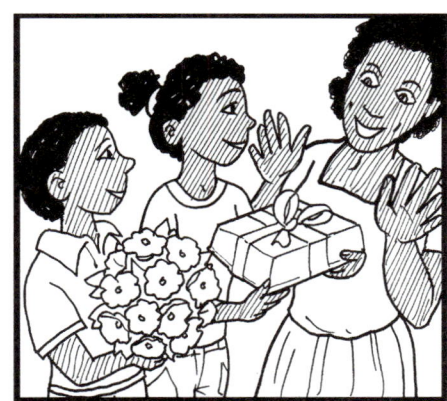

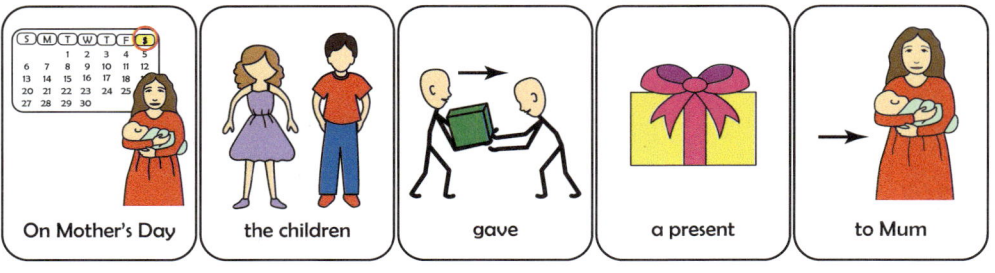

Copyright material from NHS Forth Valley (2020), *Colourful Semantics*, Routledge

Sentences including 'how'

Use these pictures alongside the 'When, Who, Doing, What, How' sentence template and blank box template on page 107.

Washing the Car (*Write About the Picture 5*, page 11)

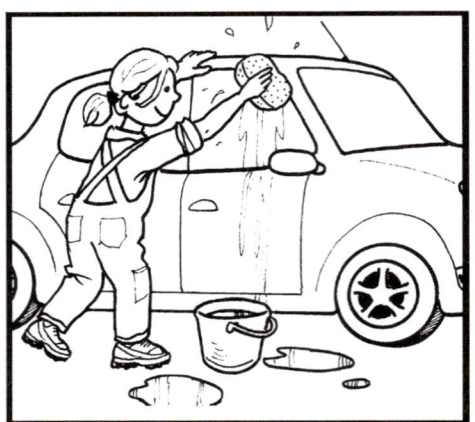

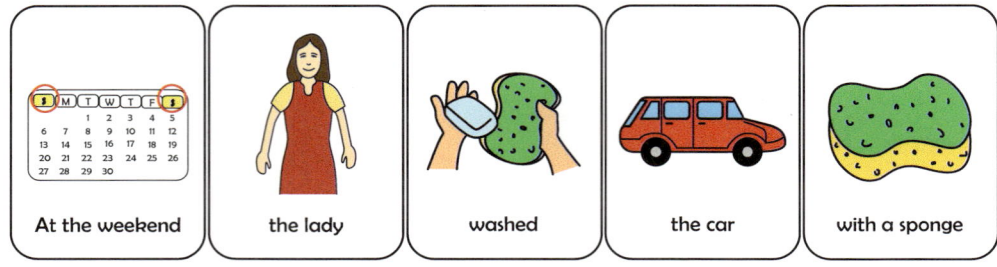

| At the weekend | the lady | washed | the car | with a sponge |

Playing Snakes and Ladders (*Write About the Picture 6*, page 15)

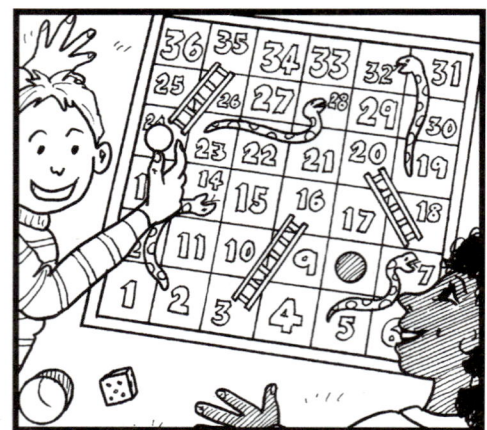

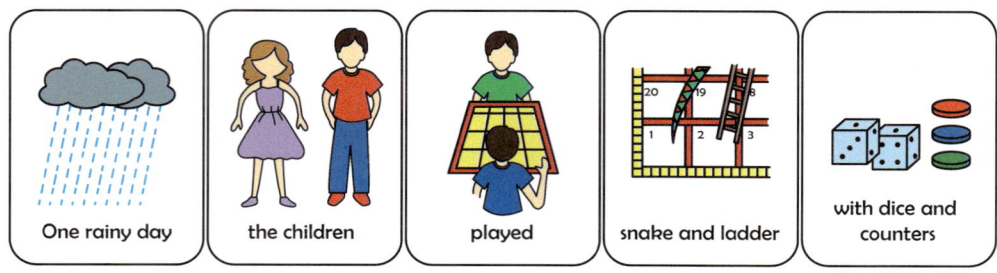

| One rainy day | the children | played | snake and ladder | with dice and counters |

Copyright material from NHS Forth Valley (2020), *Colourful Semantics*, Routledge

Example sentence templates

Cue card sentence templates and blank box templates, for use with the sentence building activities above.

Who, Doing:

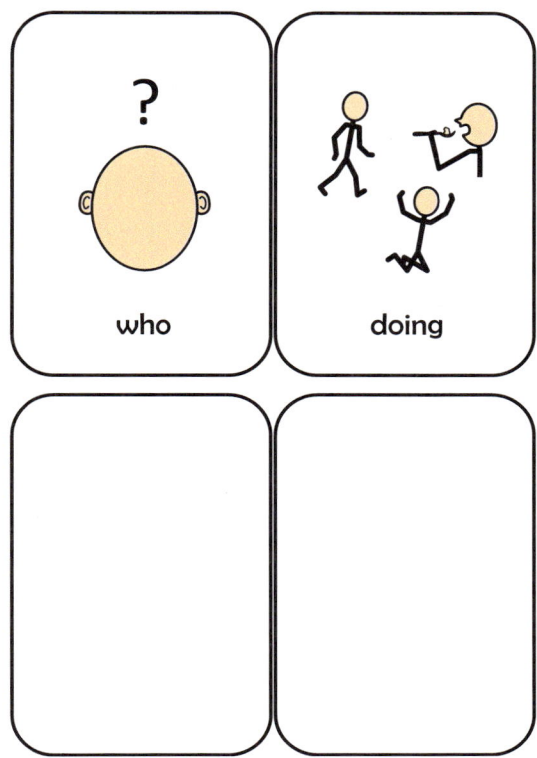

Who, Doing, What:

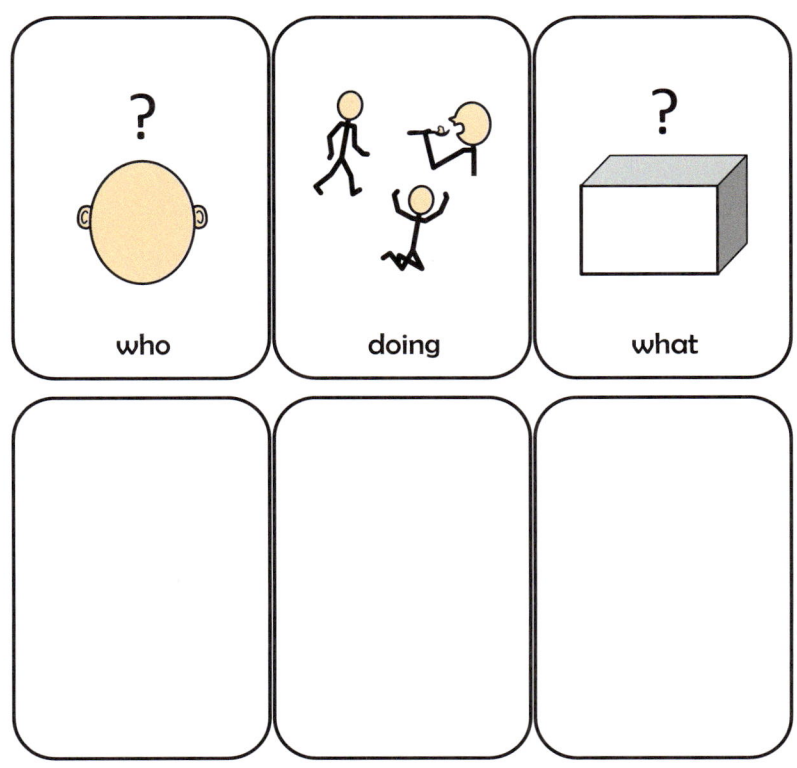

Copyright material from NHS Forth Valley (2020), *Colourful Semantics*, Routledge

Who, Doing, Where:

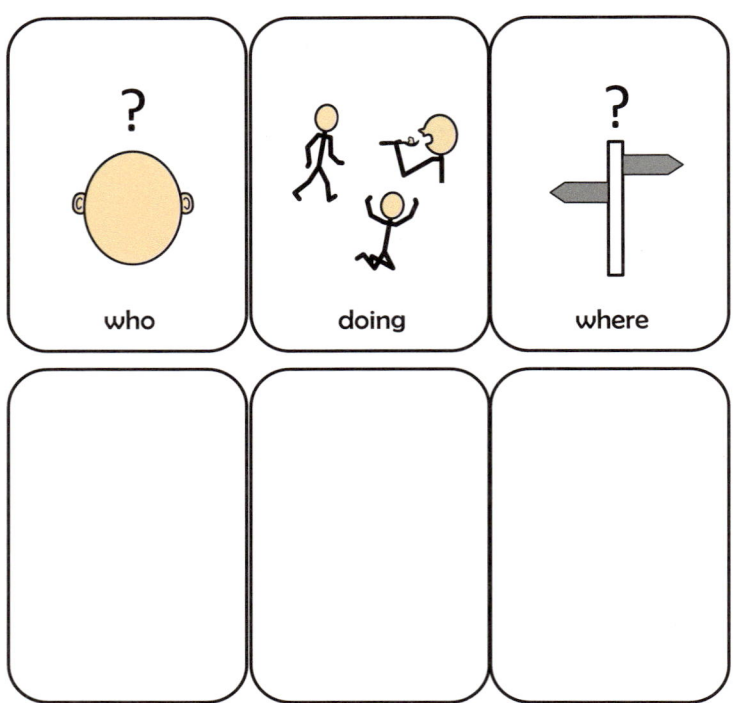

Who, Doing, What, Where:

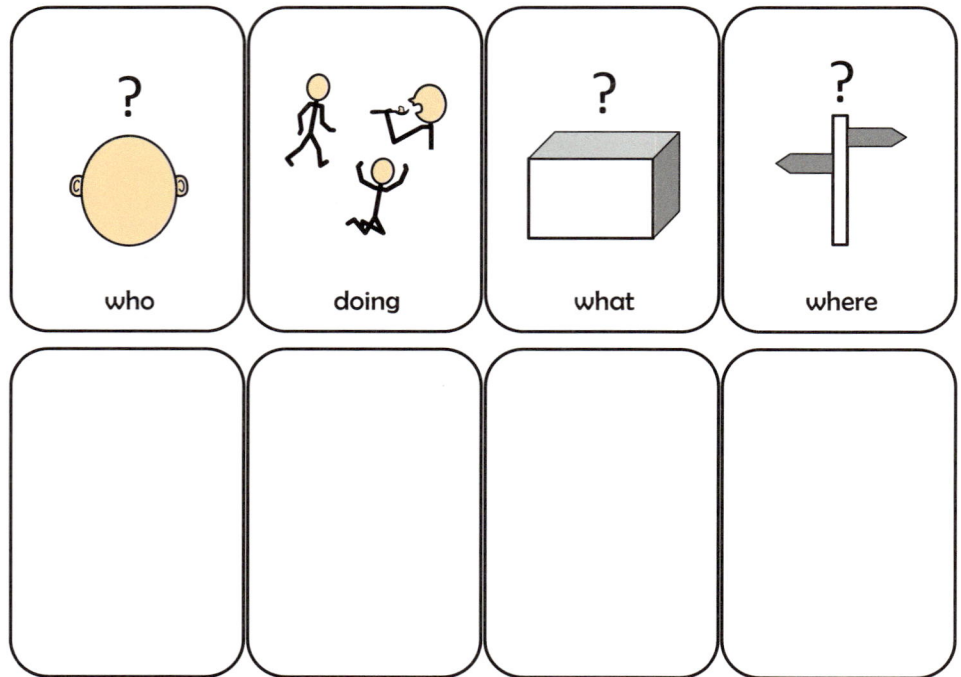

Copyright material from NHS Forth Valley (2020), *Colourful Semantics*, Routledge

When, Who, Doing, What, Where:

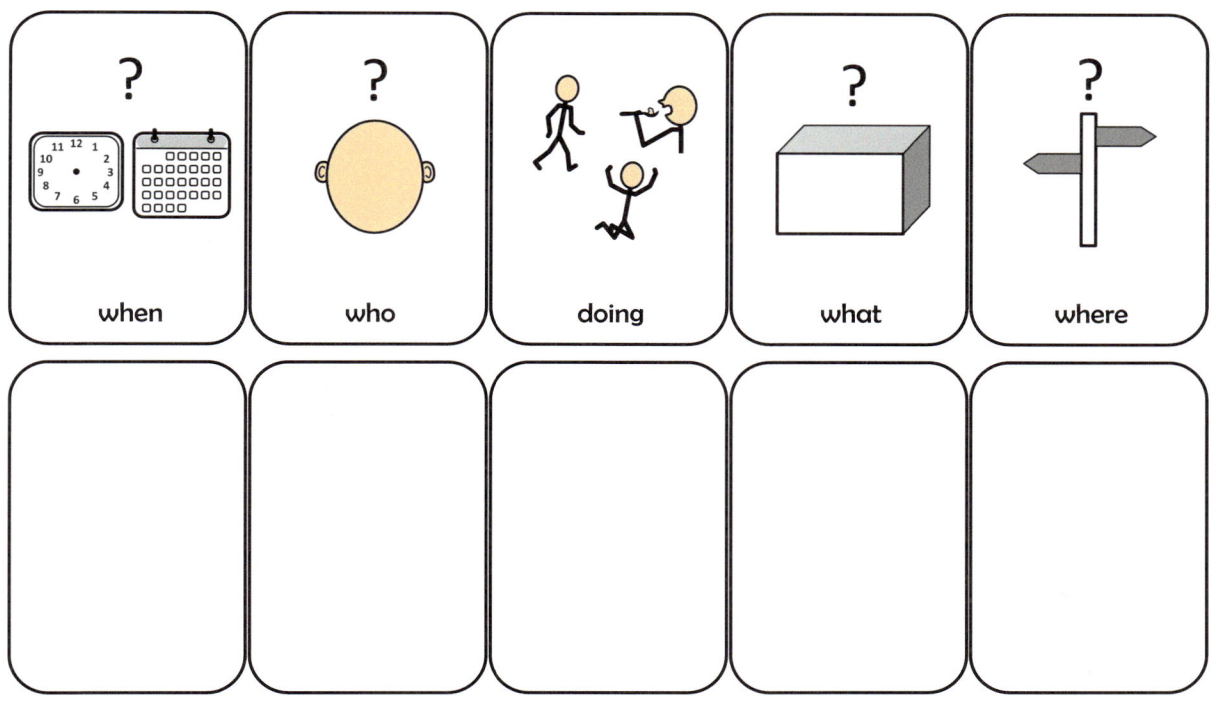

Who, Doing, What, Where, When:

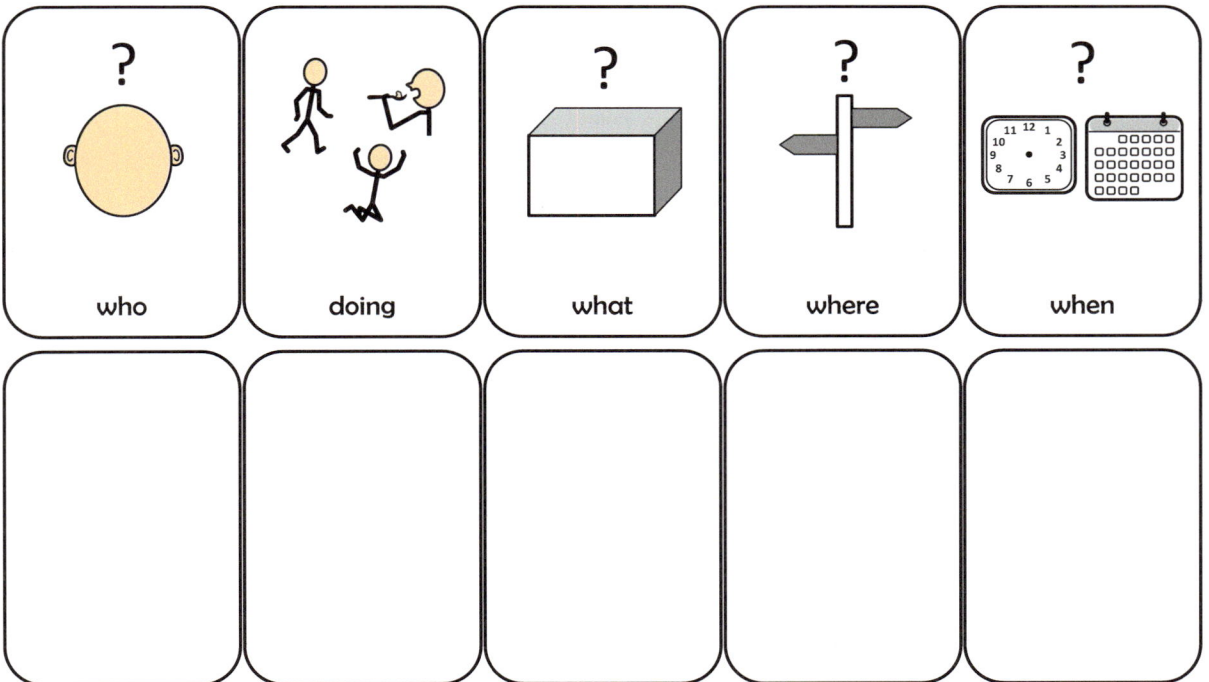

Copyright material from NHS Forth Valley (2020), *Colourful Semantics*, Routledge

Who, Doing, What, Why:

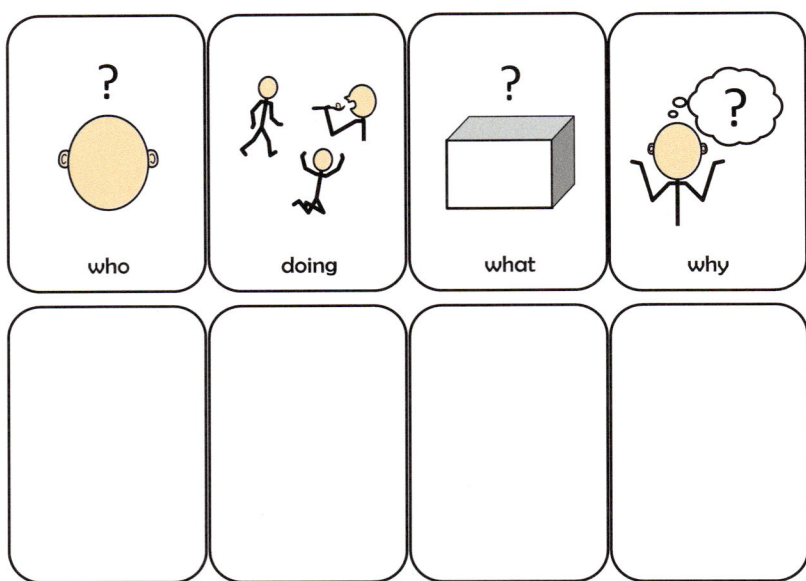

Who, Doing, What, Where, Why:

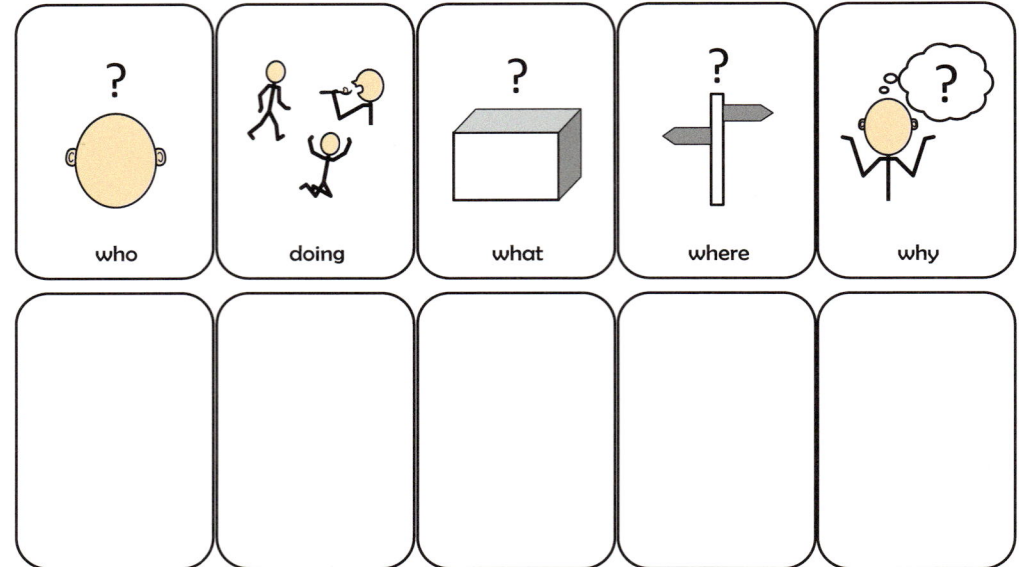

Copyright material from NHS Forth Valley (2020), *Colourful Semantics*, Routledge

Who, Doing, What, to Who:

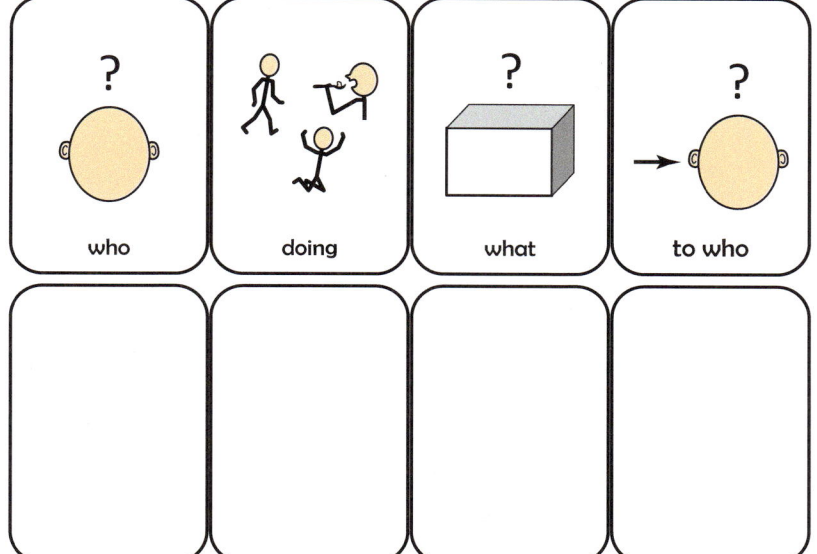

When, Who, Doing, What, to Who:

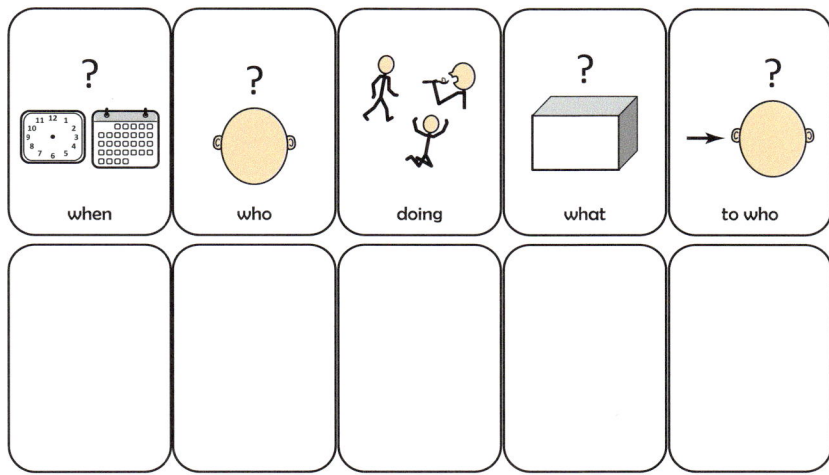

When, Who, Doing, What, How:

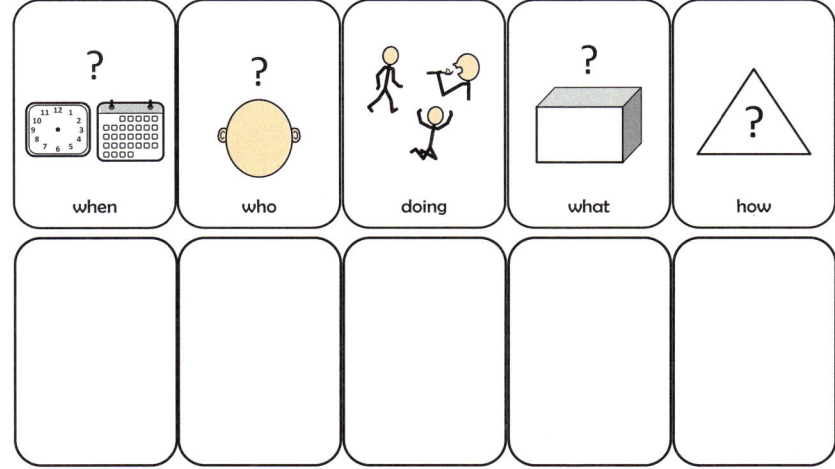

Copyright material from NHS Forth Valley (2020), *Colourful Semantics*, Routledge

Appendix 4
A5 vocabulary cards

Copyright material from NHS Forth Valley (2020), *Colourful Semantics*, Routledge

'Who' vocabulary

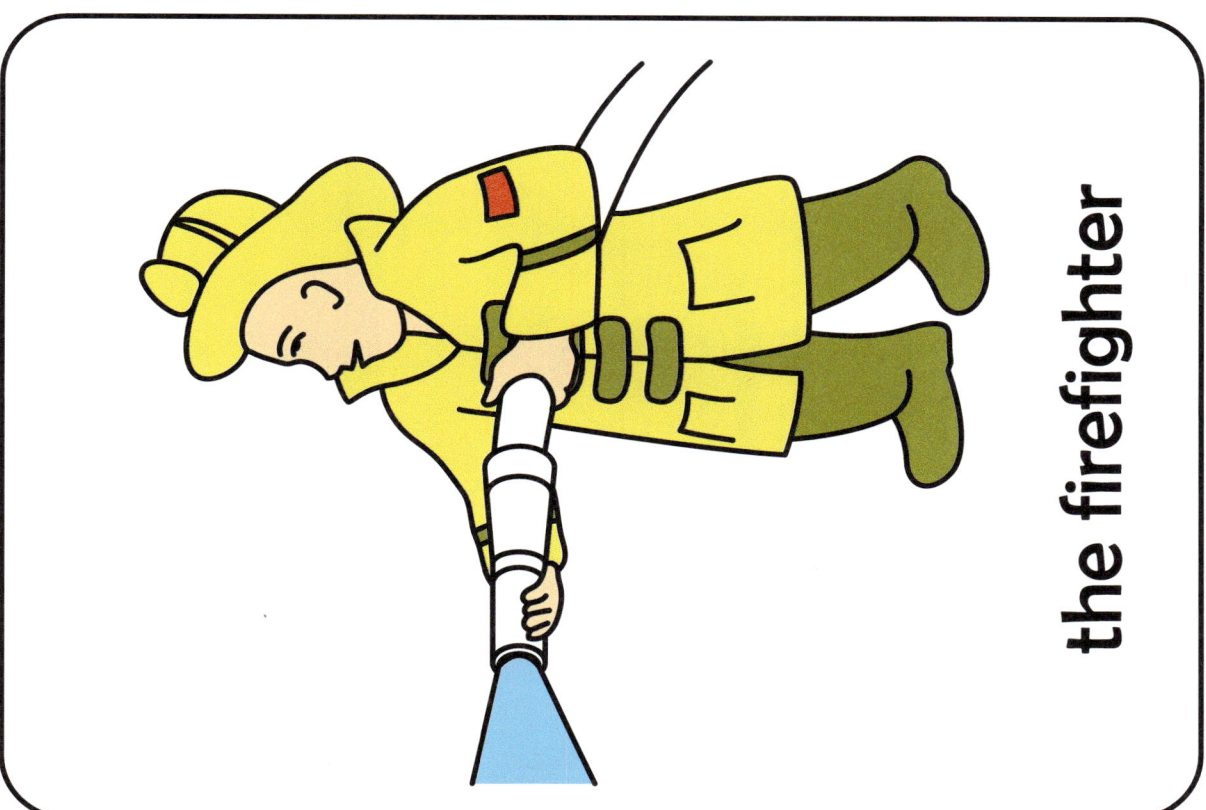

the firefighter

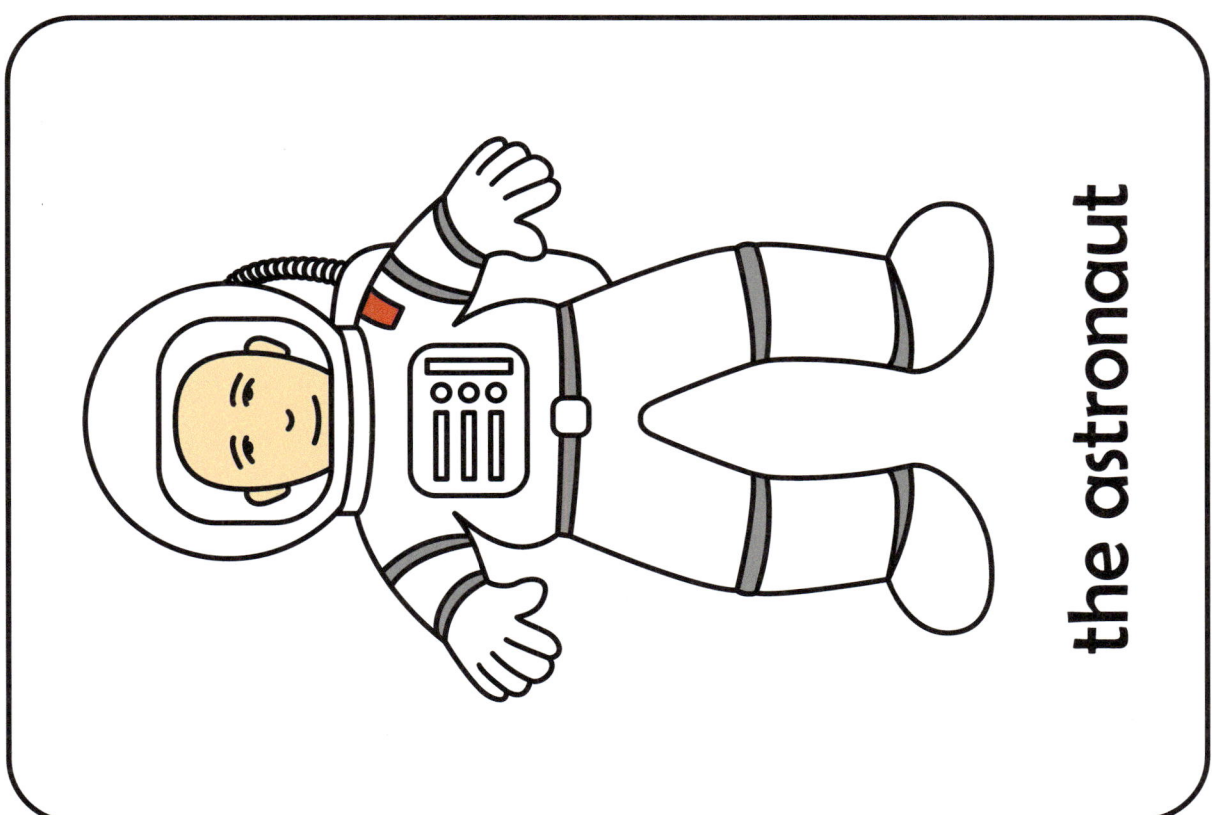

the astronaut

Copyright material from NHS Forth Valley (2020), *Colourful Semantics*, Routledge

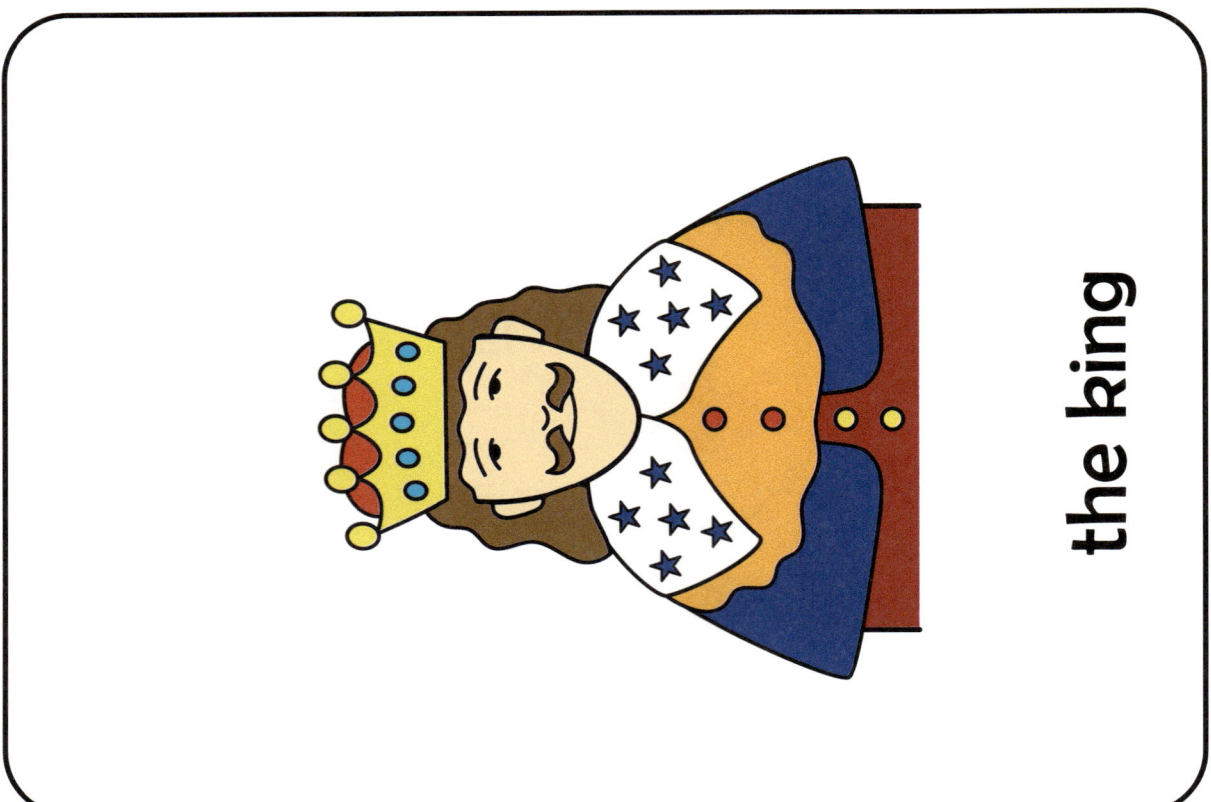

the king

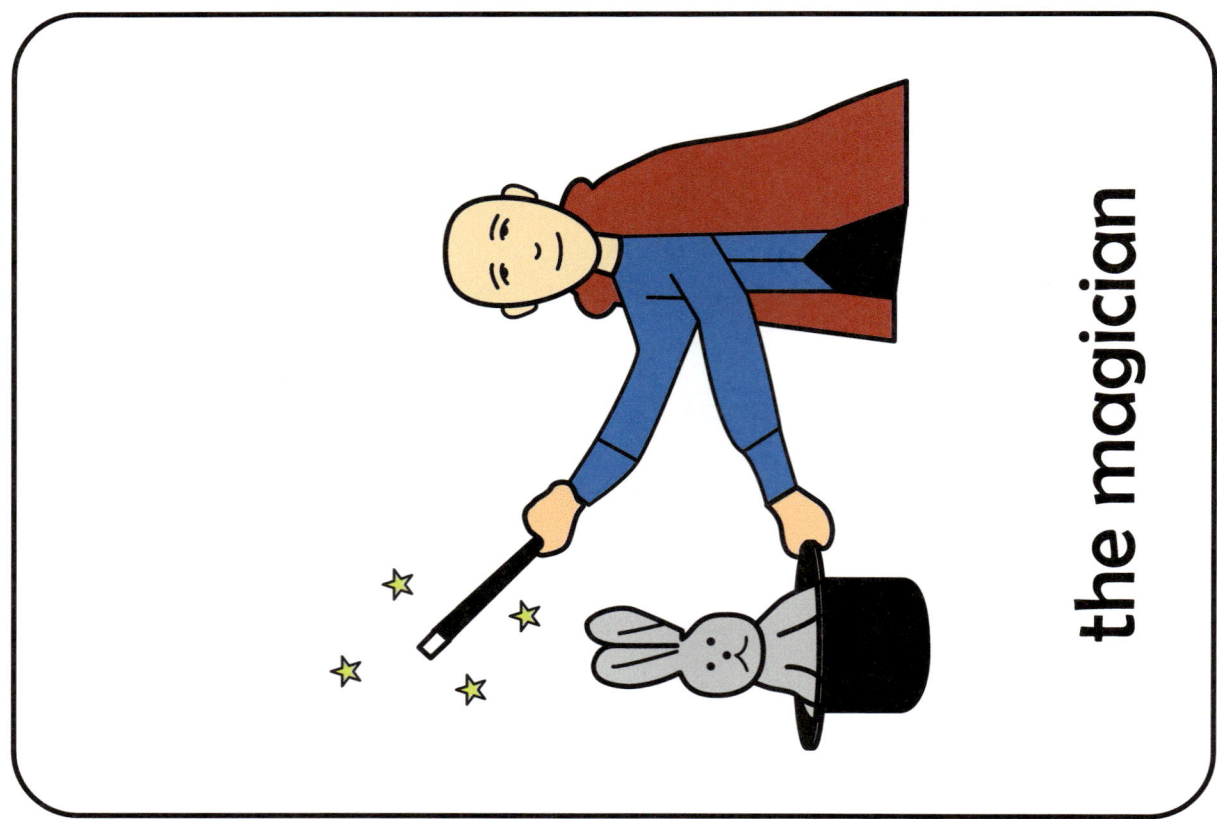

the magician

Copyright material from NHS Forth Valley (2020), *Colourful Semantics*, Routledge

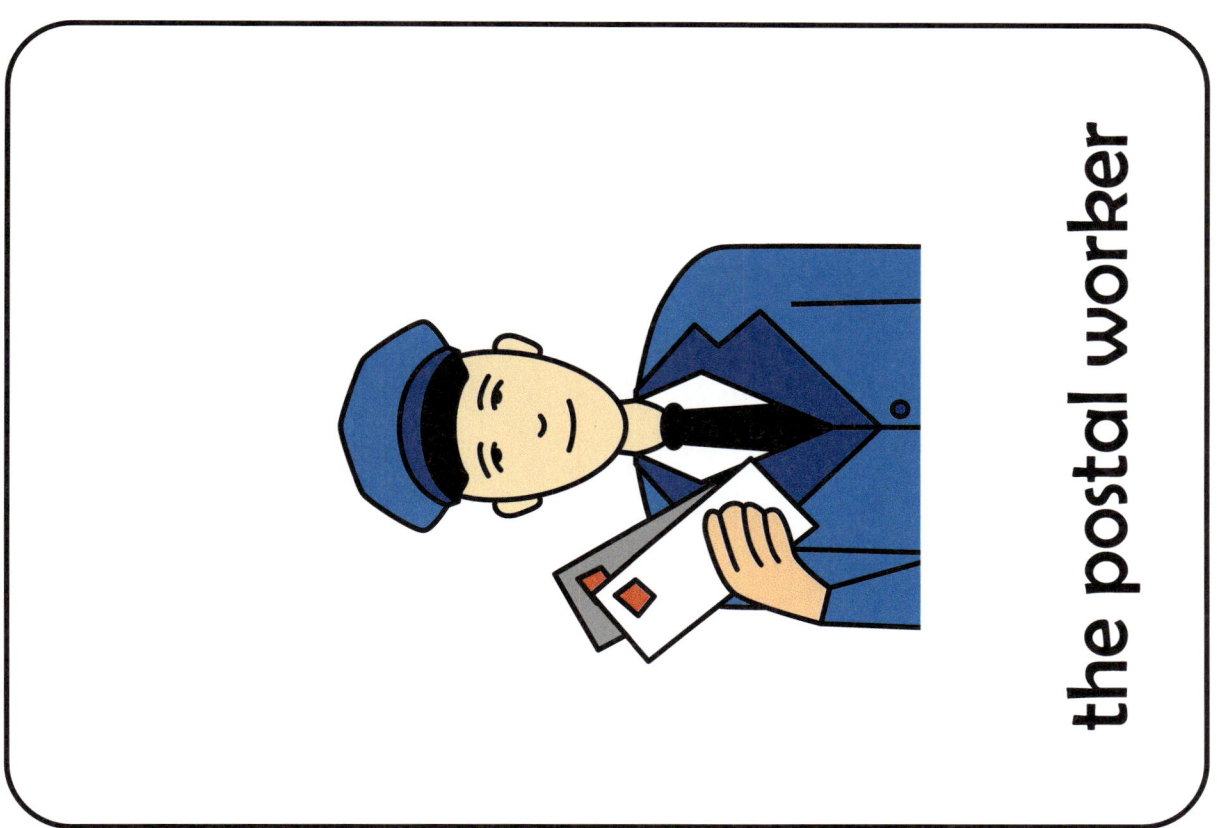

the postal worker

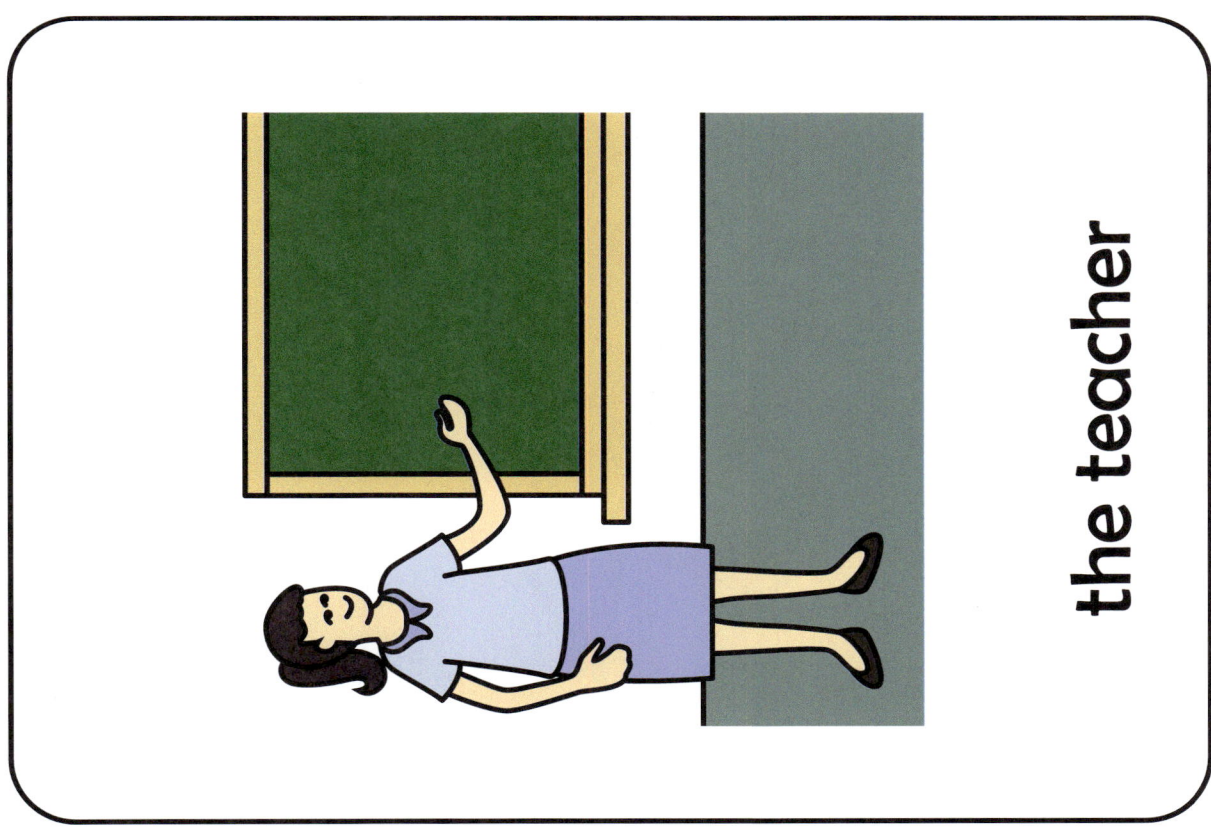

the teacher

Copyright material from NHS Forth Valley (2020), *Colourful Semantics*, Routledge

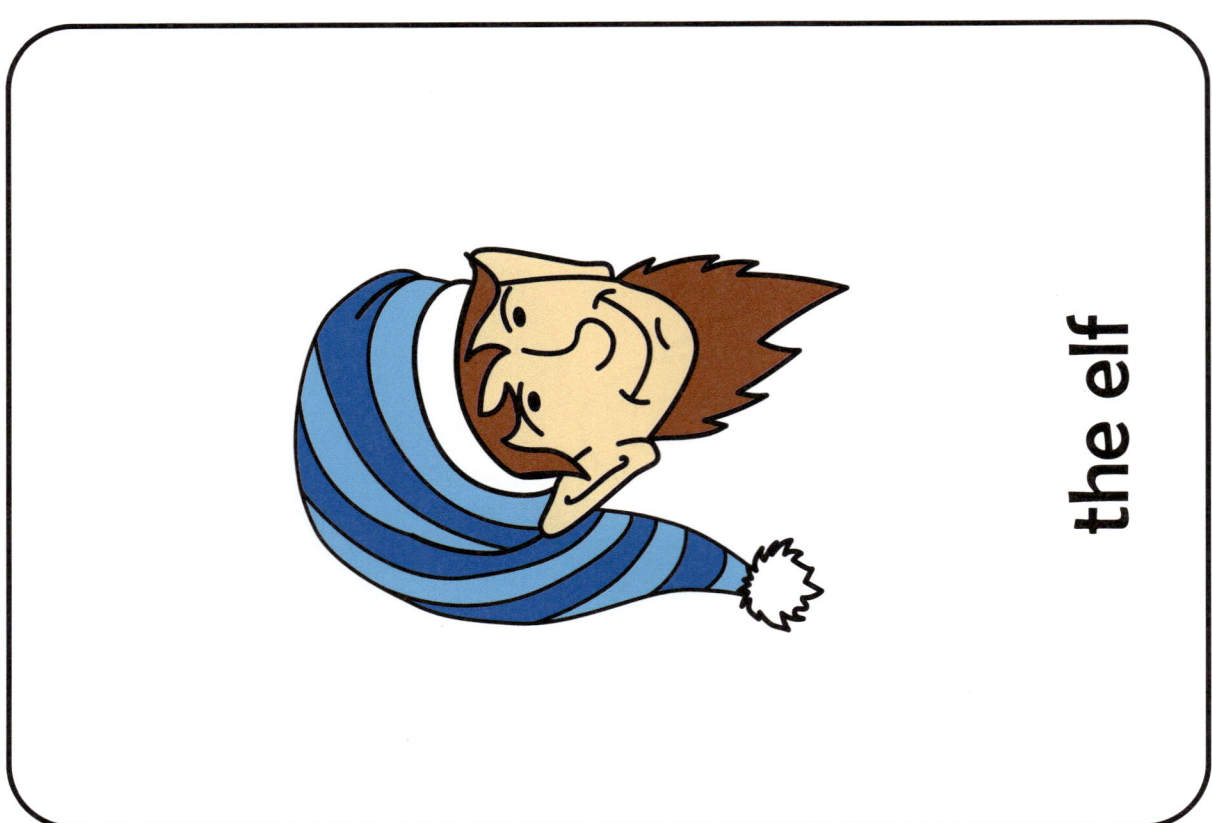

the elf

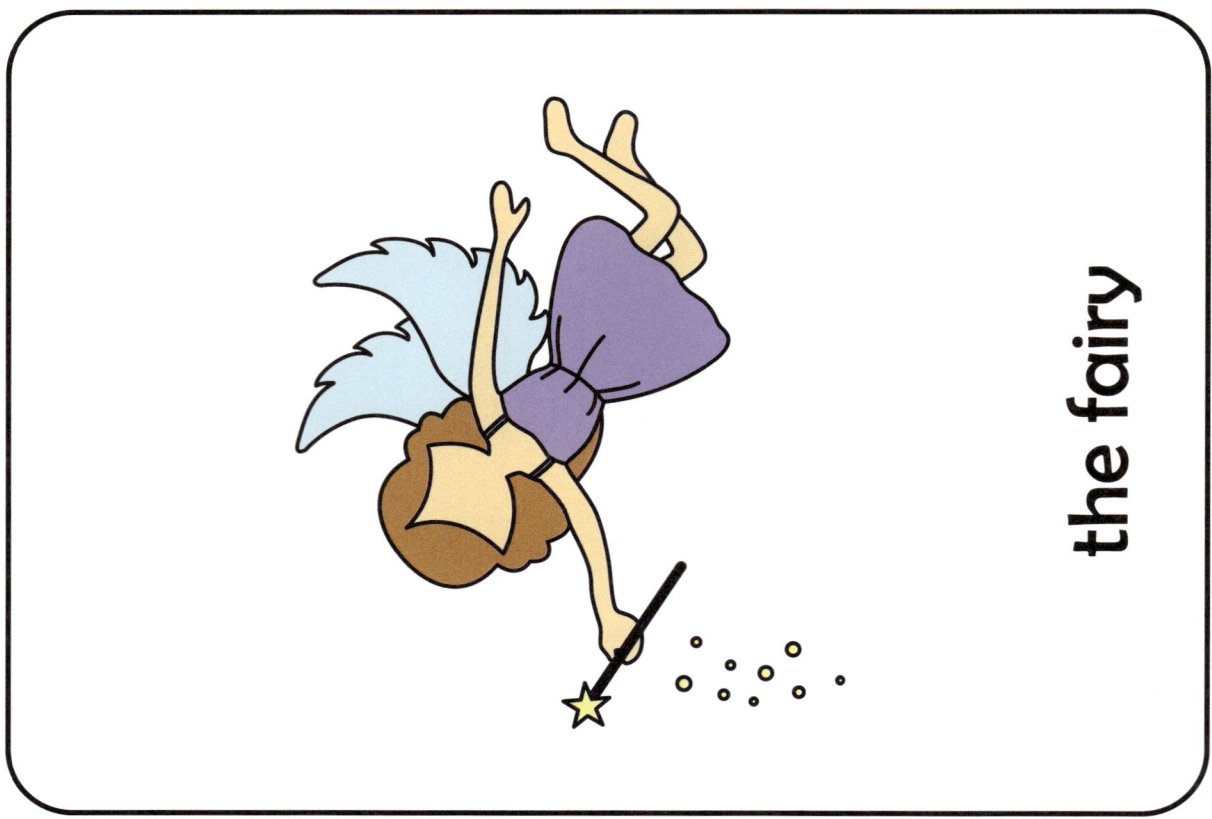

the fairy

Copyright material from NHS Forth Valley (2020), *Colourful Semantics*, Routledge

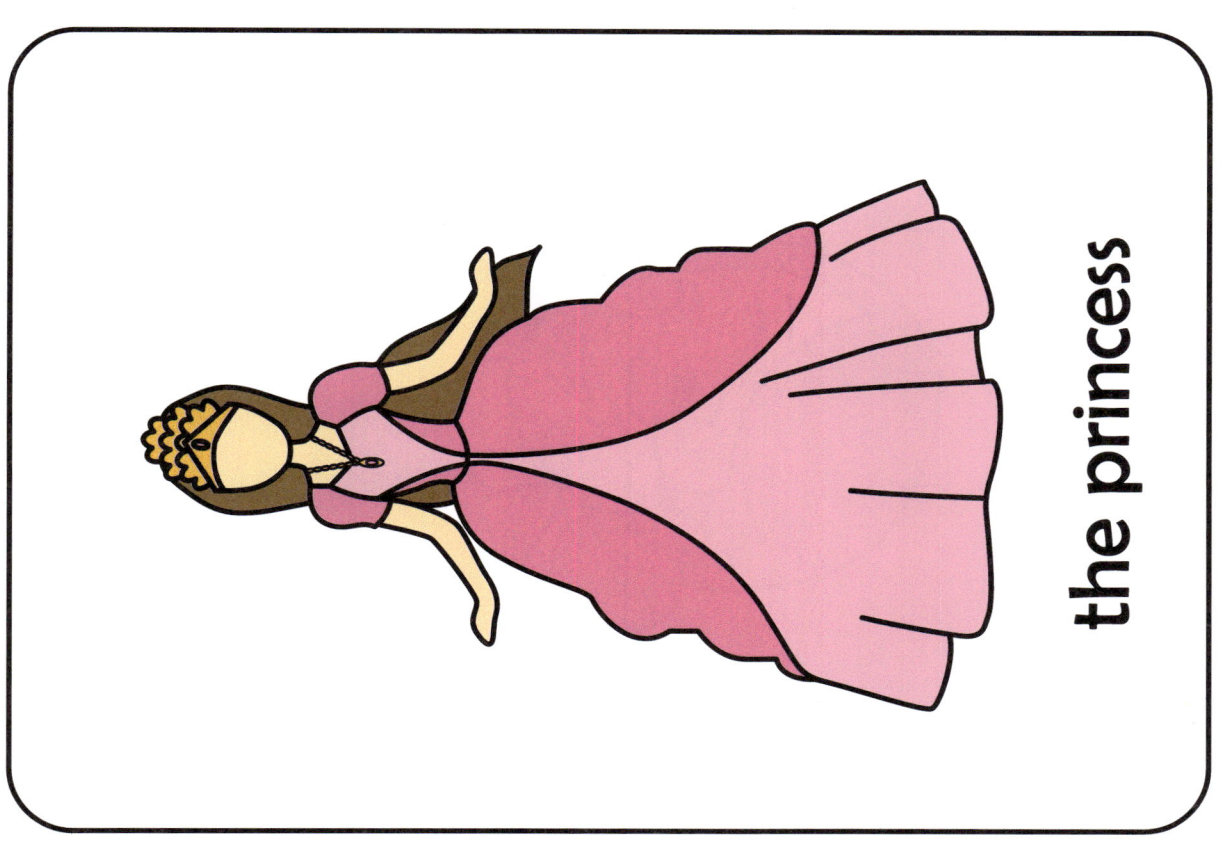

the princess

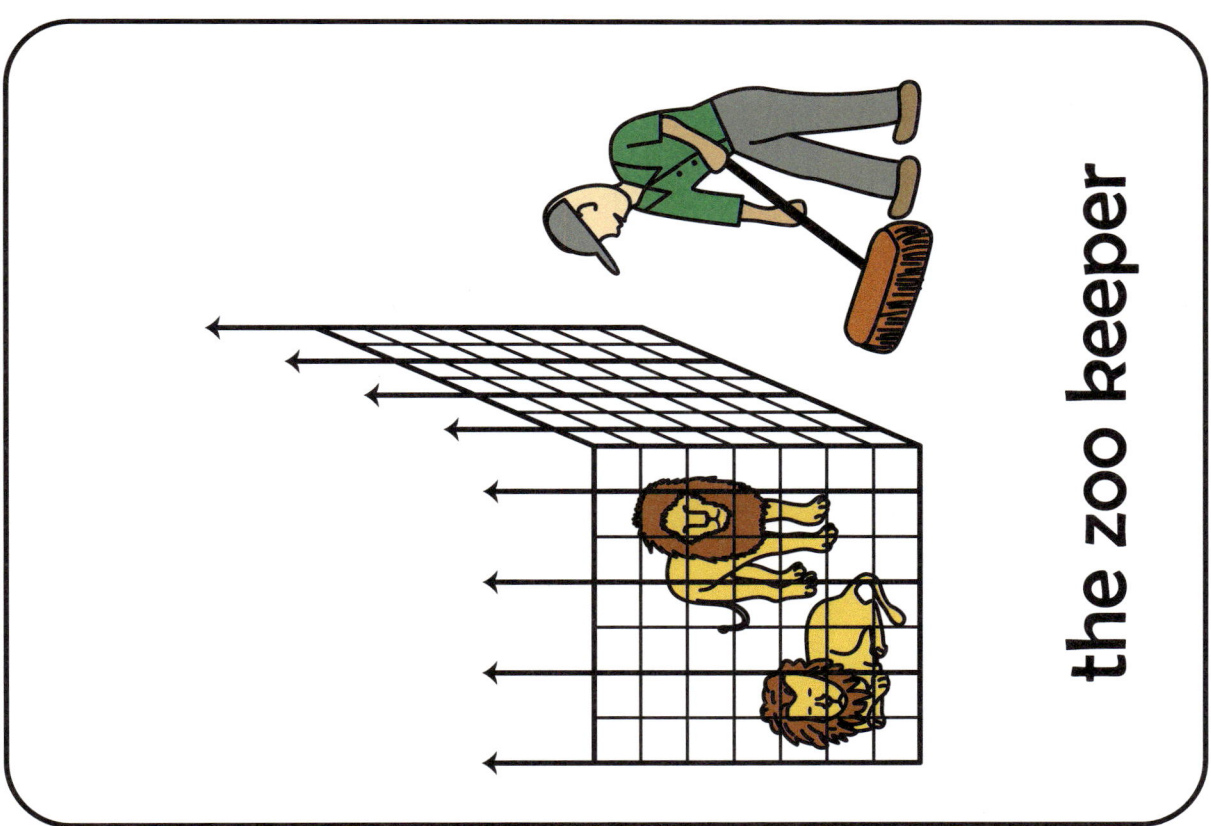

the zoo keeper

Copyright material from NHS Forth Valley (2020), *Colourful Semantics*, Routledge

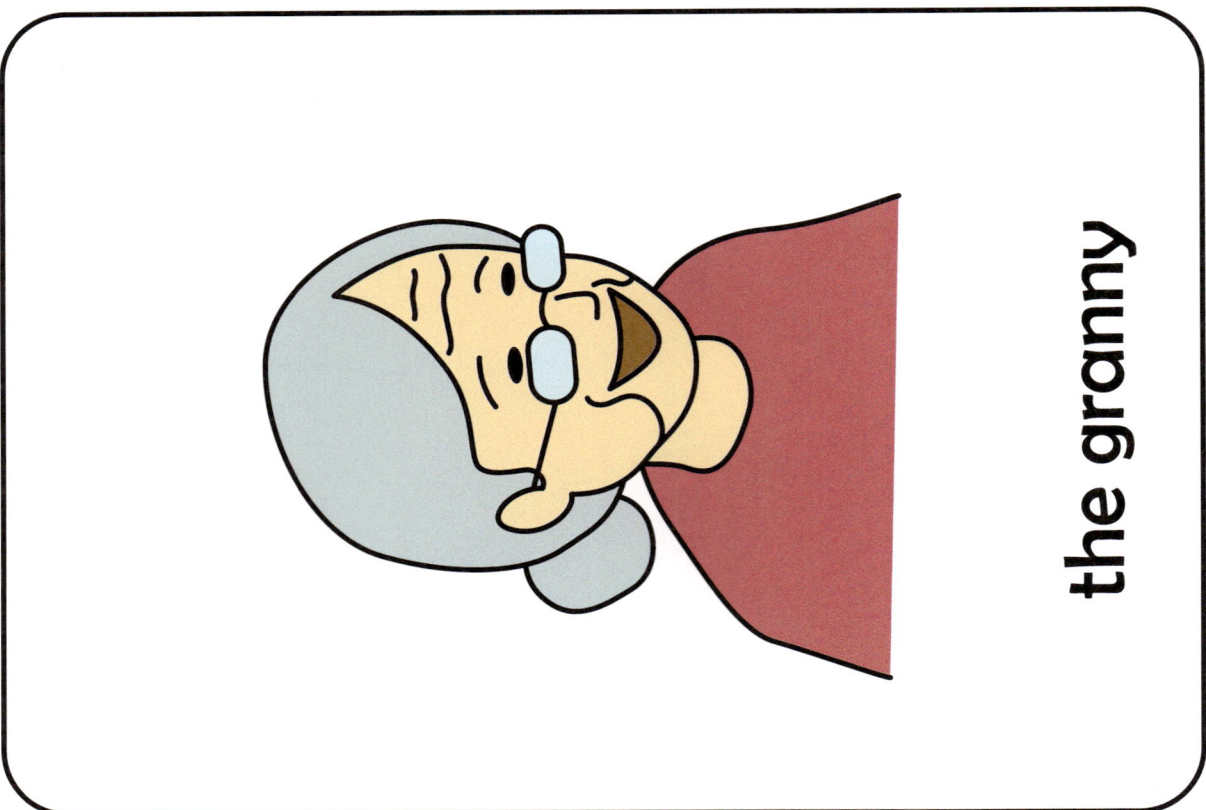

the granny

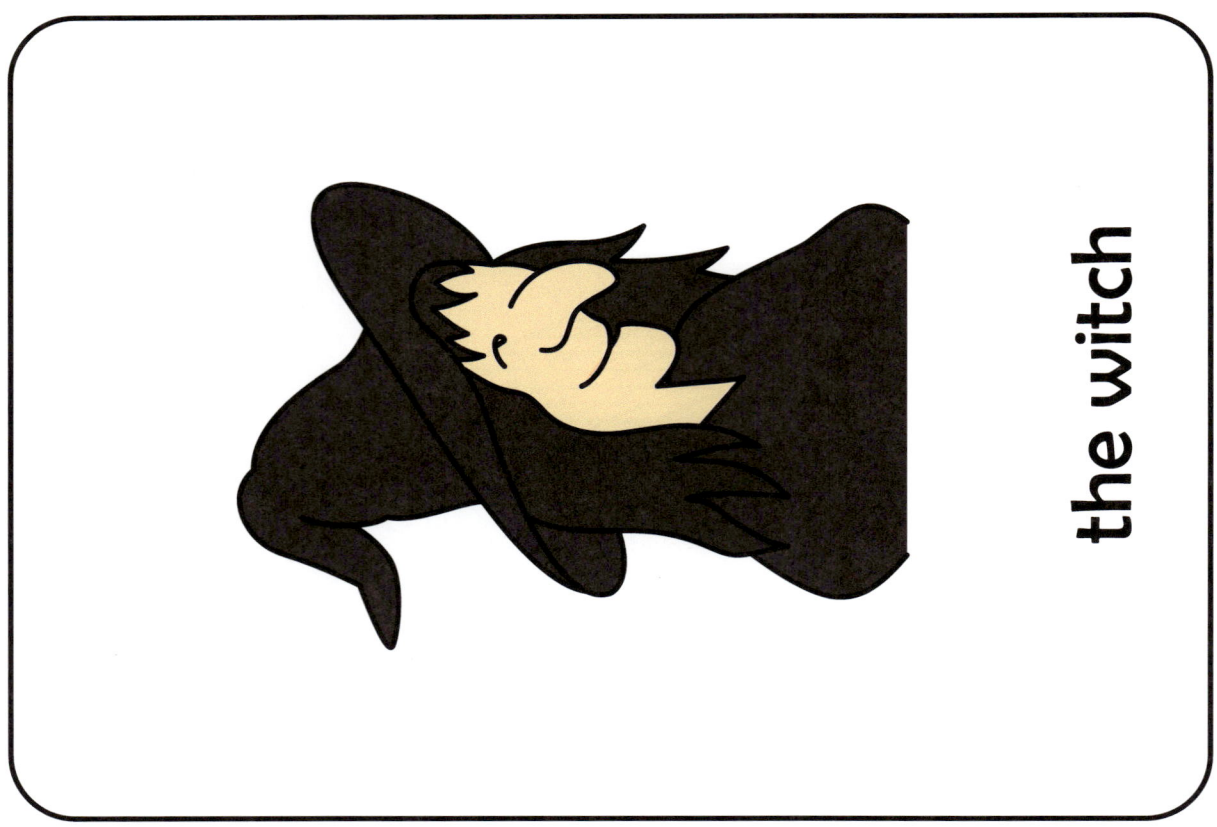

the witch

Copyright material from NHS Forth Valley (2020), *Colourful Semantics*, Routledge

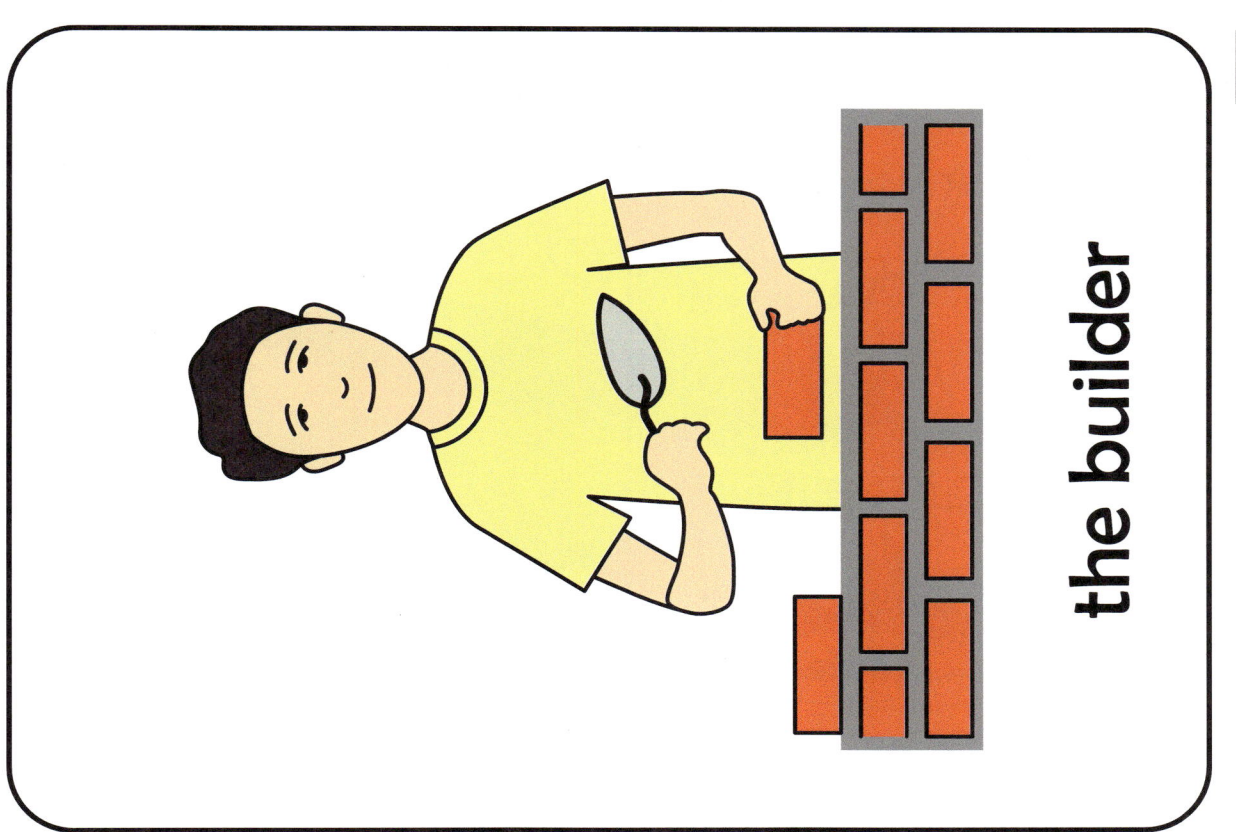

the builder

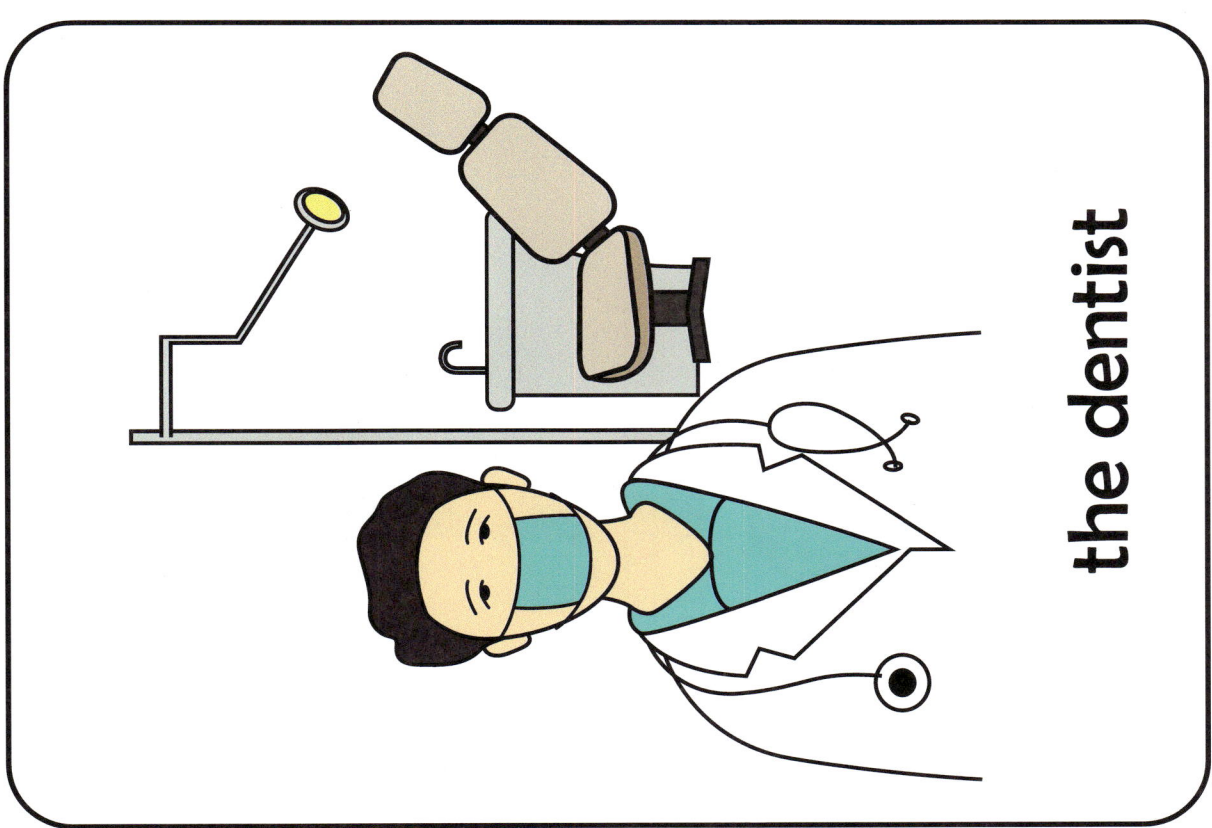

the dentist

Copyright material from NHS Forth Valley (2020), *Colourful Semantics*, Routledge

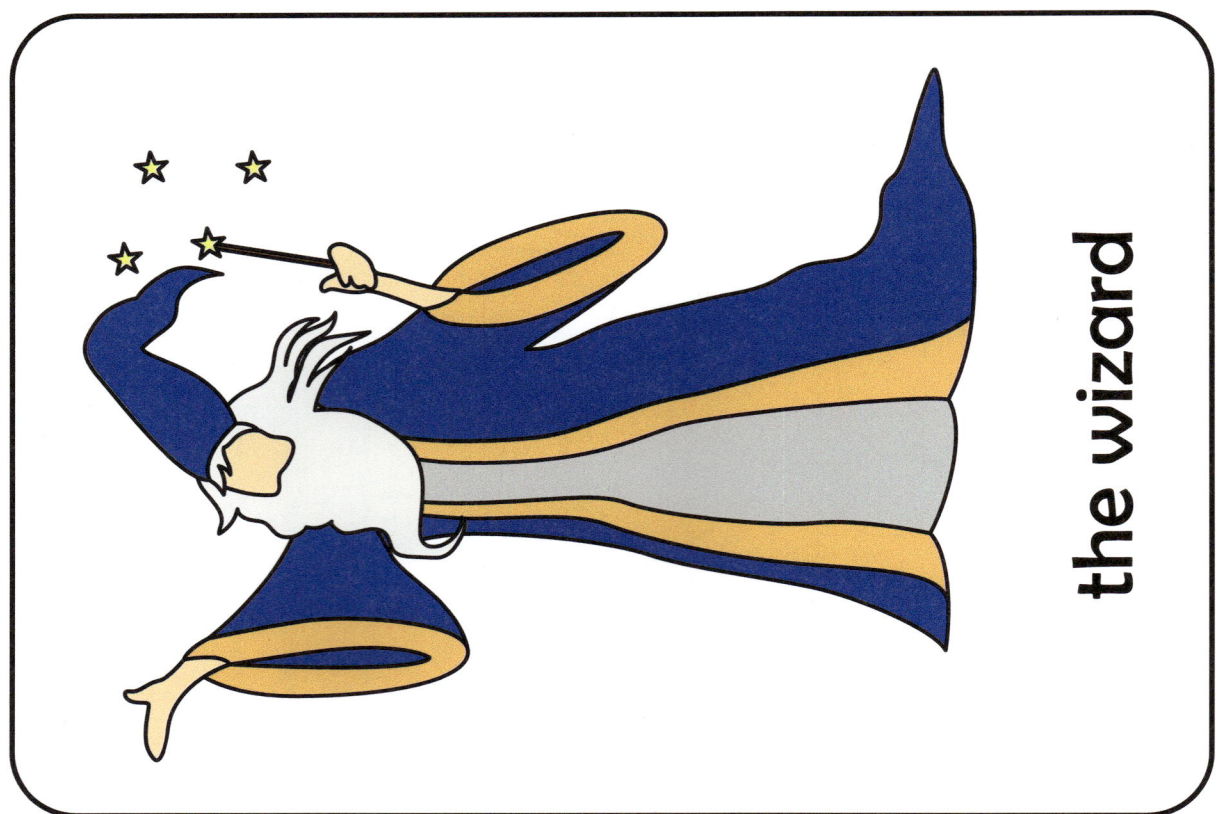

the wizard

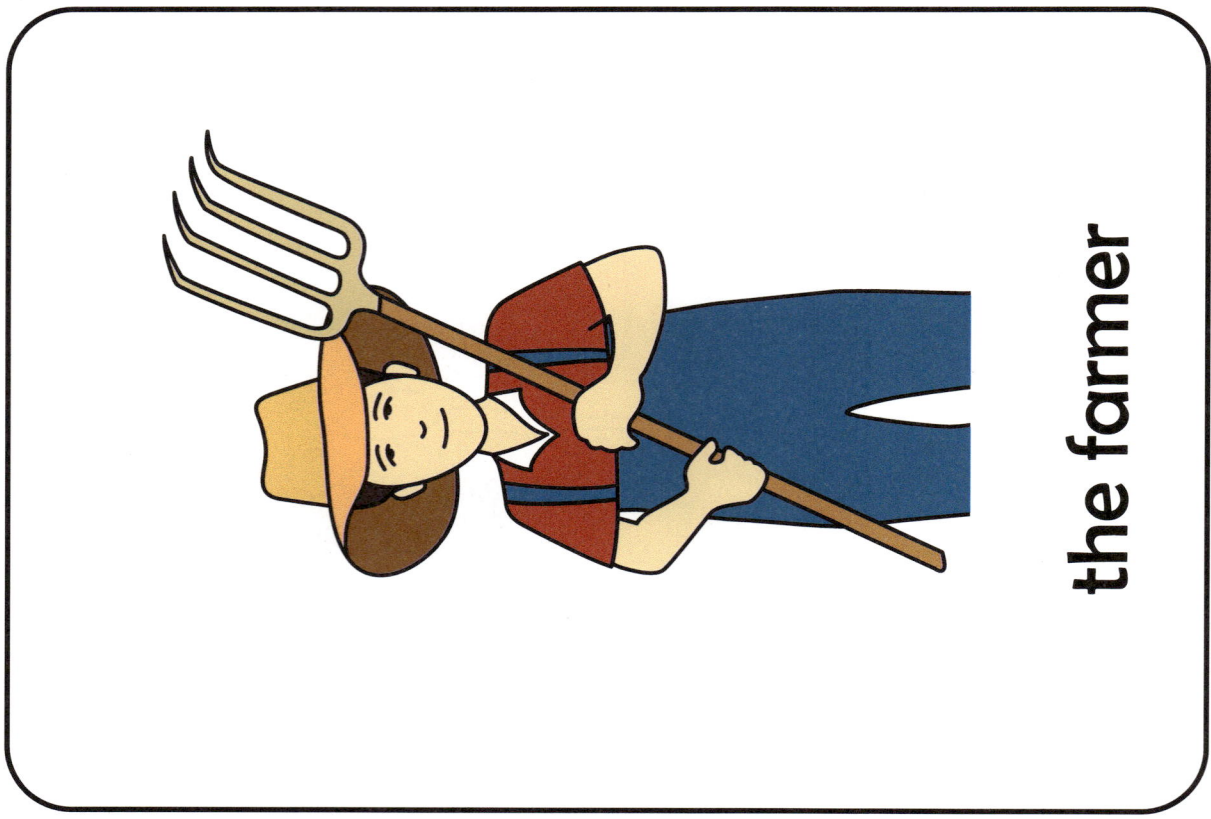

the farmer

Copyright material from NHS Forth Valley (2020), *Colourful Semantics*, Routledge

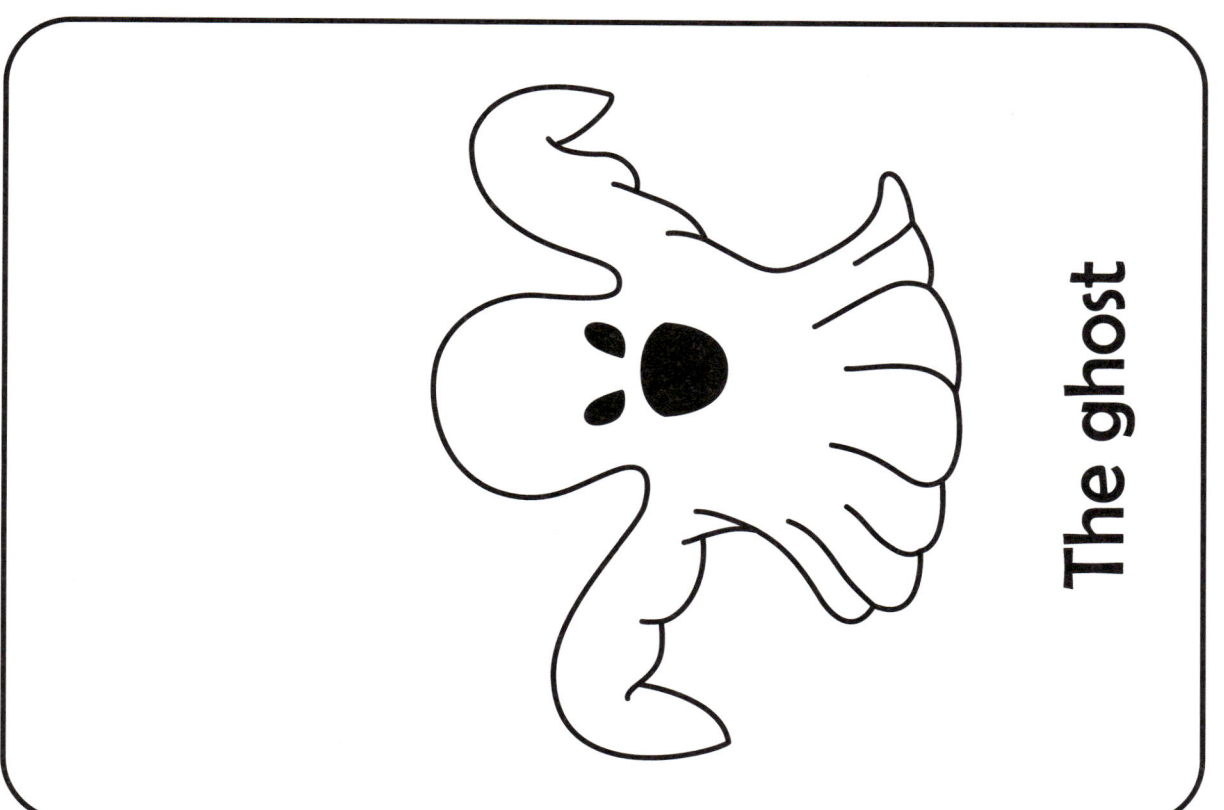

The ghost

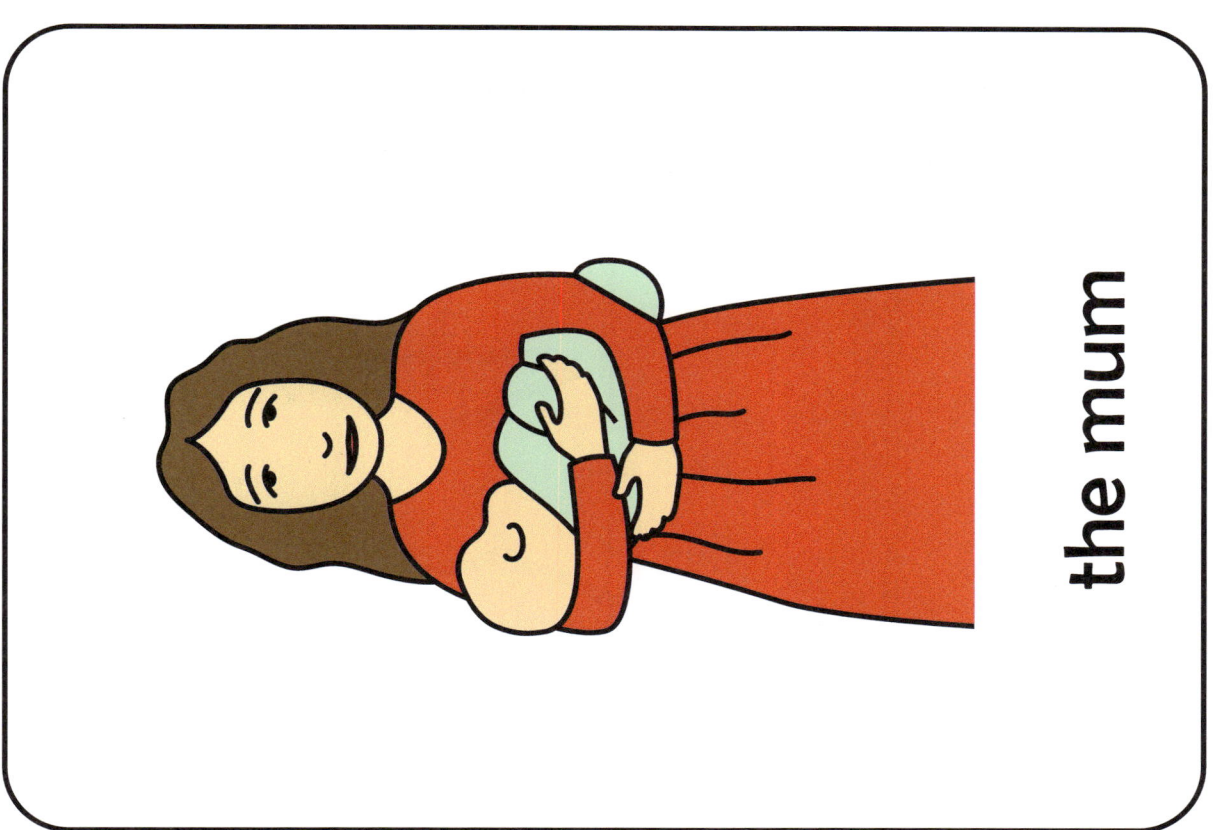

the mum

Copyright material from NHS Forth Valley (2020), *Colourful Semantics*, Routledge

'Doing' vocabulary

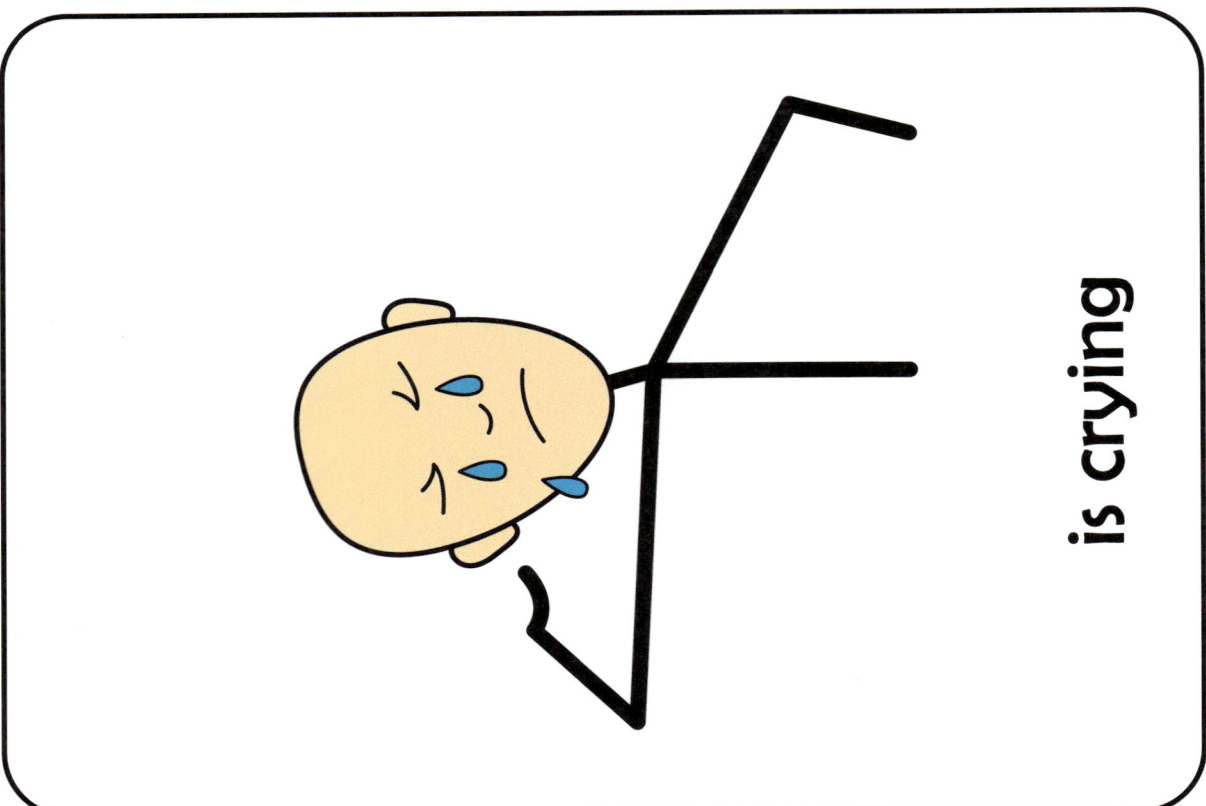

is crying

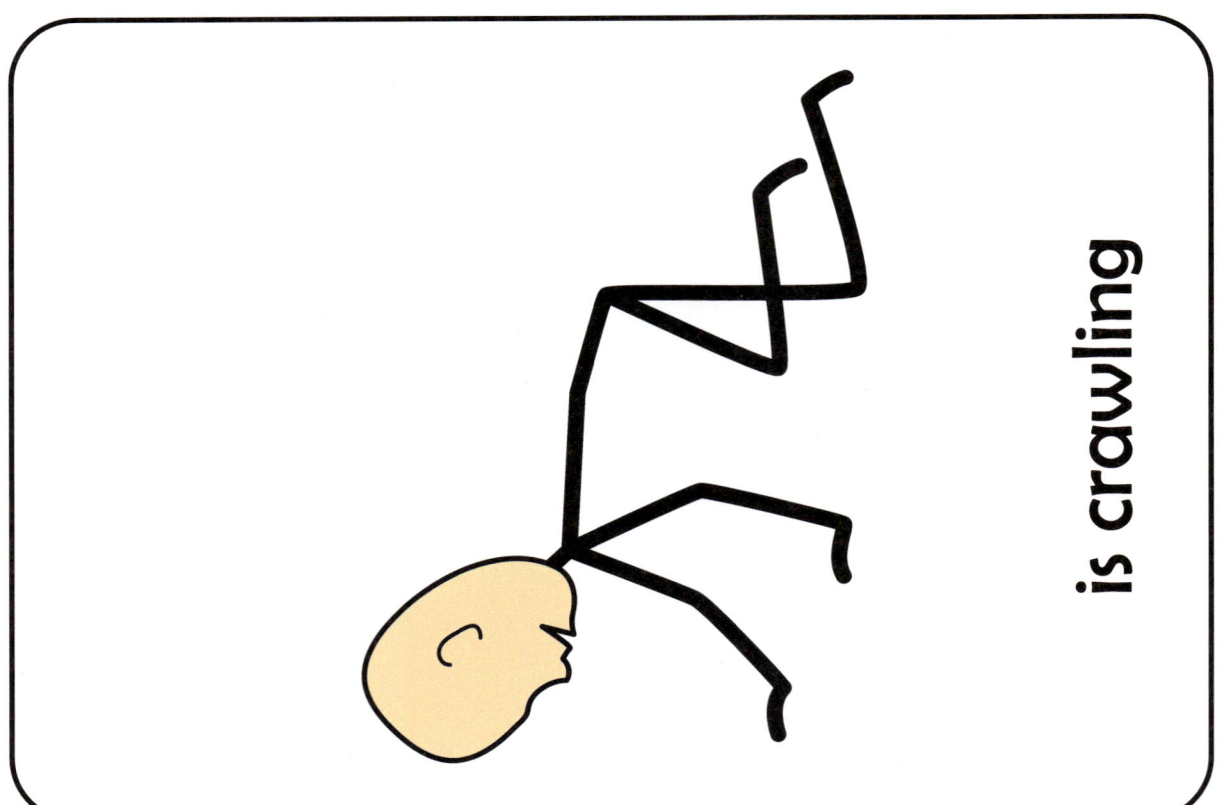

is crawling

Copyright material from NHS Forth Valley (2020), *Colourful Semantics*, Routledge

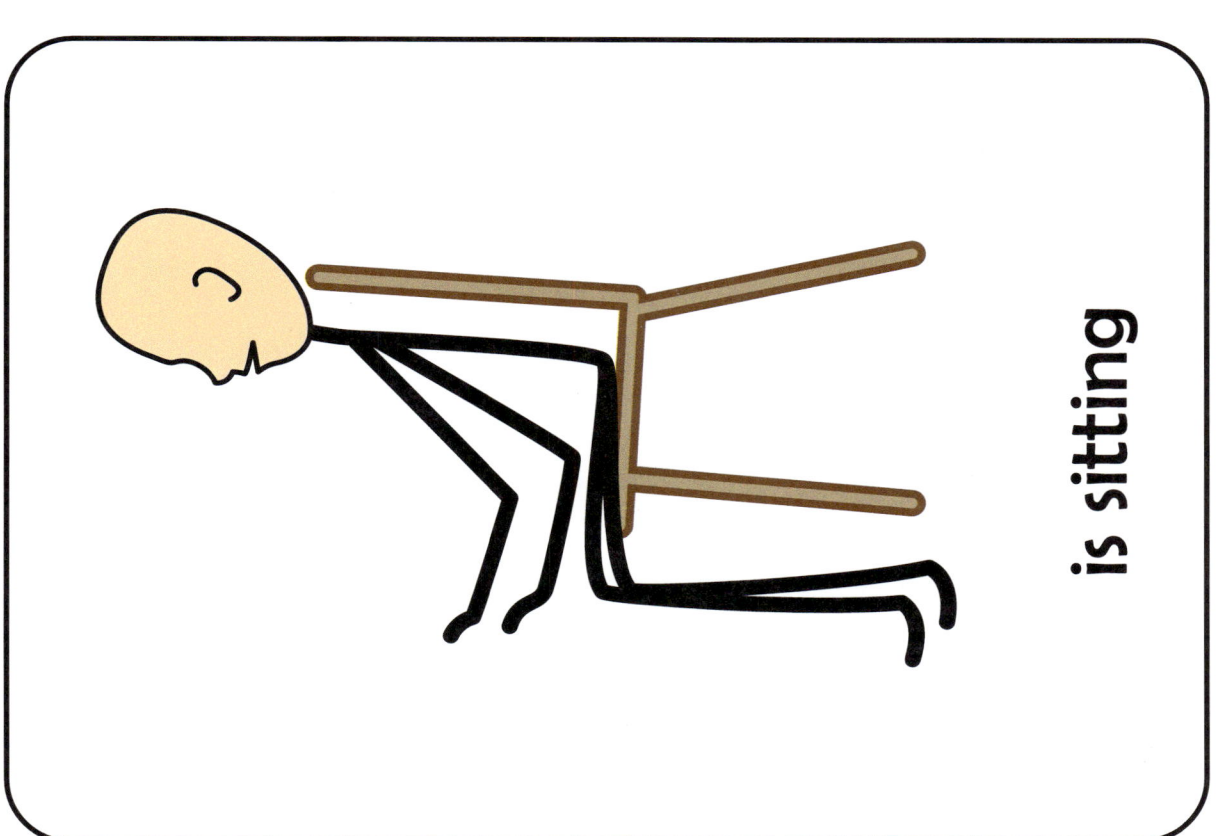

is sitting

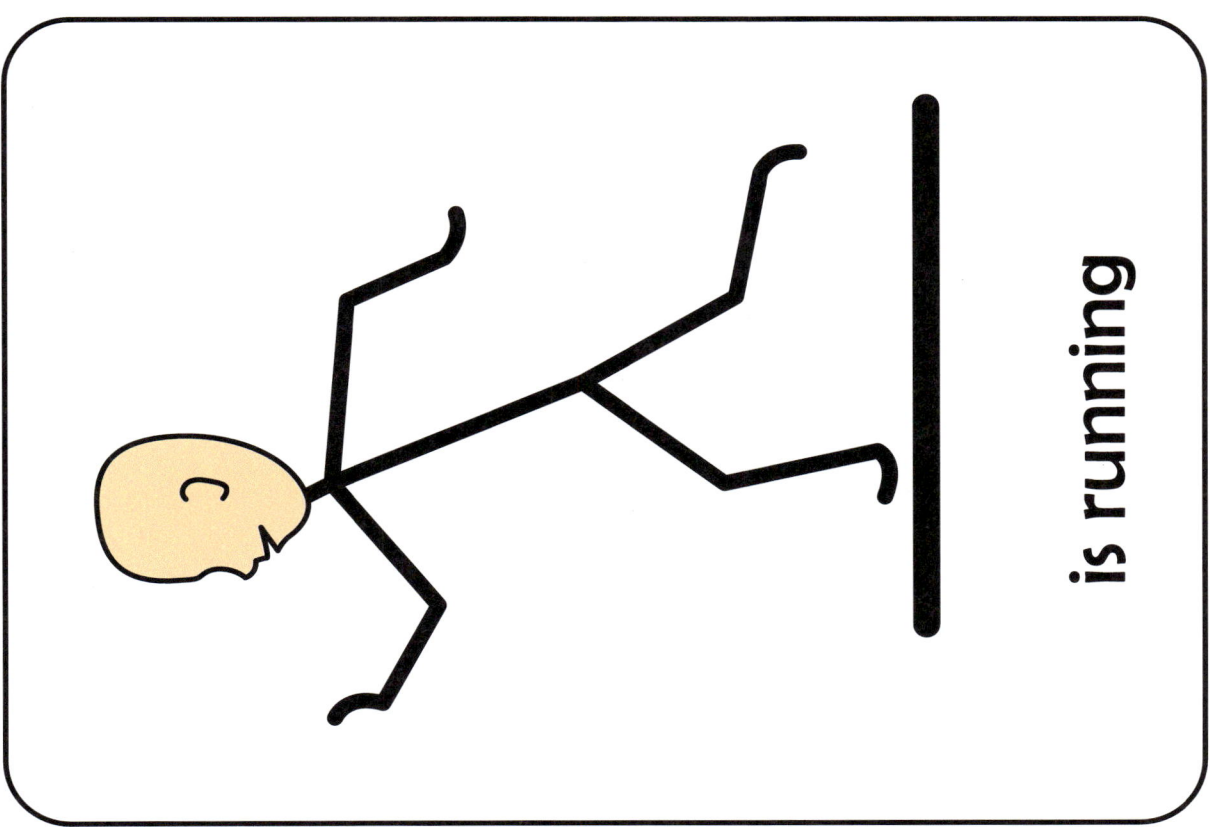

is running

Copyright material from NHS Forth Valley (2020), *Colourful Semantics*, Routledge

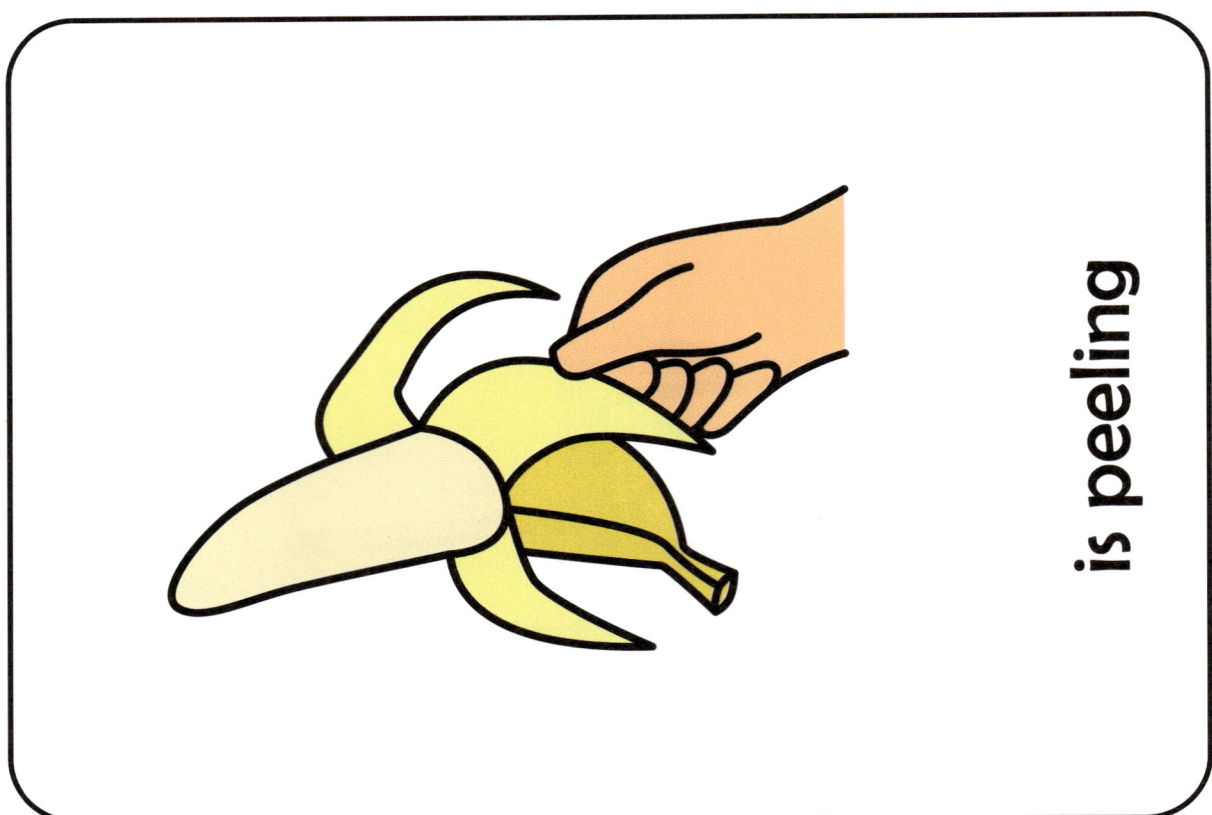

is peeling

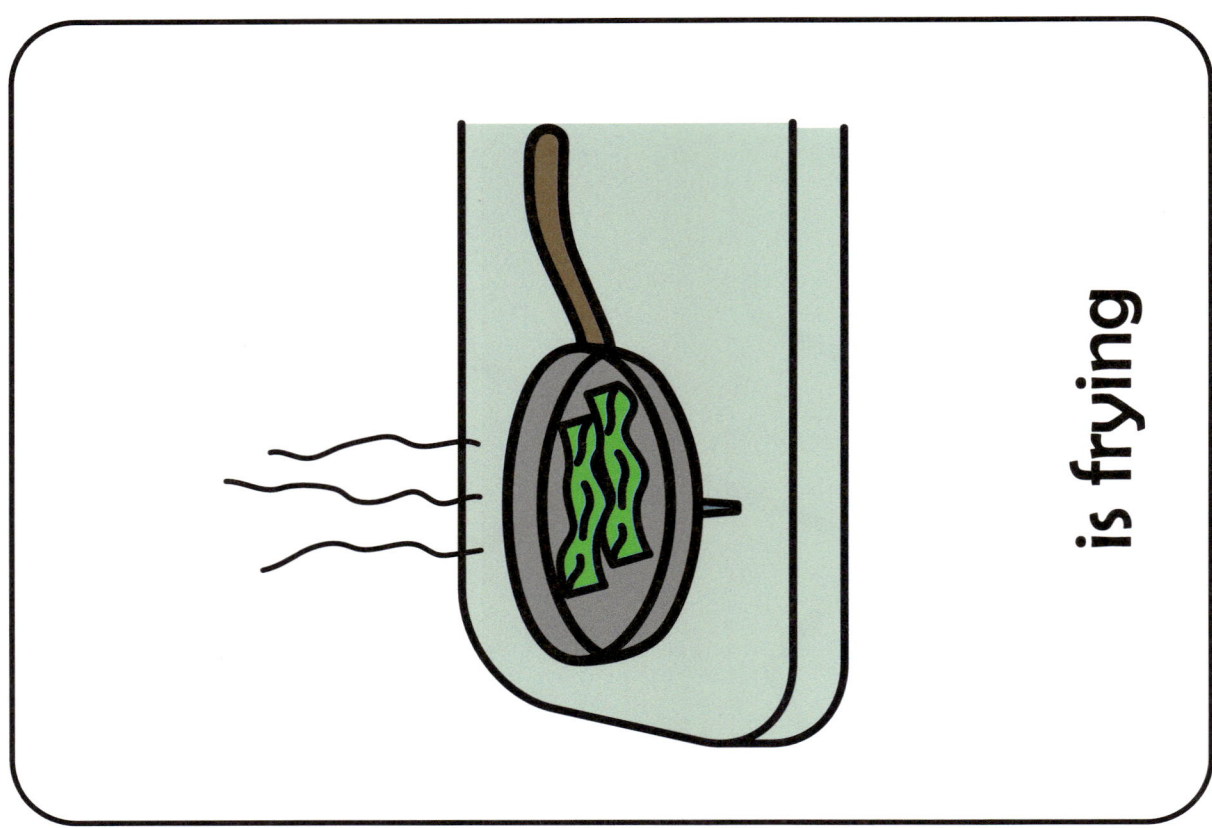

is frying

Copyright material from NHS Forth Valley (2020), *Colourful Semantics*, Routledge

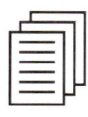

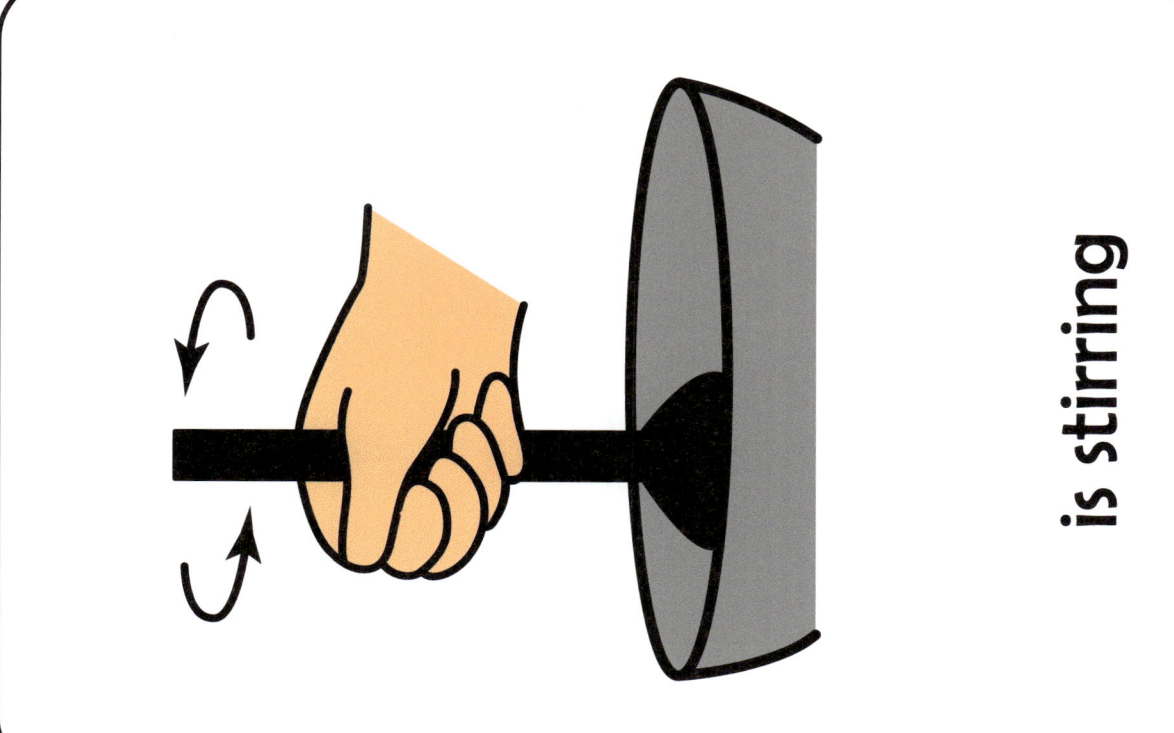

is stirring

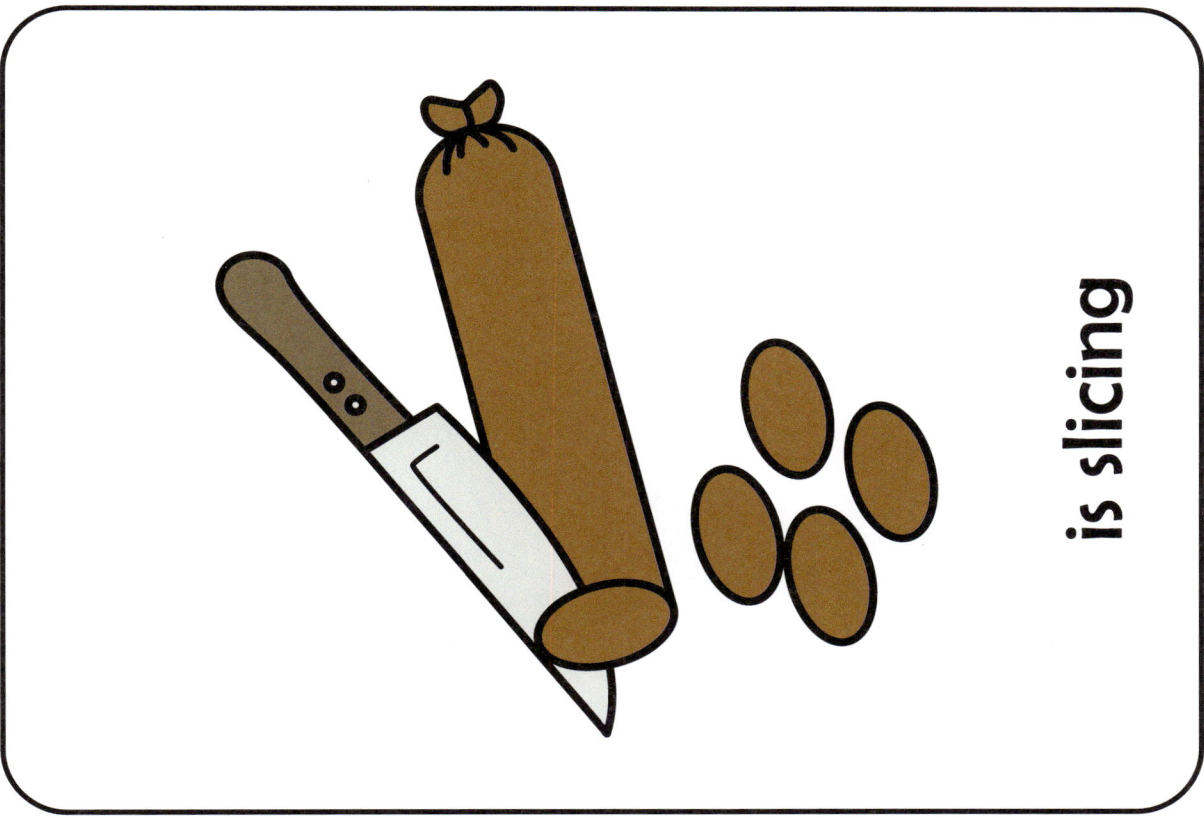

is slicing

Copyright material from NHS Forth Valley (2020), *Colourful Semantics*, Routledge

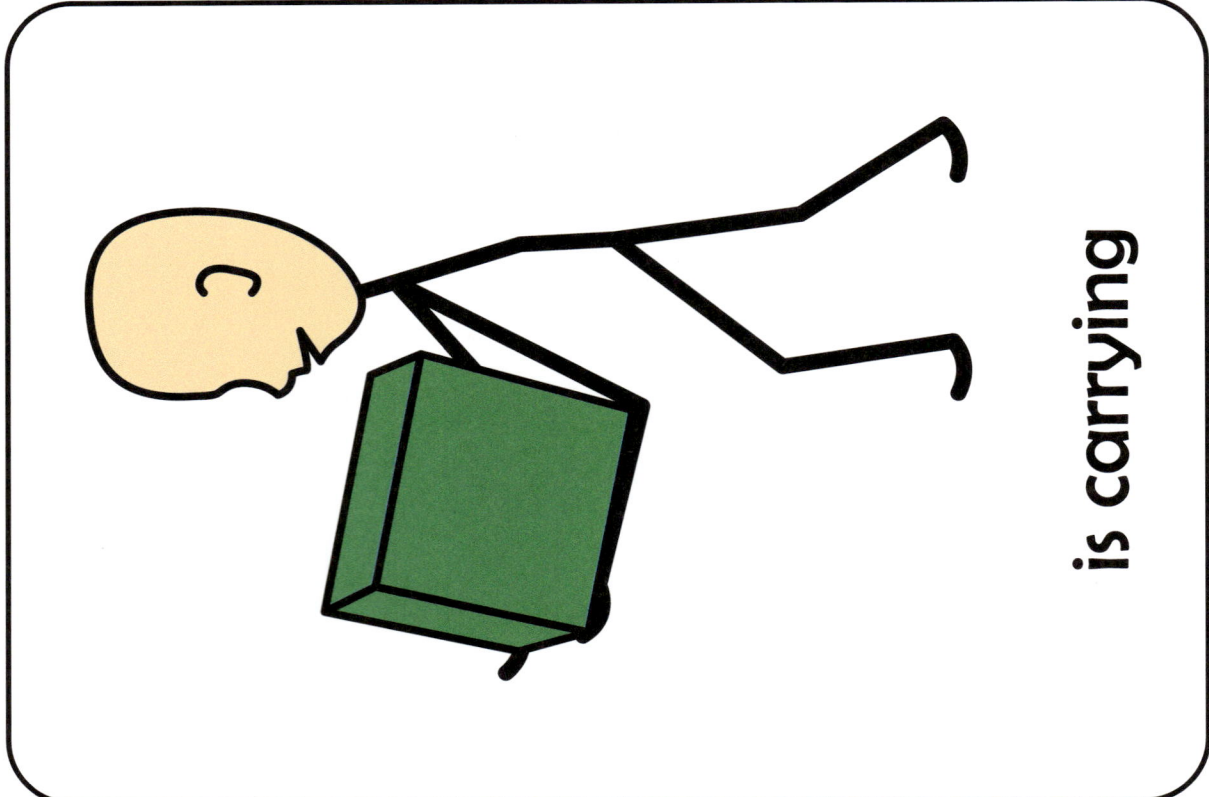

is carrying

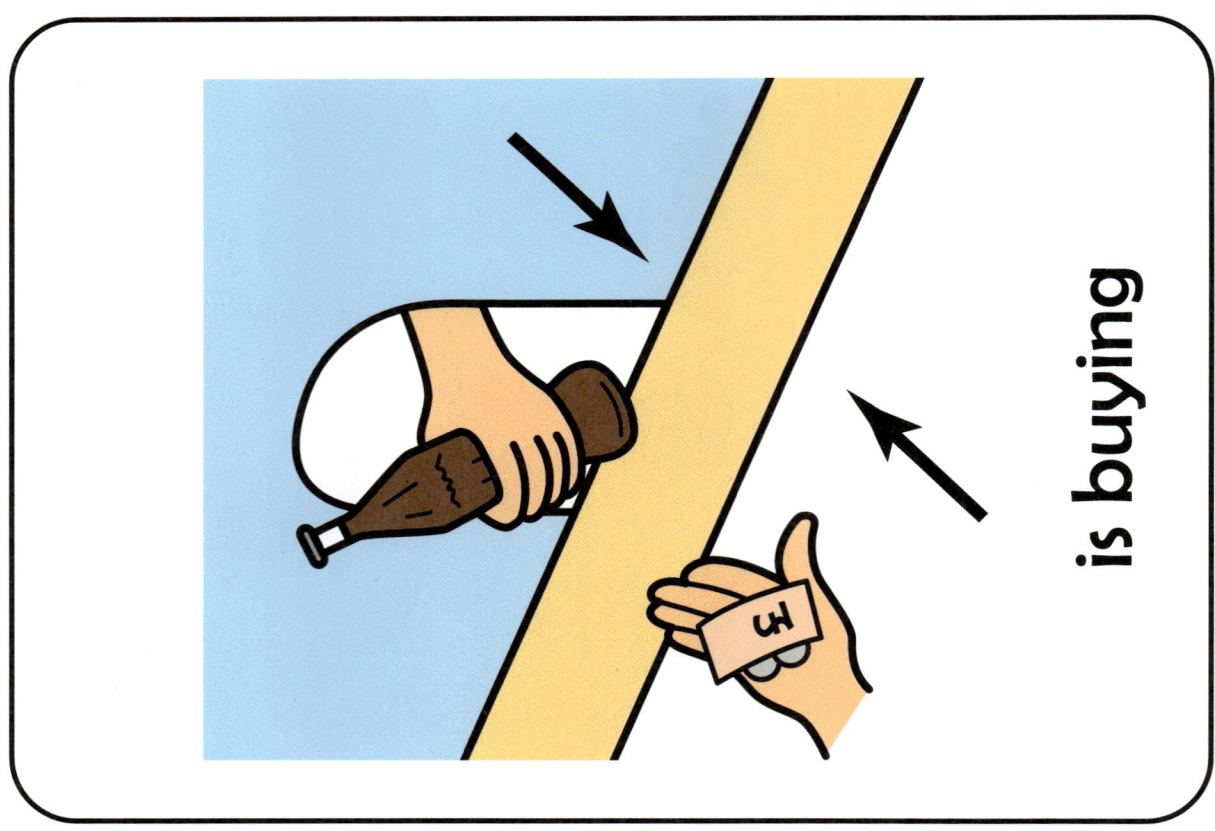

is buying

Copyright material from NHS Forth Valley (2020), *Colourful Semantics*, Routledge

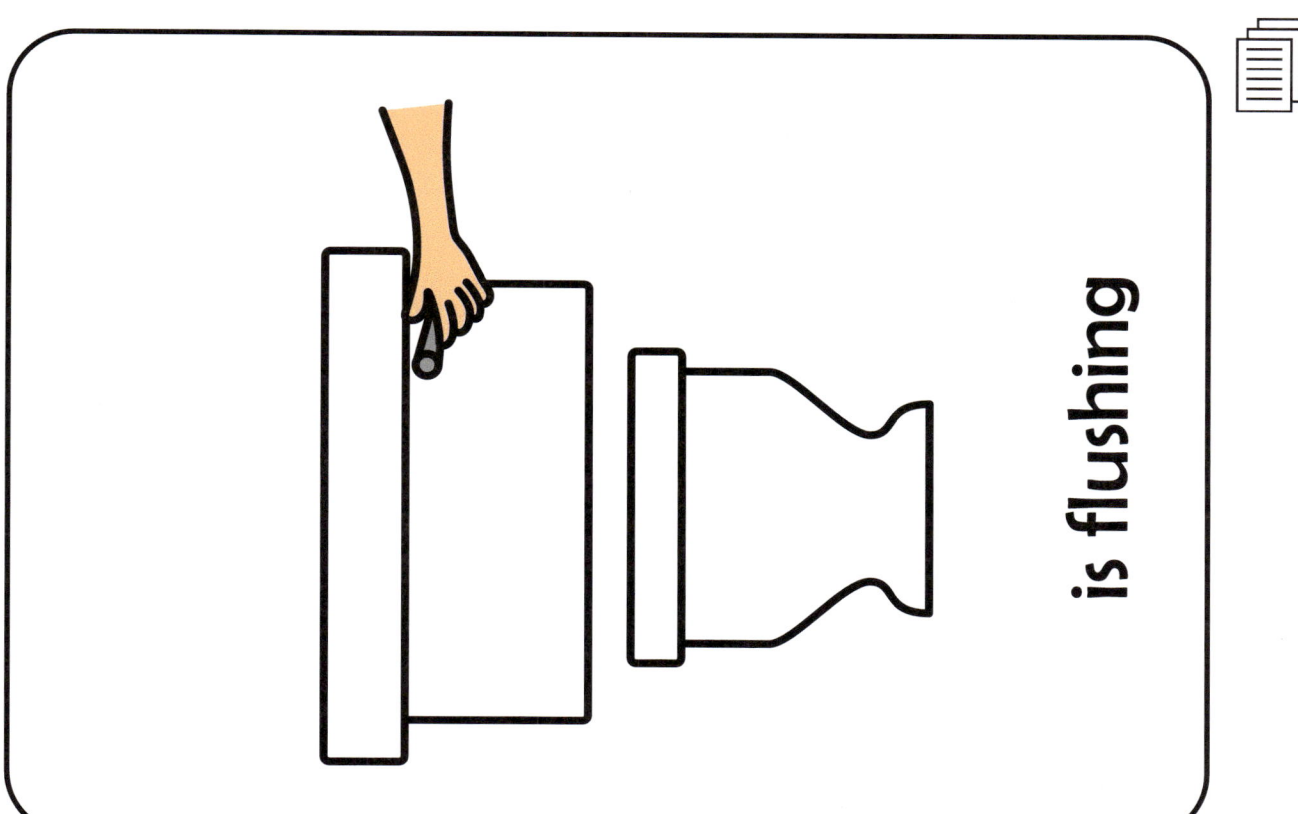

is flushing

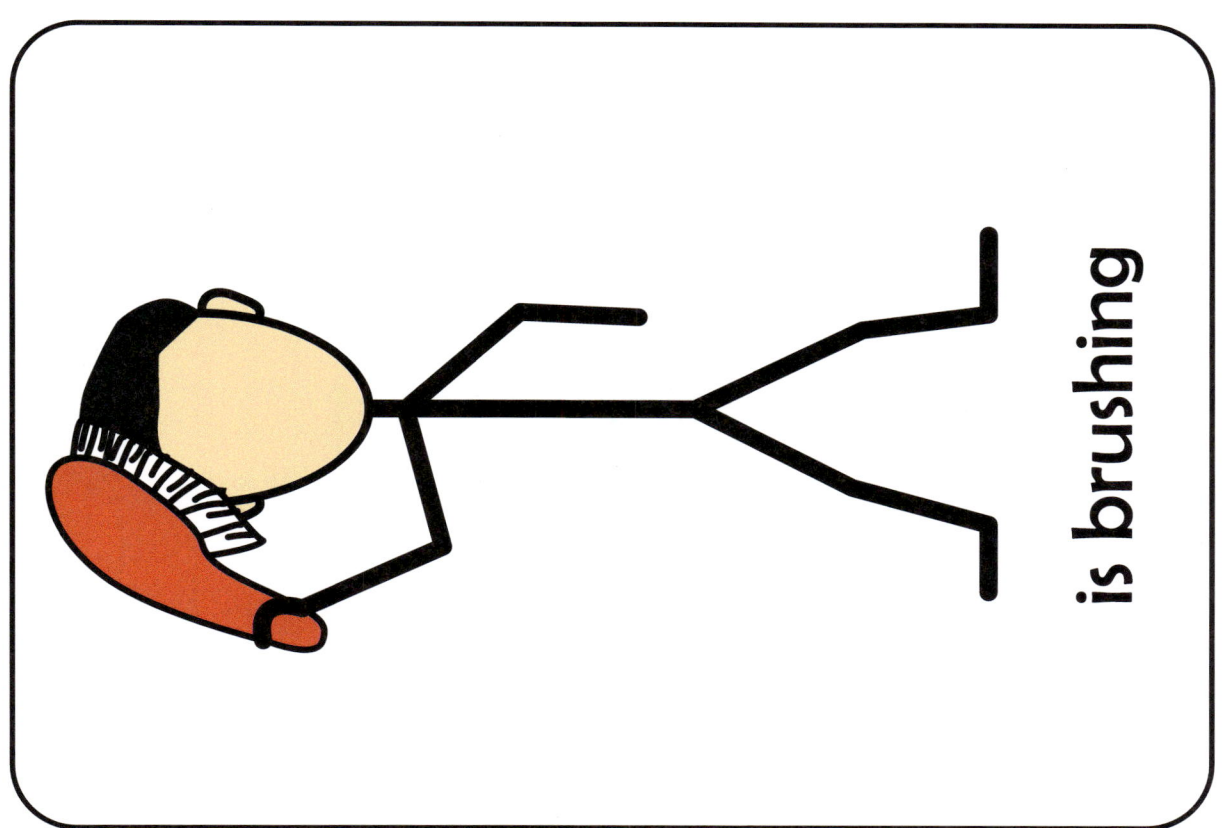

is brushing

Copyright material from NHS Forth Valley (2020), *Colourful Semantics*, Routledge

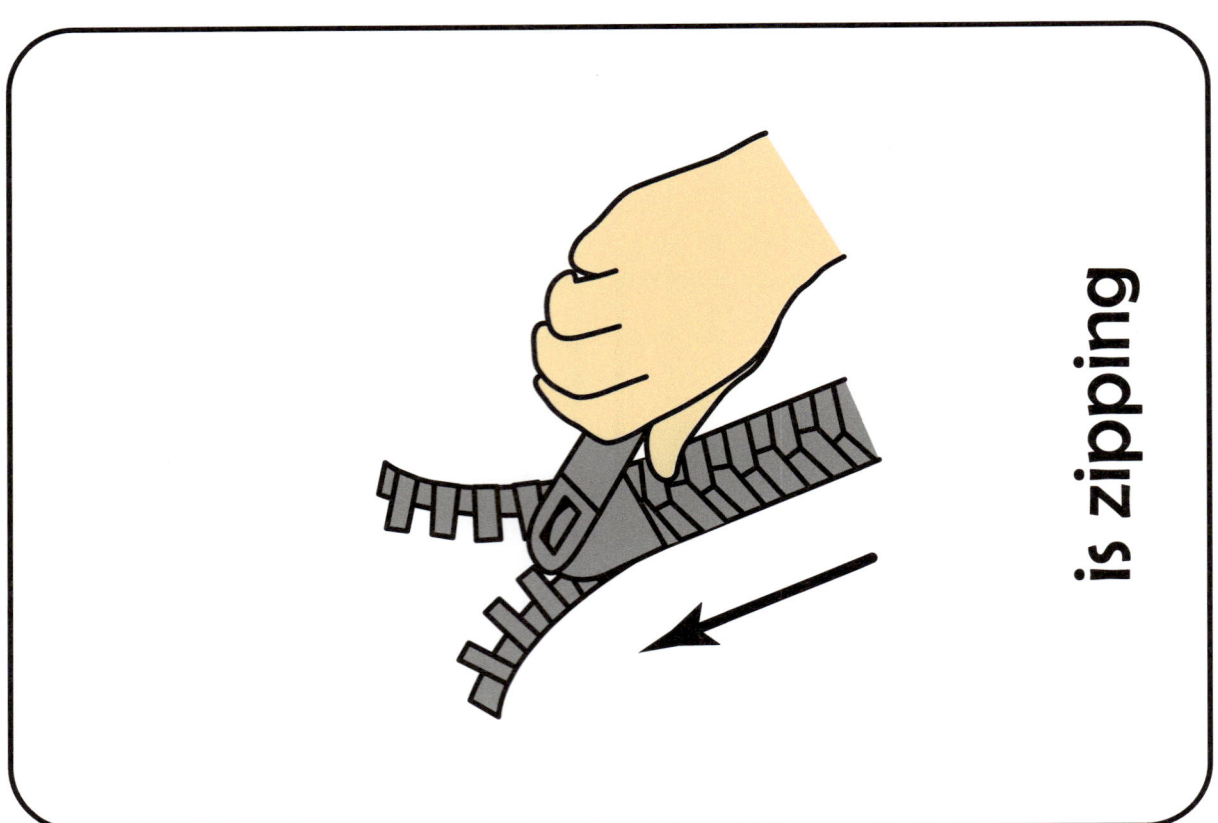

is zipping

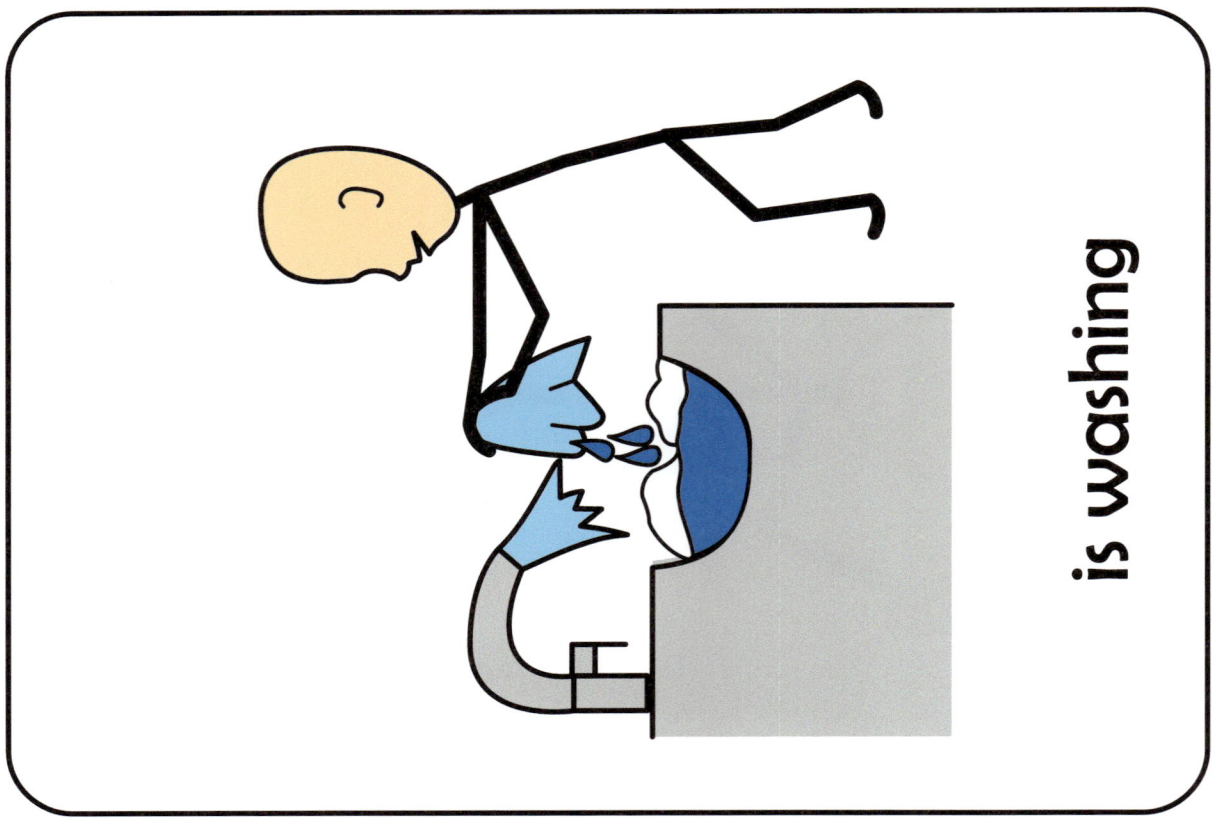

is washing

Copyright material from NHS Forth Valley (2020), *Colourful Semantics*, Routledge

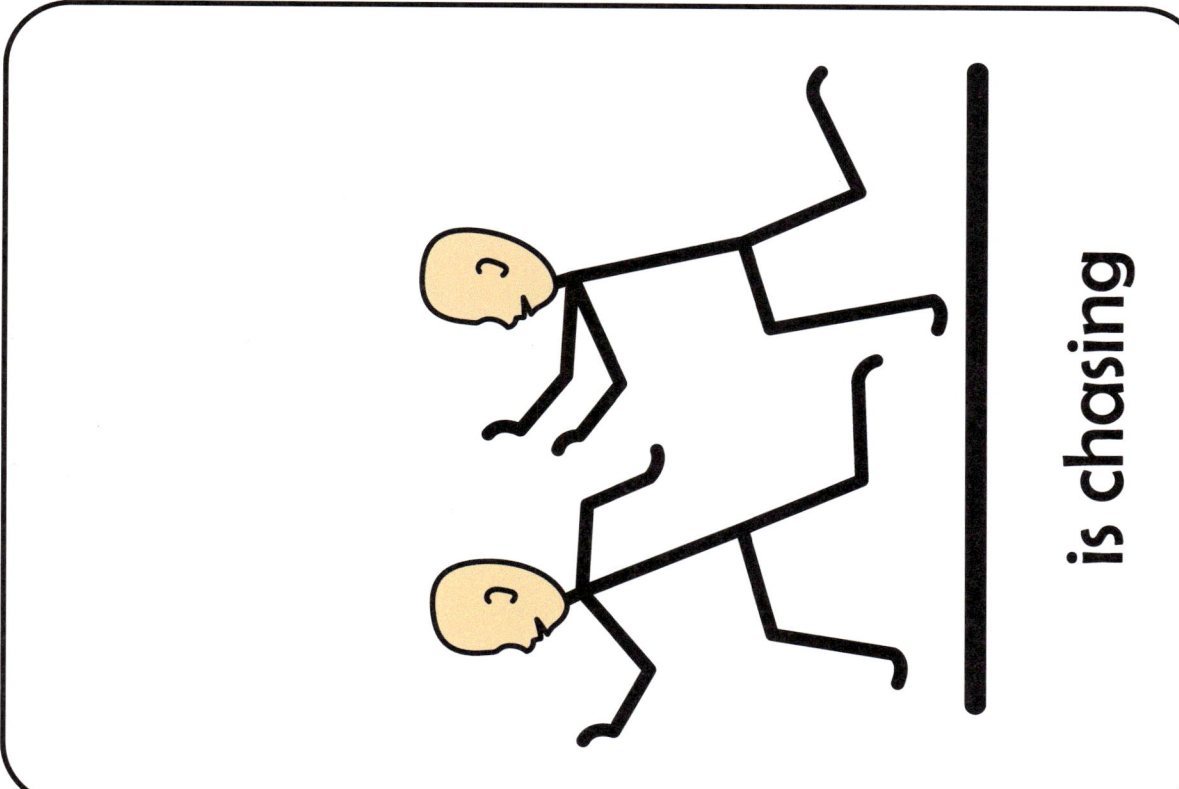

is chasing

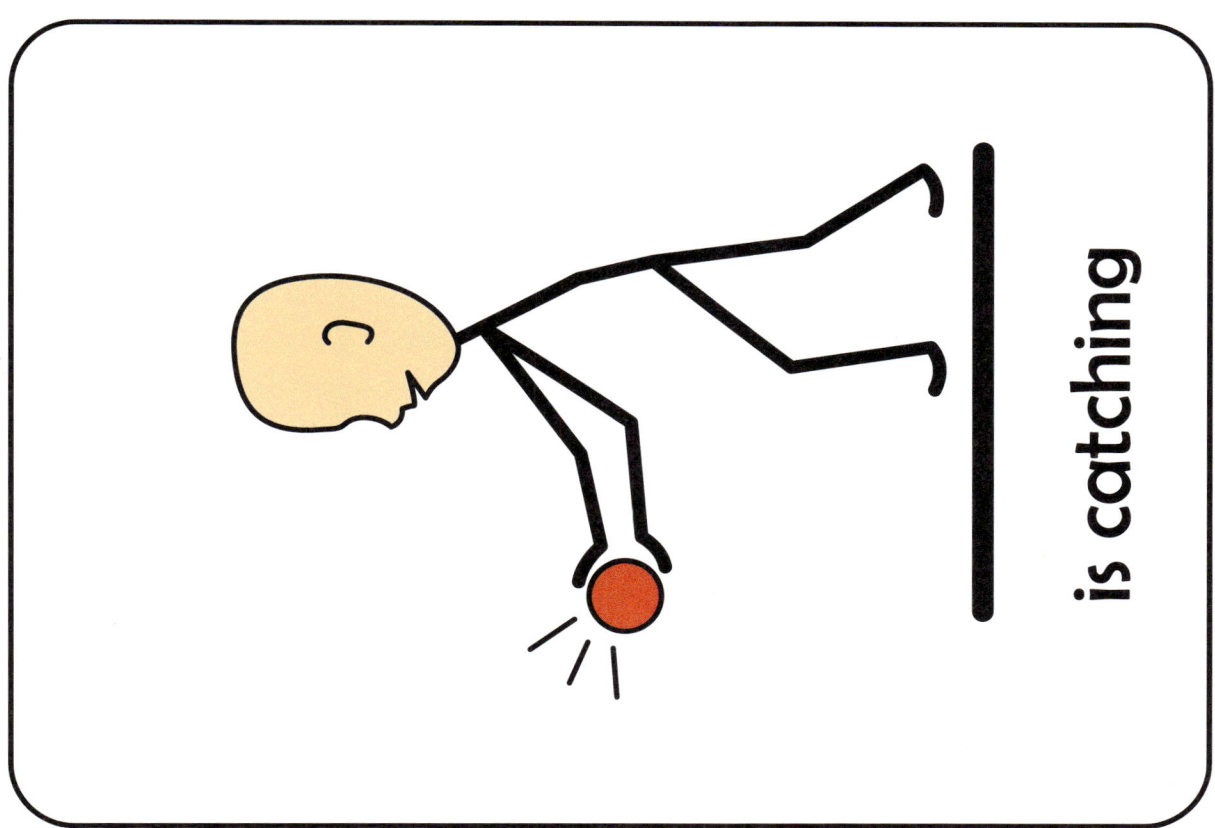

is catching

Copyright material from NHS Forth Valley (2020), *Colourful Semantics*, Routledge

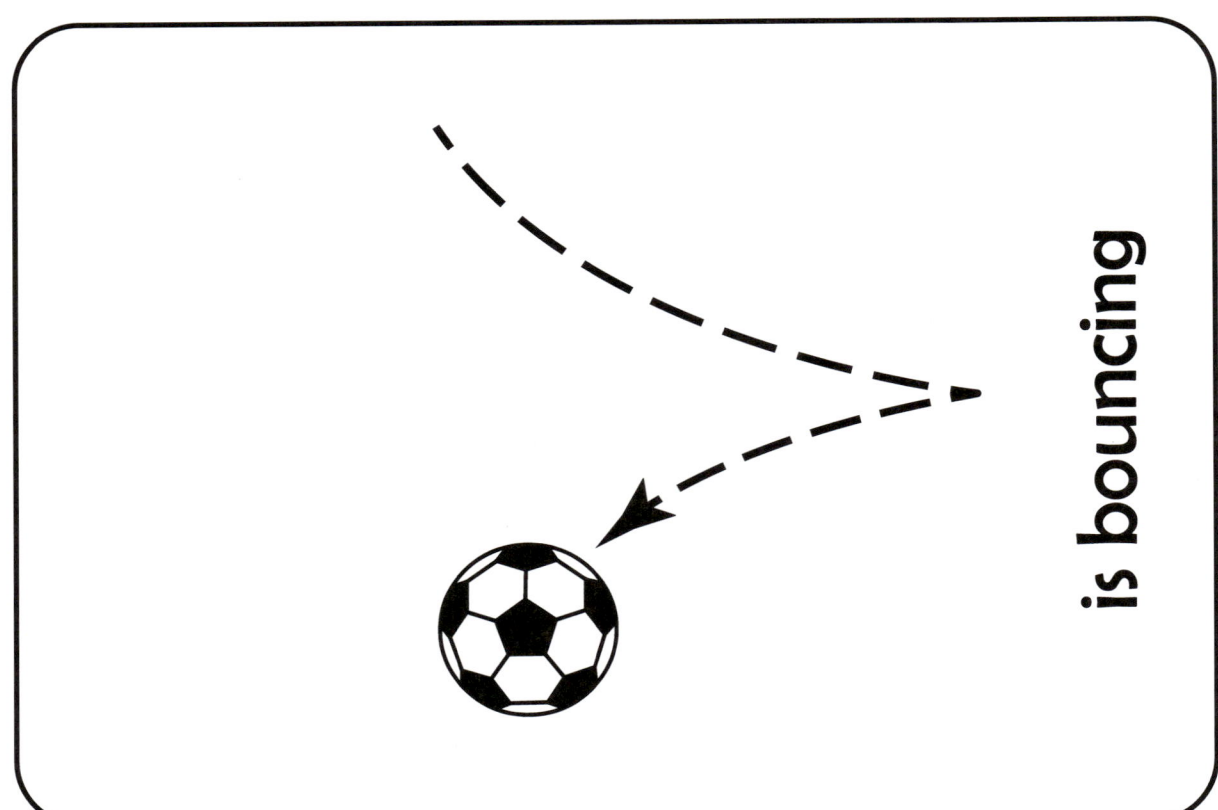

is bouncing

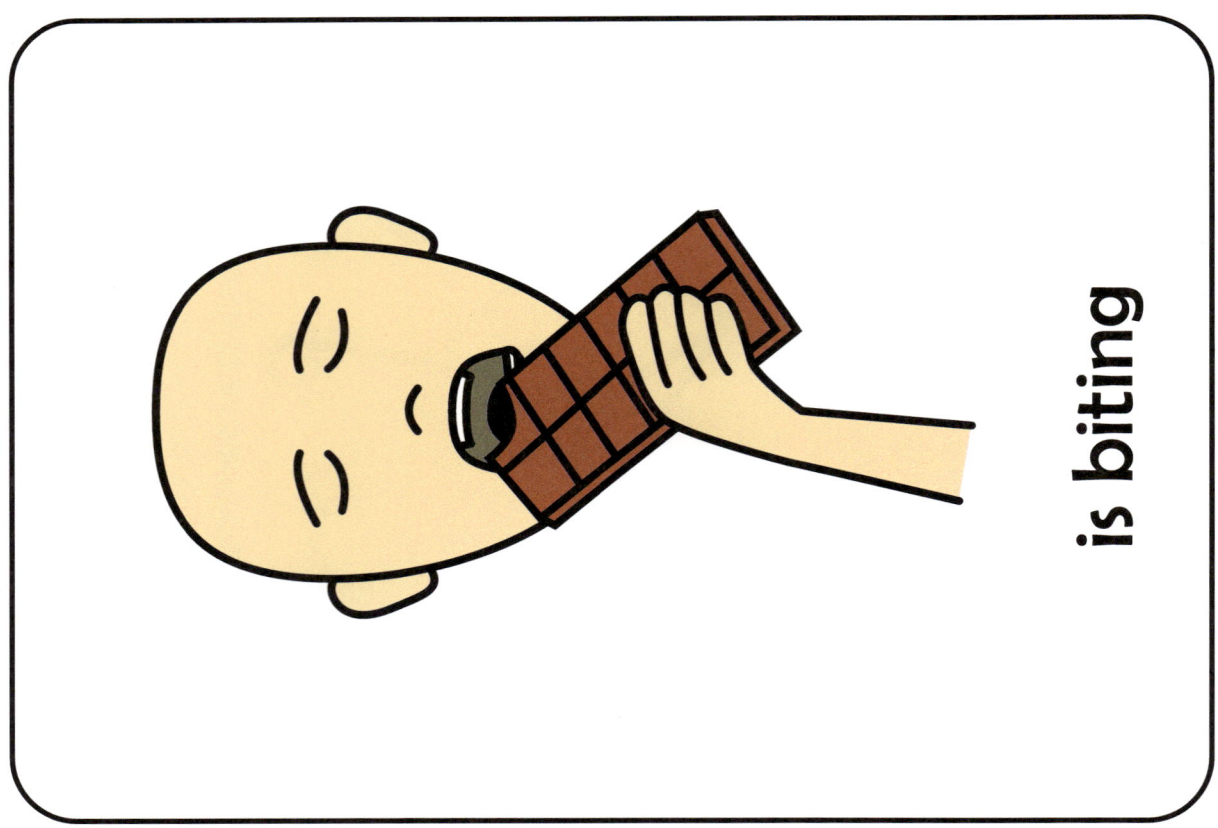

is biting

Copyright material from NHS Forth Valley (2020), *Colourful Semantics*, Routledge

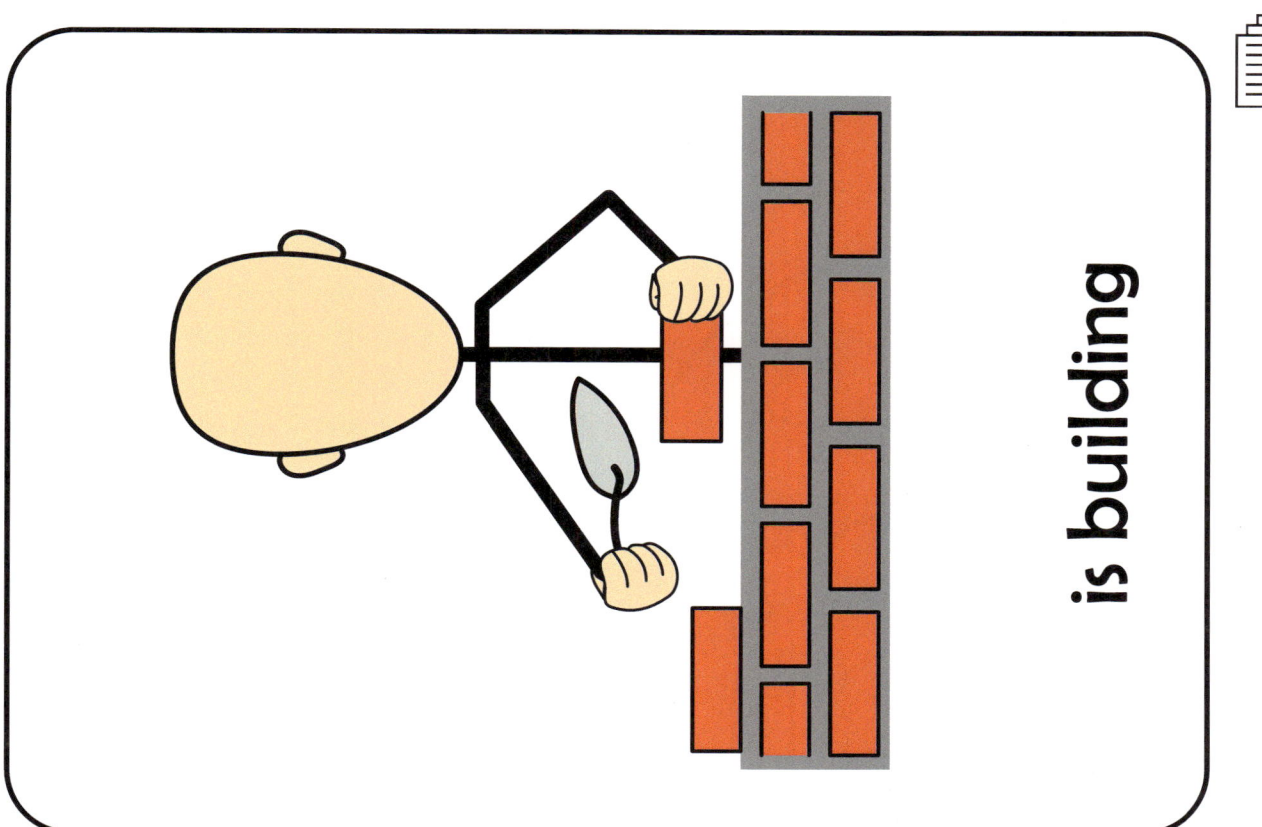

is building

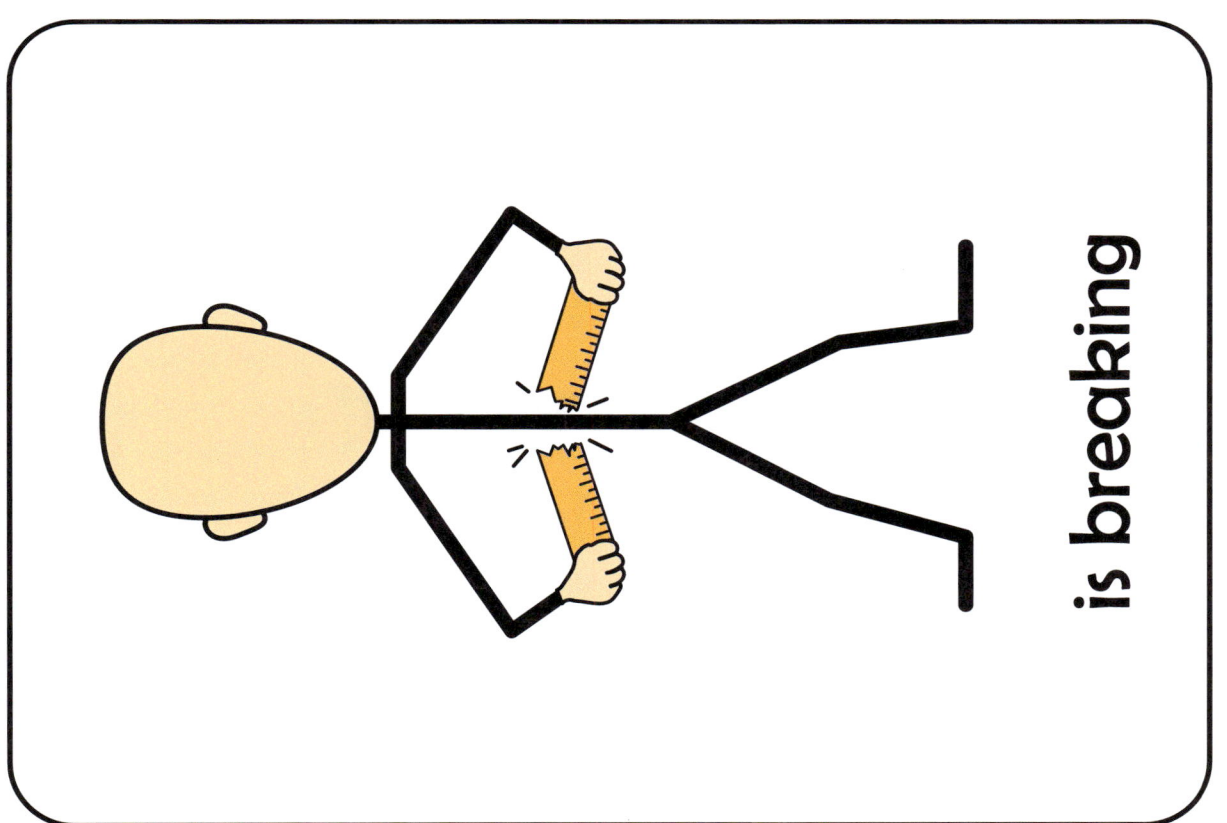

is breaking

Copyright material from NHS Forth Valley (2020), *Colourful Semantics*, Routledge

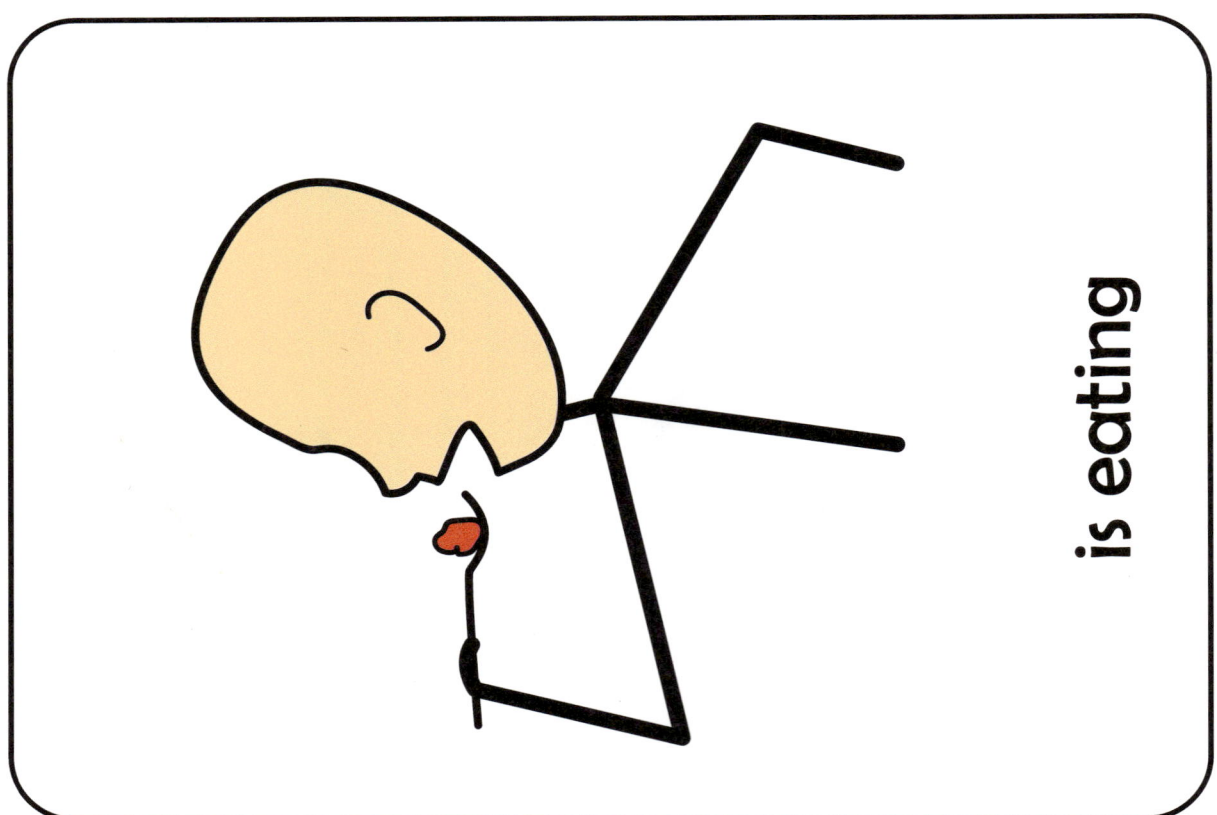

is eating

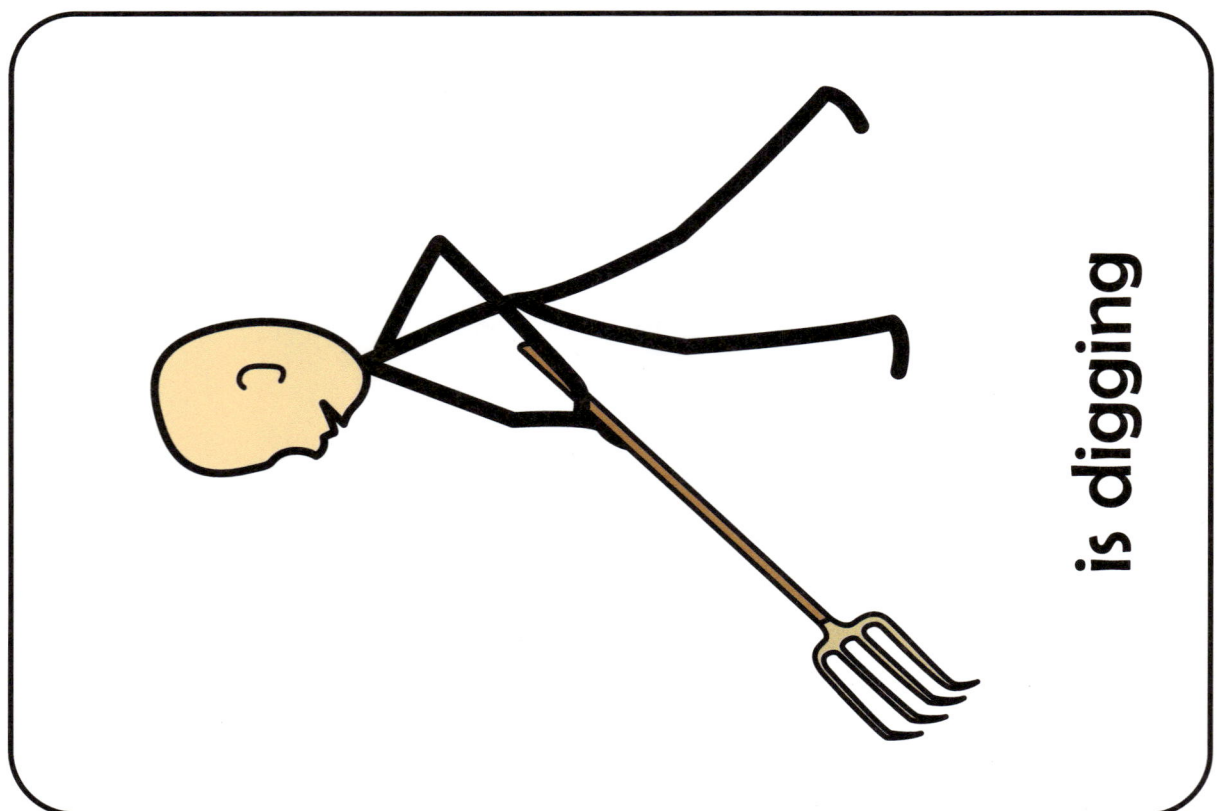

is digging

Copyright material from NHS Forth Valley (2020), *Colourful Semantics*, Routledge

Doing words for sentences with a '*to who*'

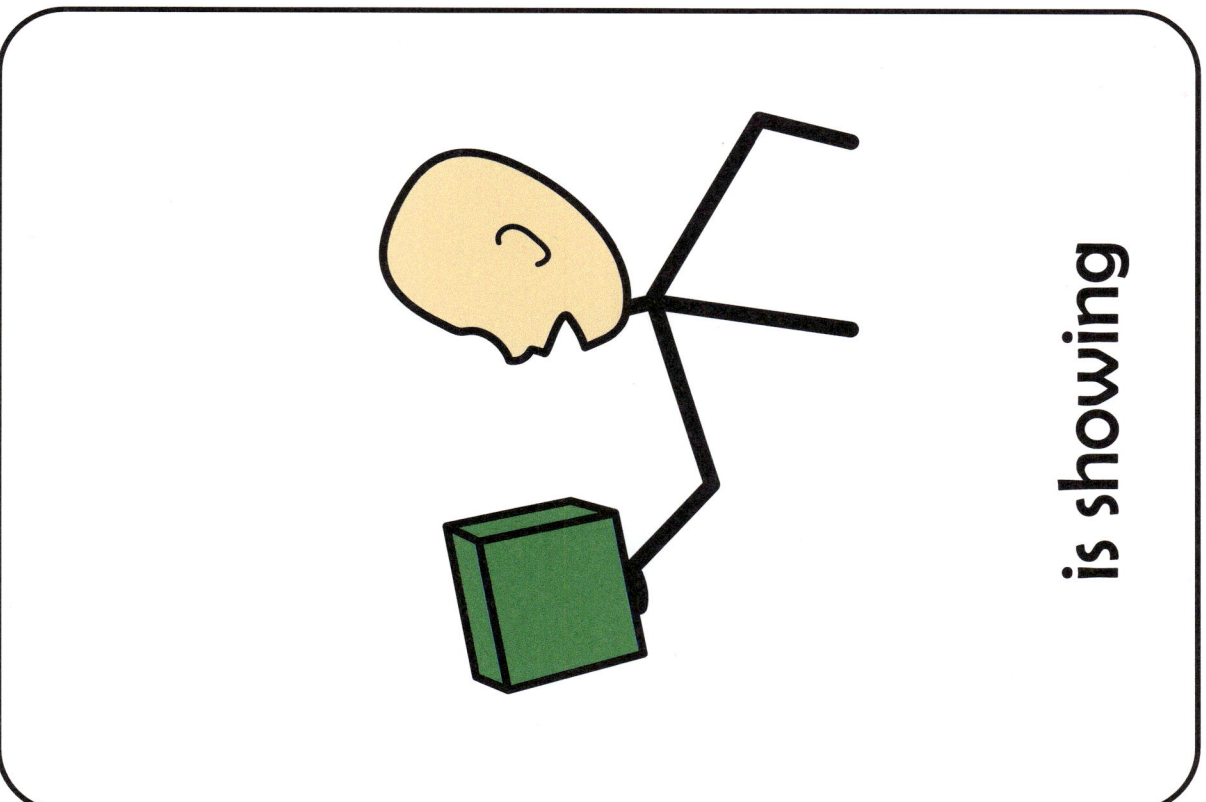

is showing

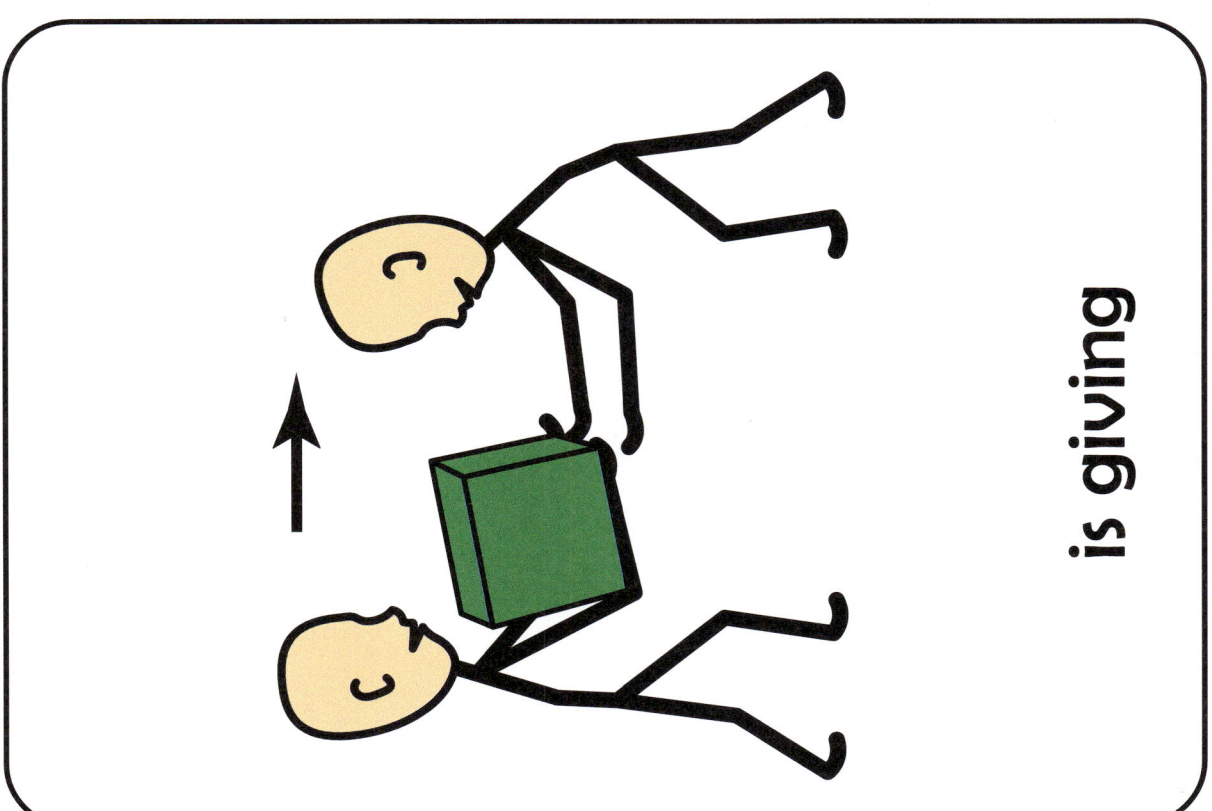

is giving

Copyright material from NHS Forth Valley (2020), *Colourful Semantics*, Routledge

'What' vocabulary

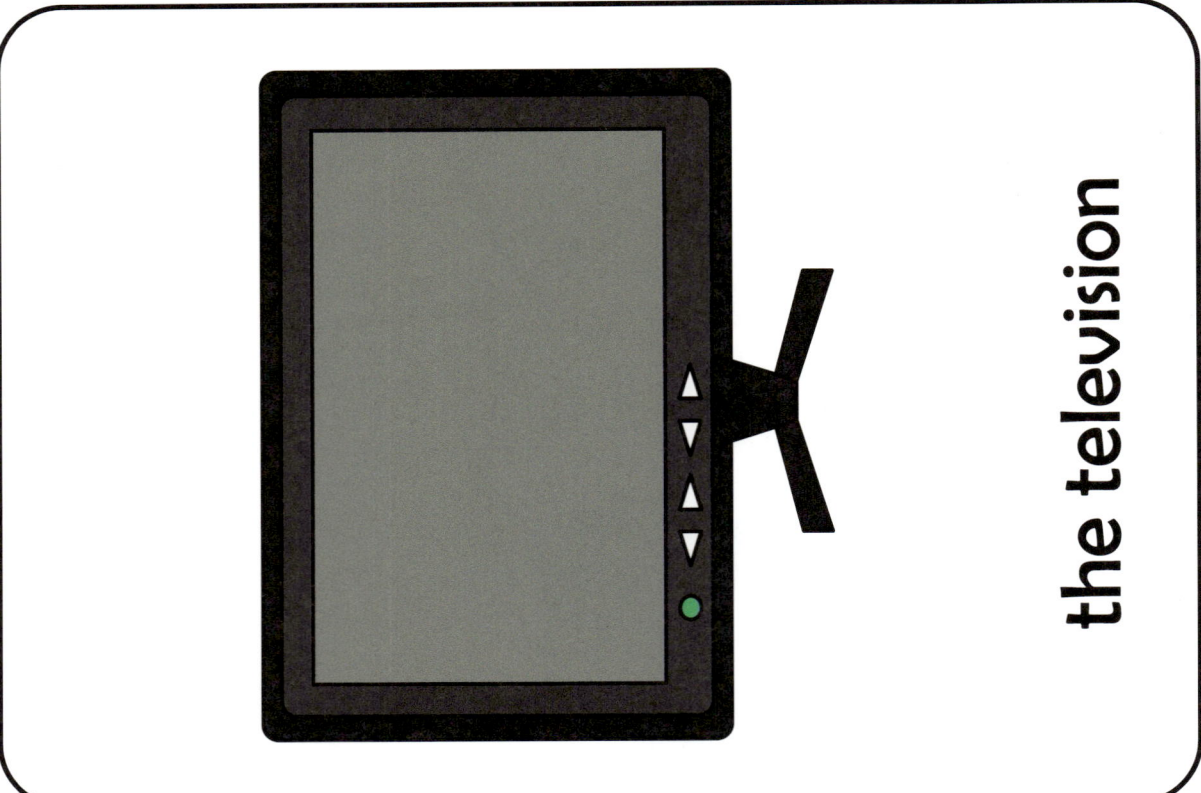

the television

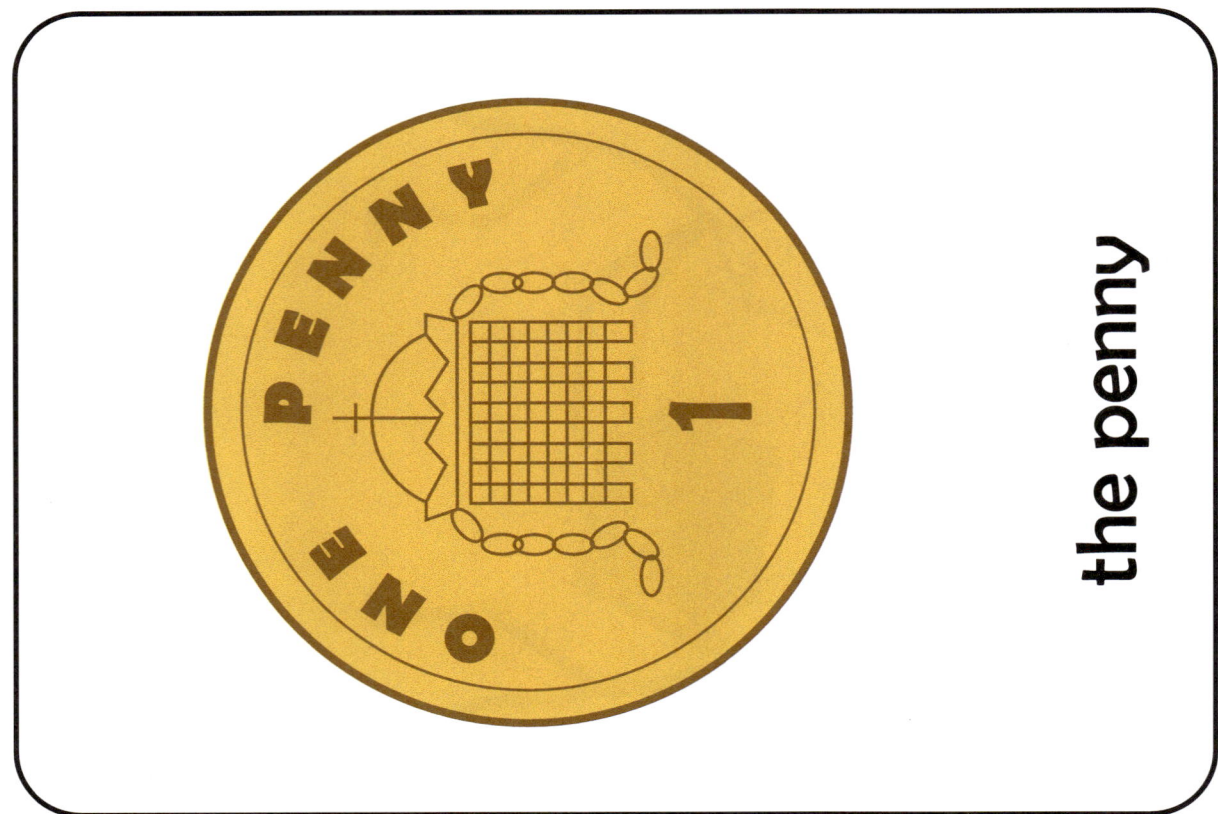

the penny

Copyright material from NHS Forth Valley (2020), *Colourful Semantics*, Routledge

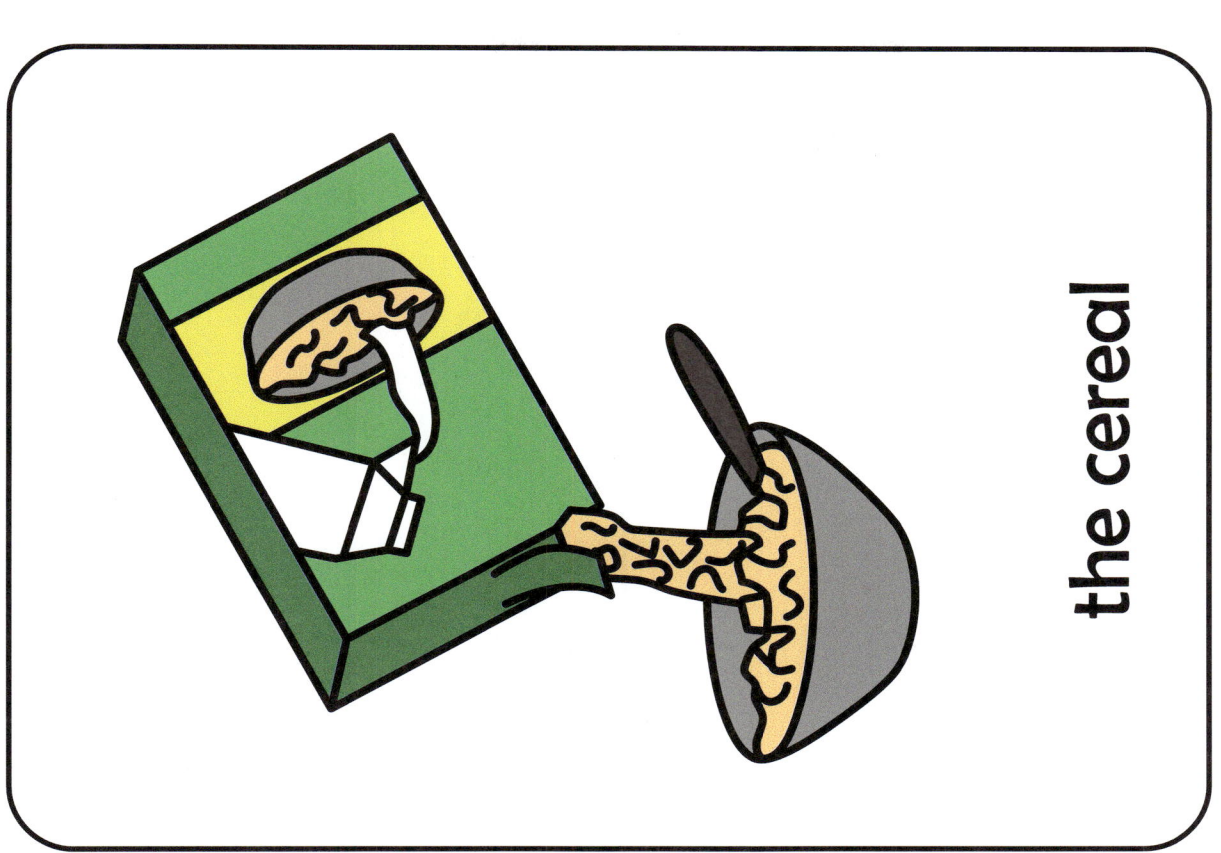

the cereal

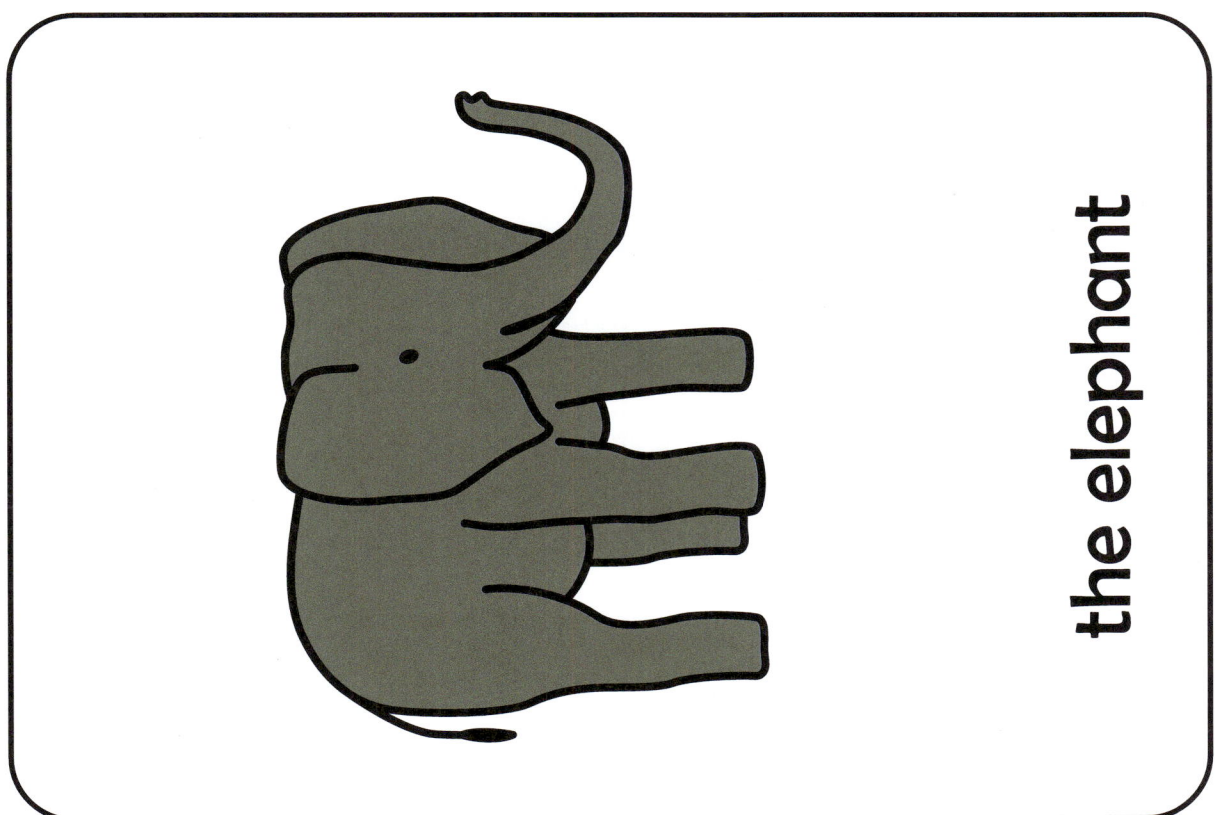

the elephant

Copyright material from NHS Forth Valley (2020), *Colourful Semantics*, Routledge

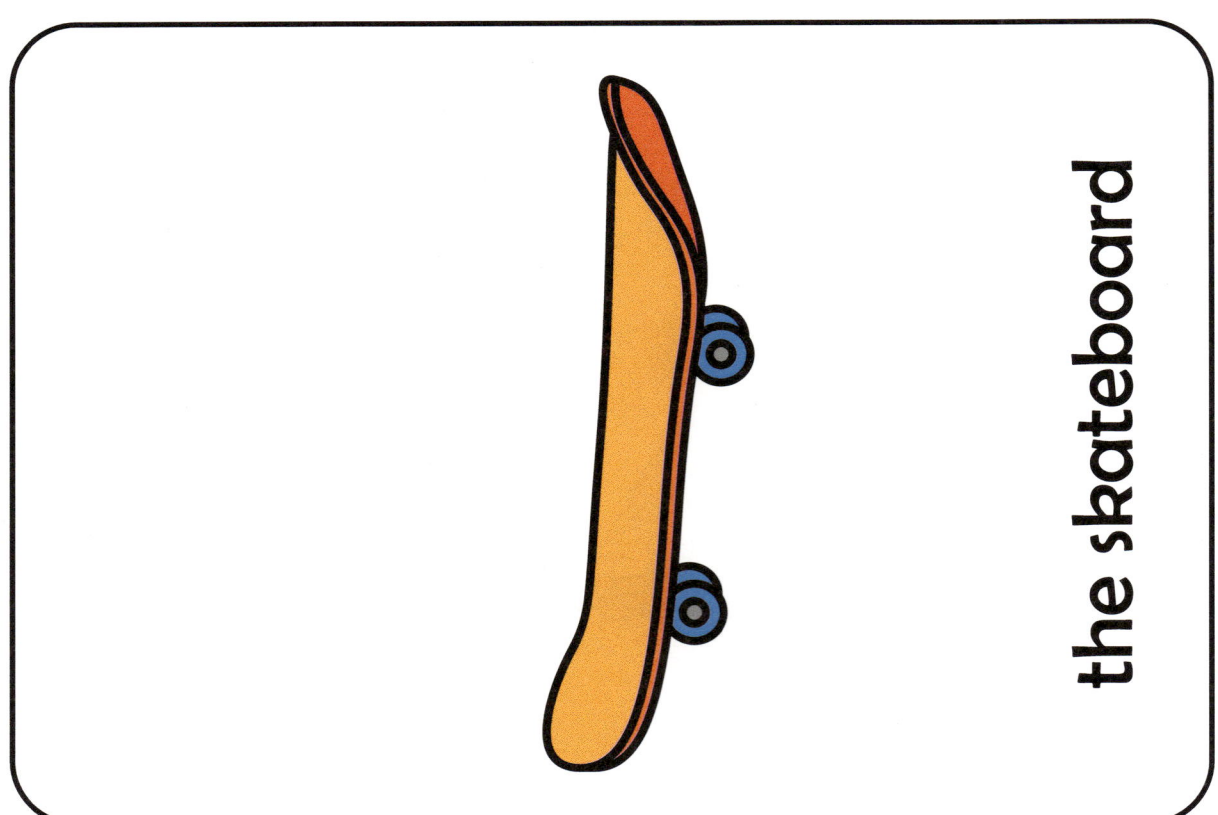

the skateboard

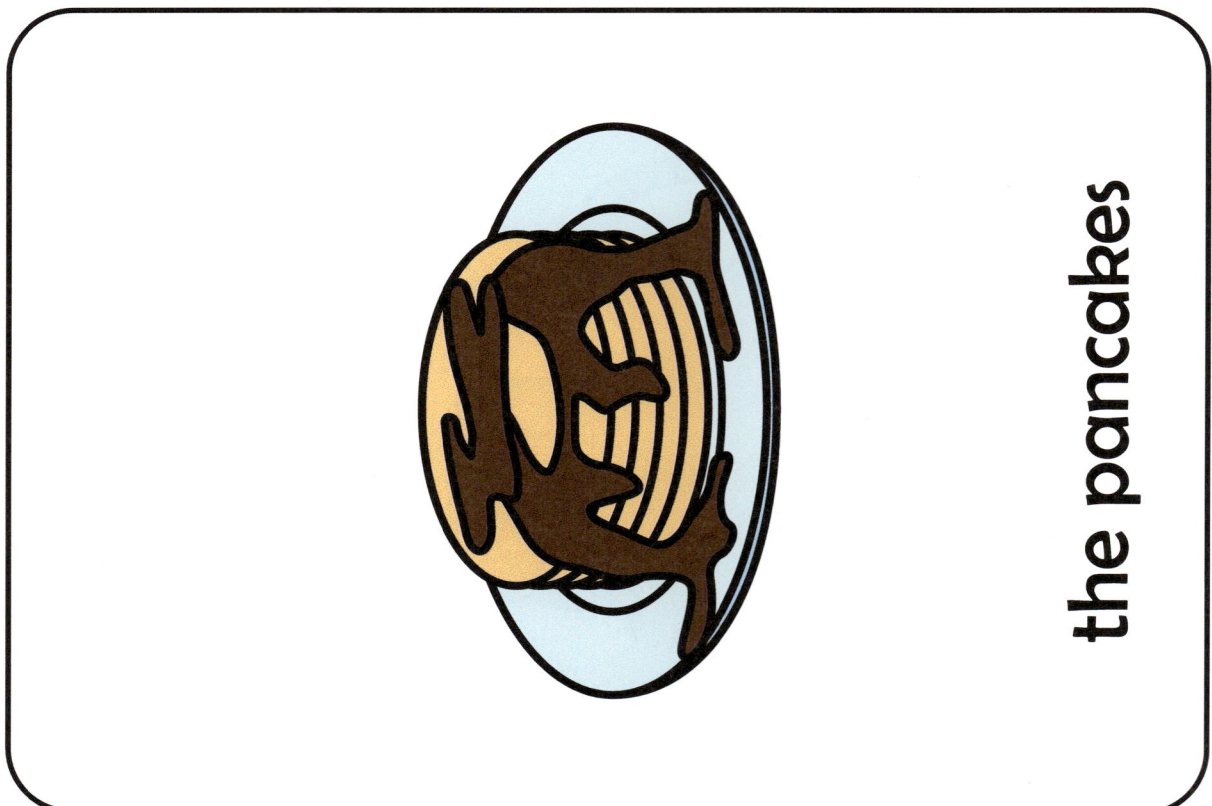

the pancakes

Copyright material from NHS Forth Valley (2020), *Colourful Semantics*, Routledge

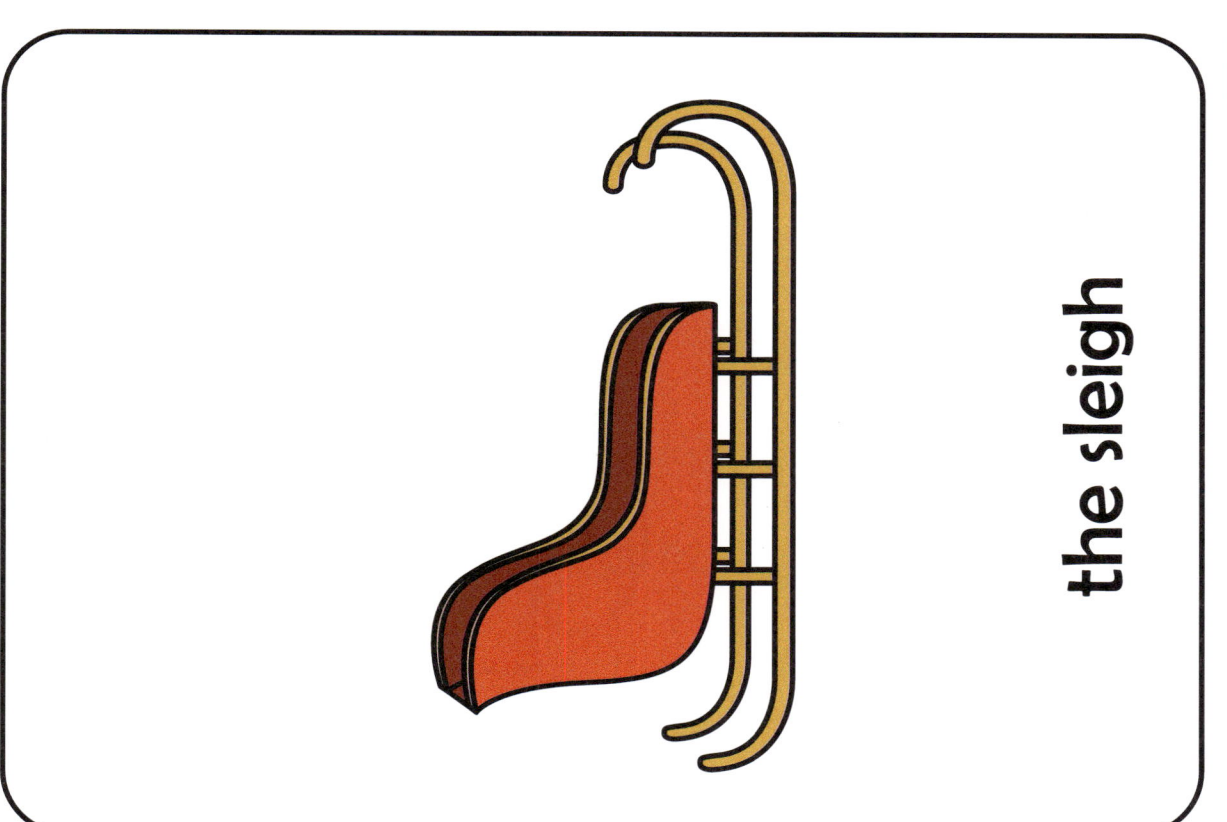

the sleigh

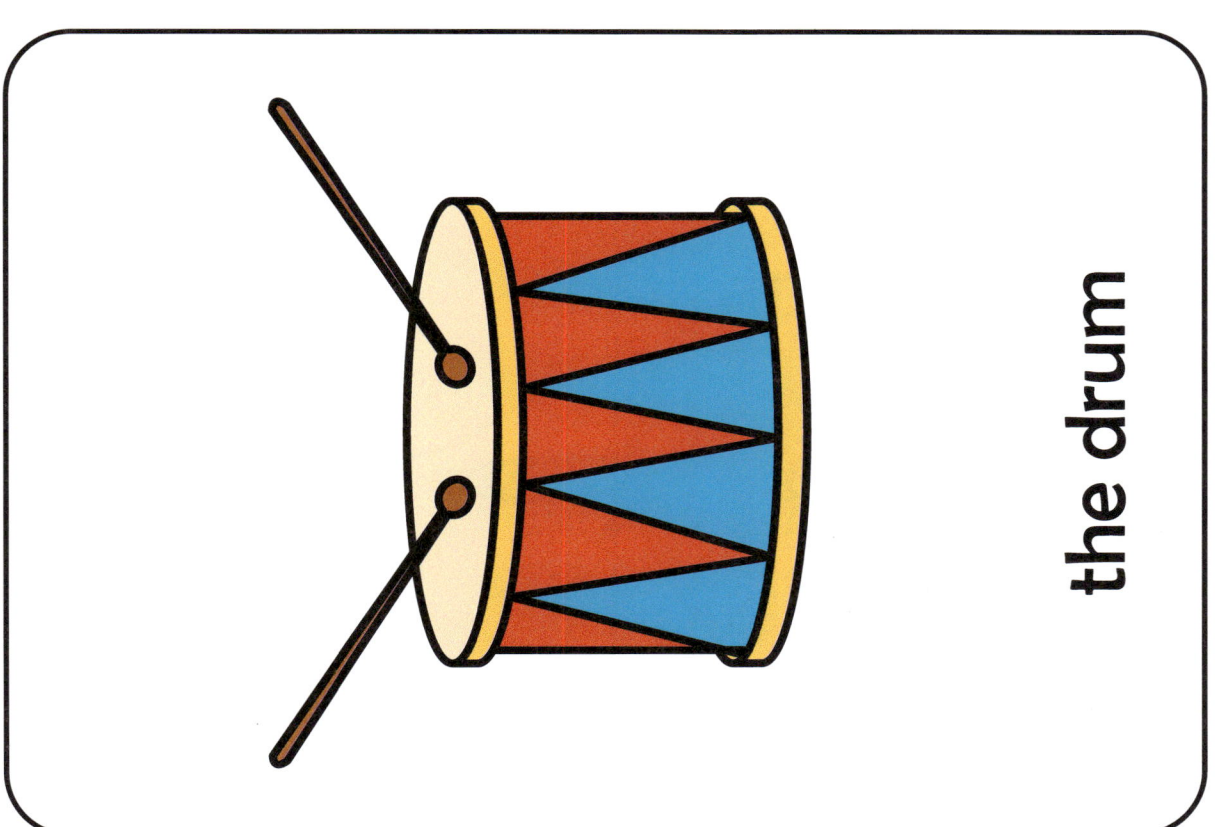

the drum

Copyright material from NHS Forth Valley (2020), *Colourful Semantics*, Routledge

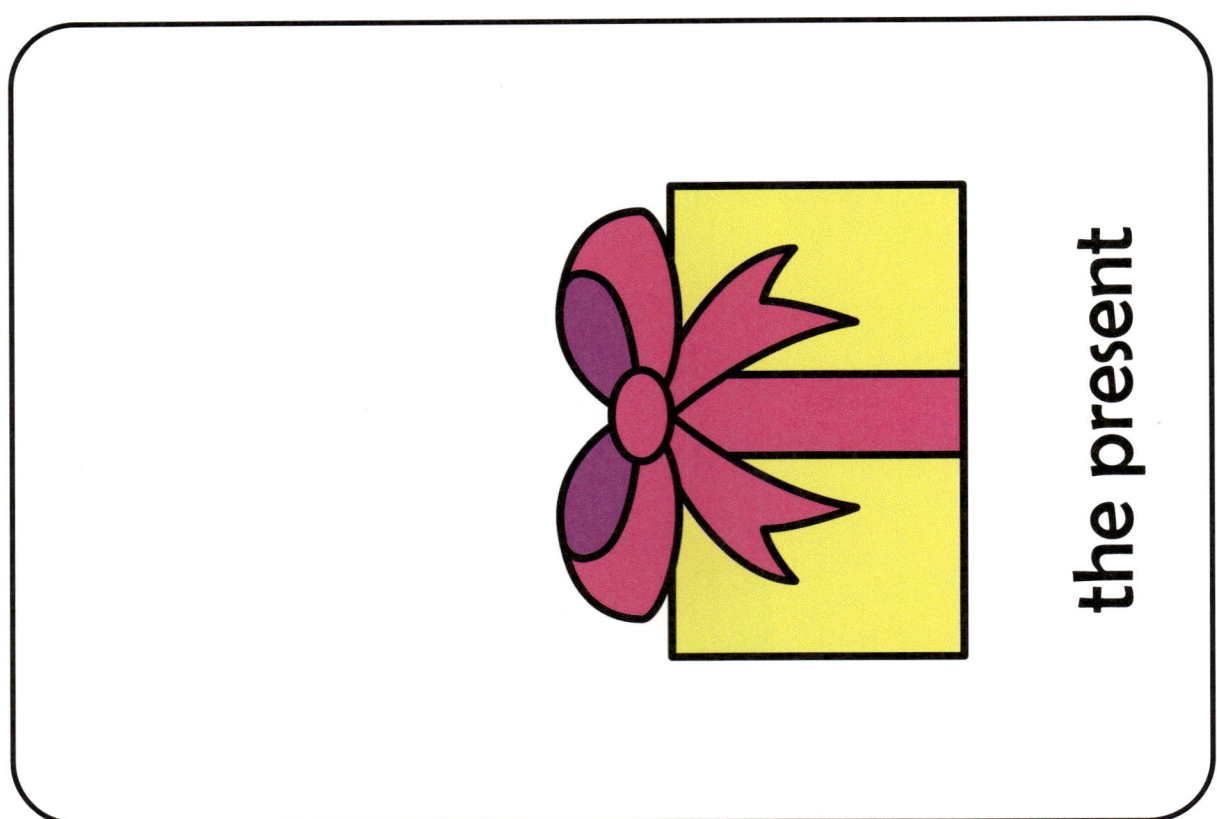

the present

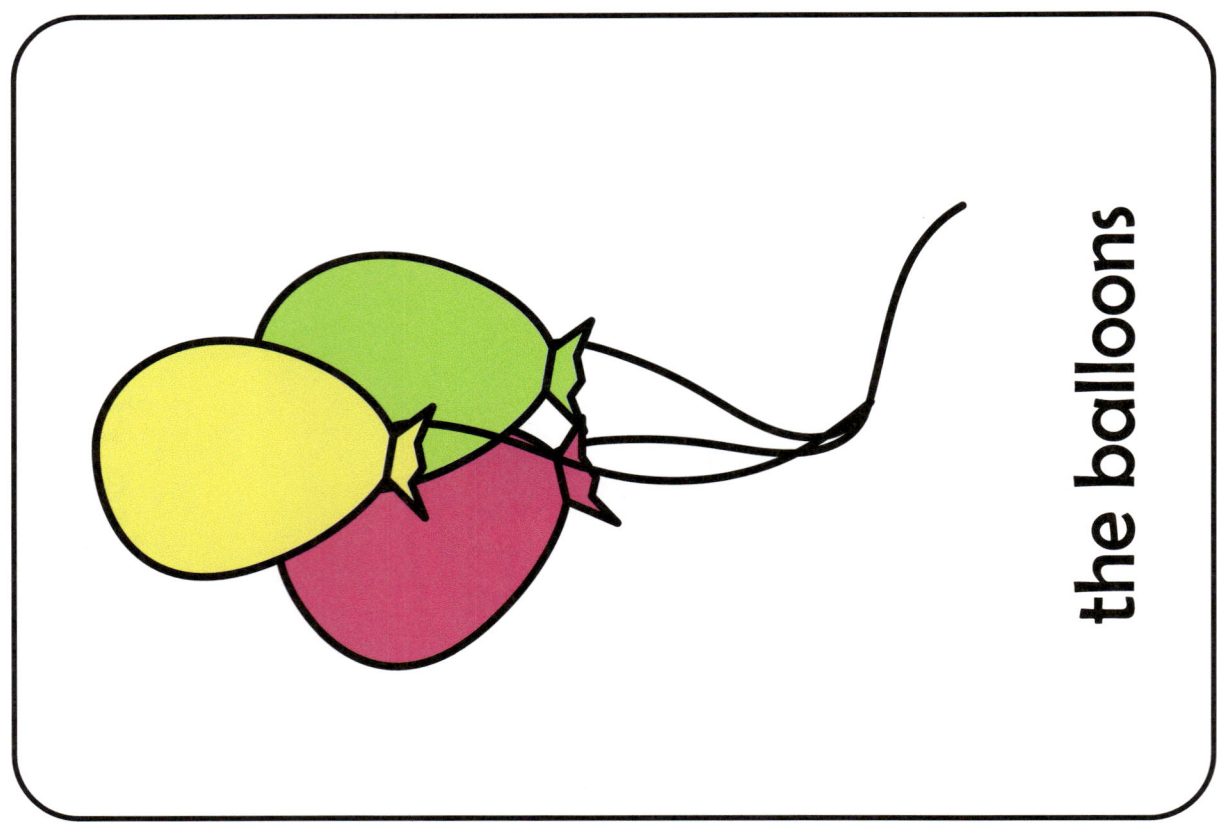

the balloons

Copyright material from NHS Forth Valley (2020), *Colourful Semantics*, Routledge

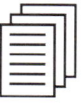

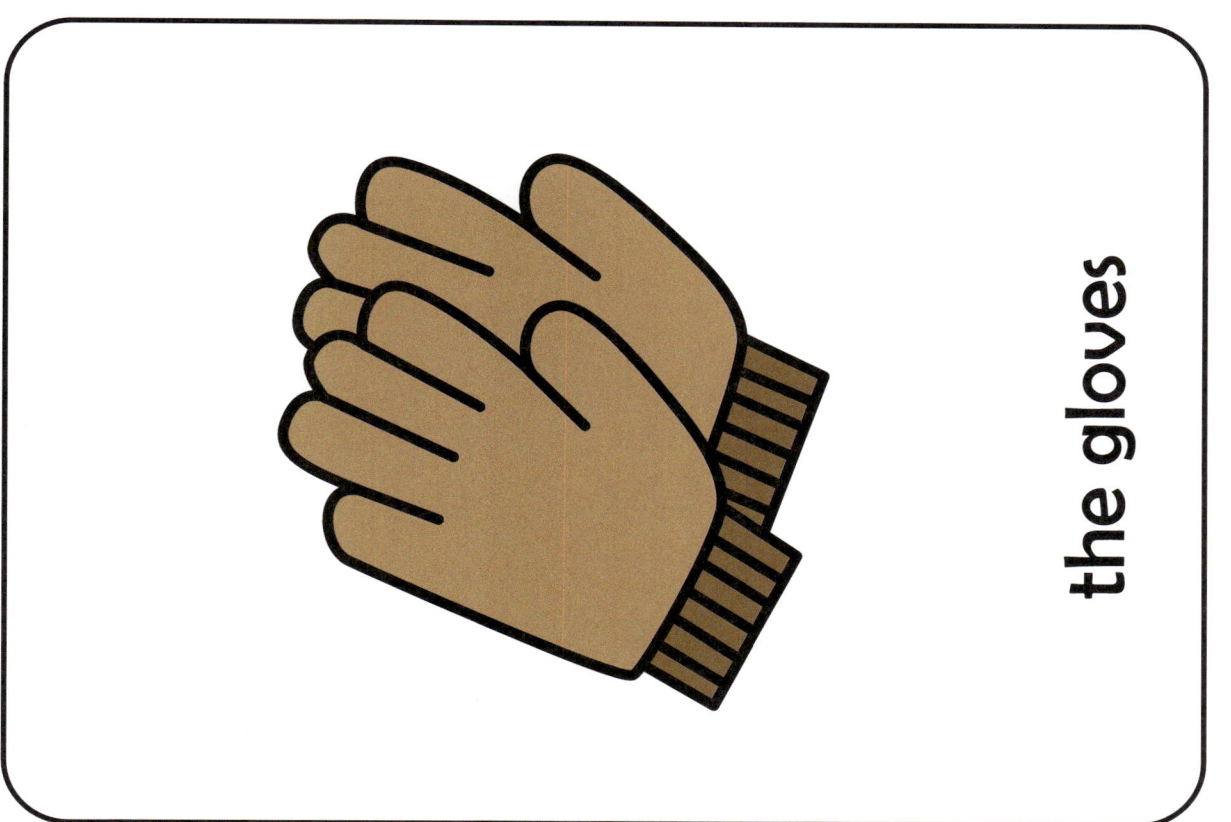

the gloves

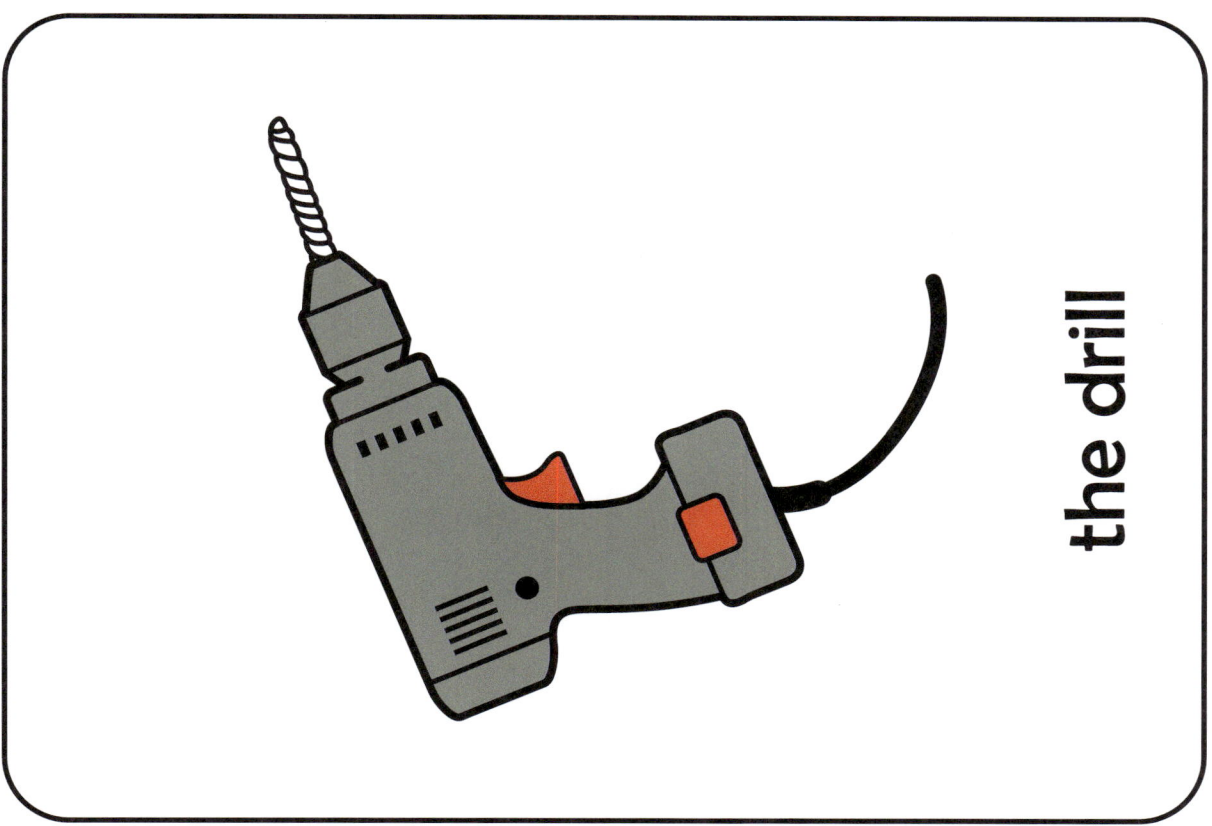

the drill

Copyright material from NHS Forth Valley (2020), *Colourful Semantics*, Routledge

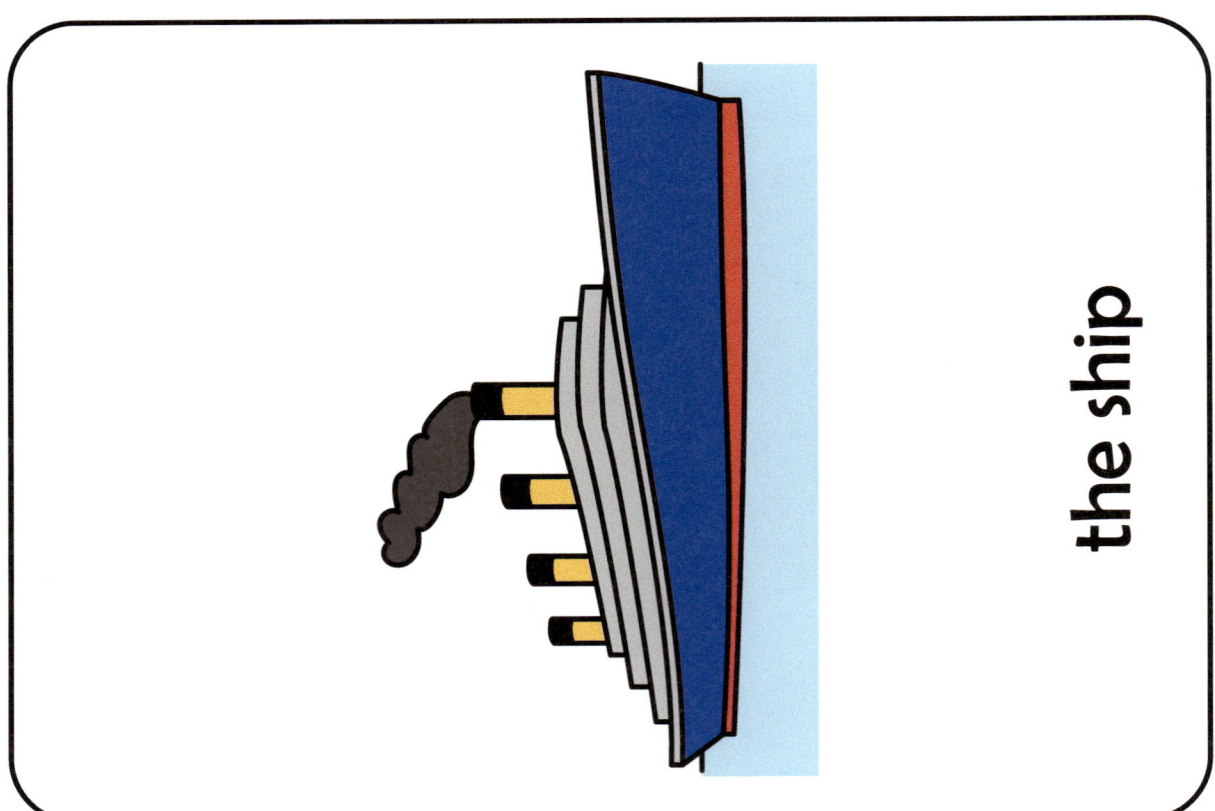

the ship

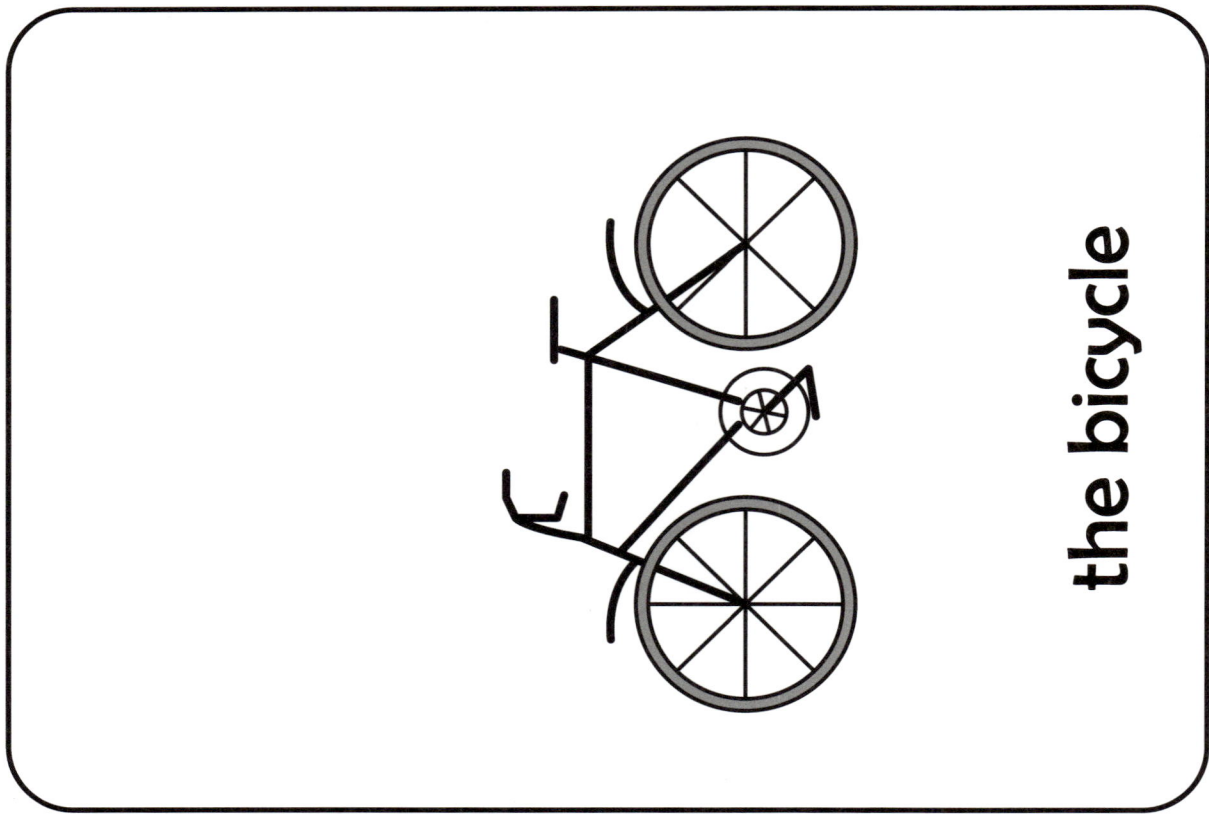

the bicycle

Copyright material from NHS Forth Valley (2020), *Colourful Semantics*, Routledge

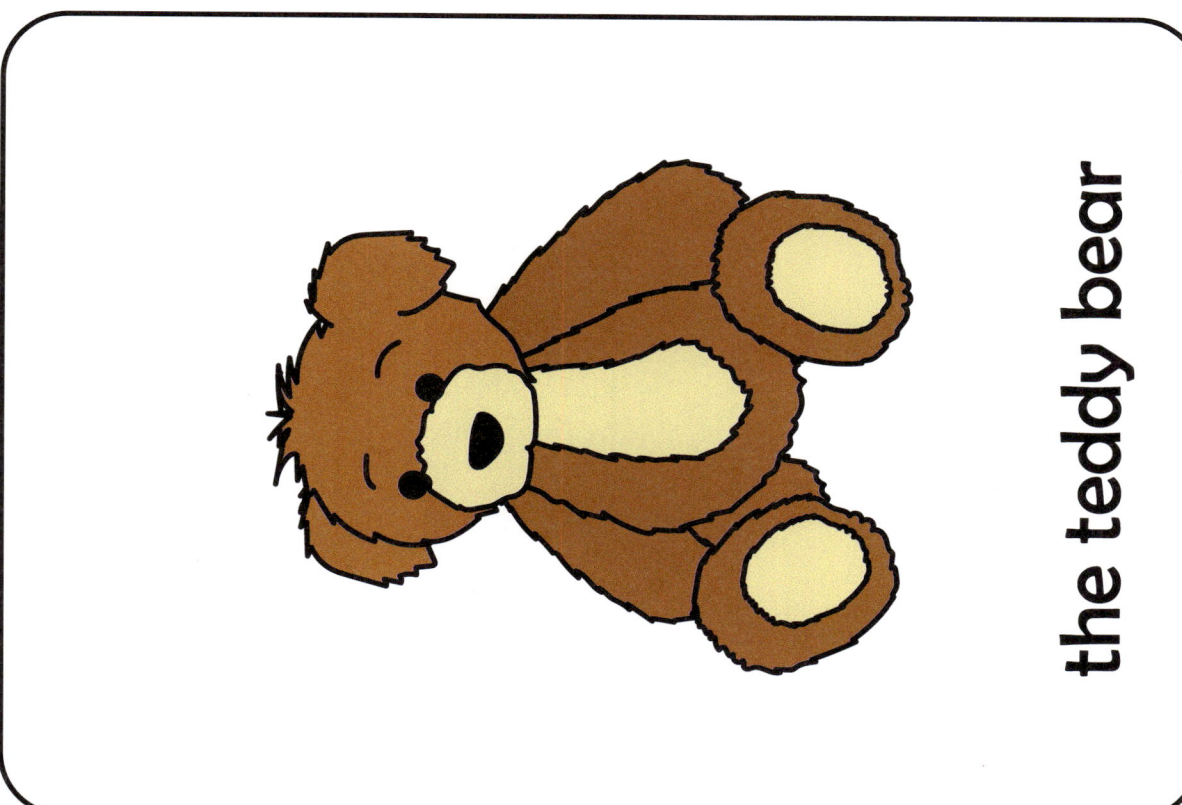

the teddy bear

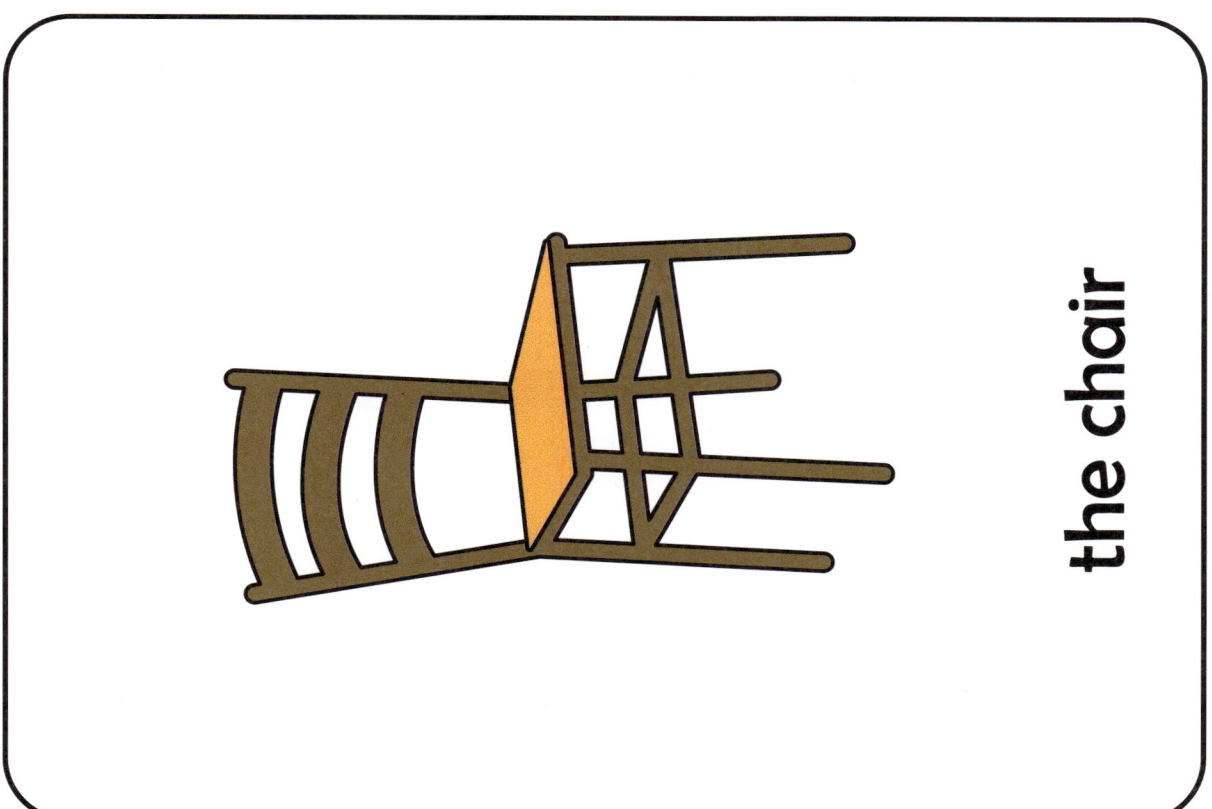

the chair

Copyright material from NHS Forth Valley (2020), *Colourful Semantics*, Routledge

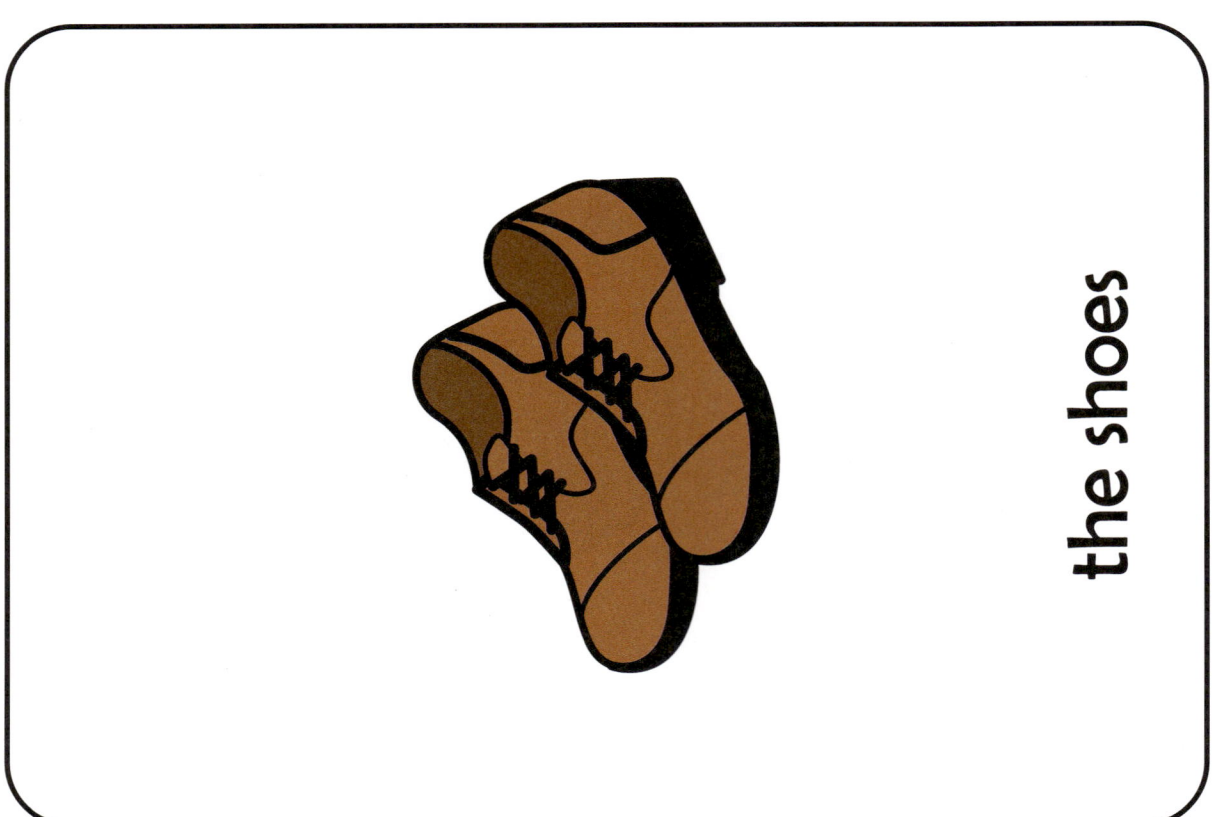

the shoes

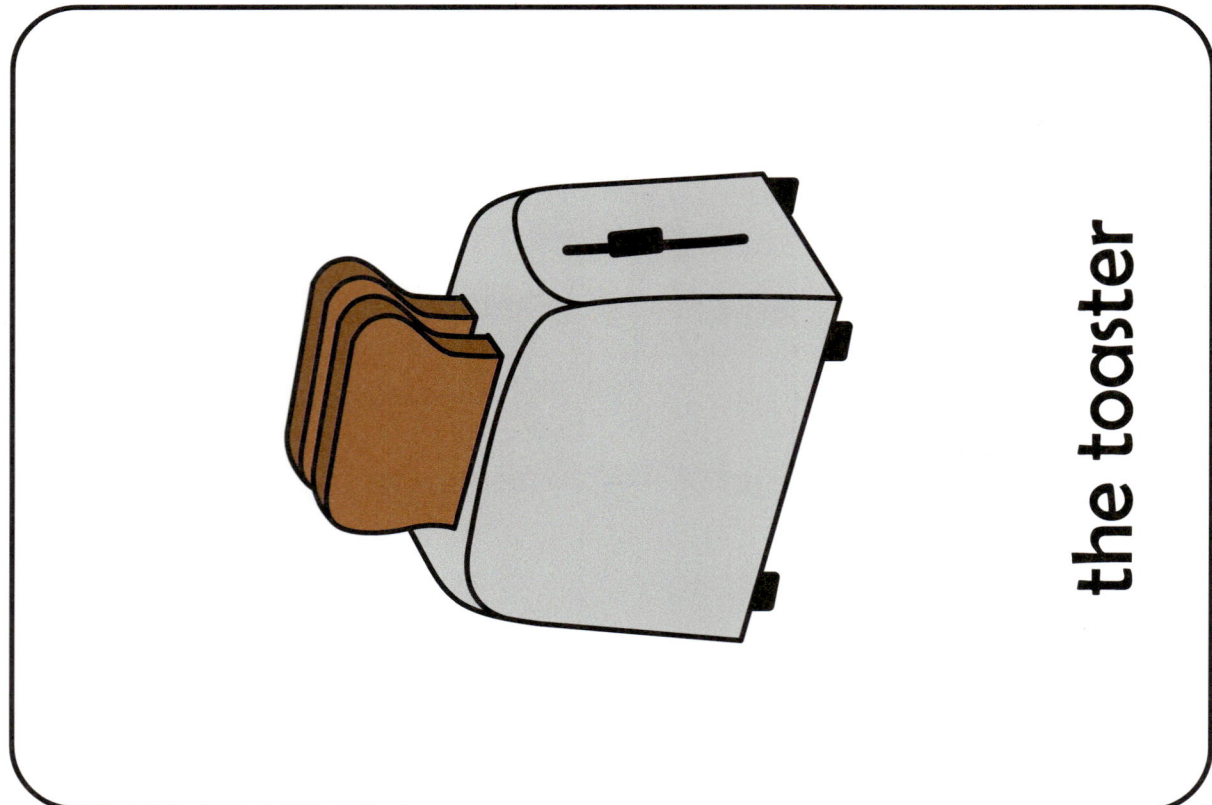

the toaster

Copyright material from NHS Forth Valley (2020), *Colourful Semantics*, Routledge

'Where' vocabulary

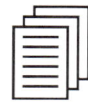

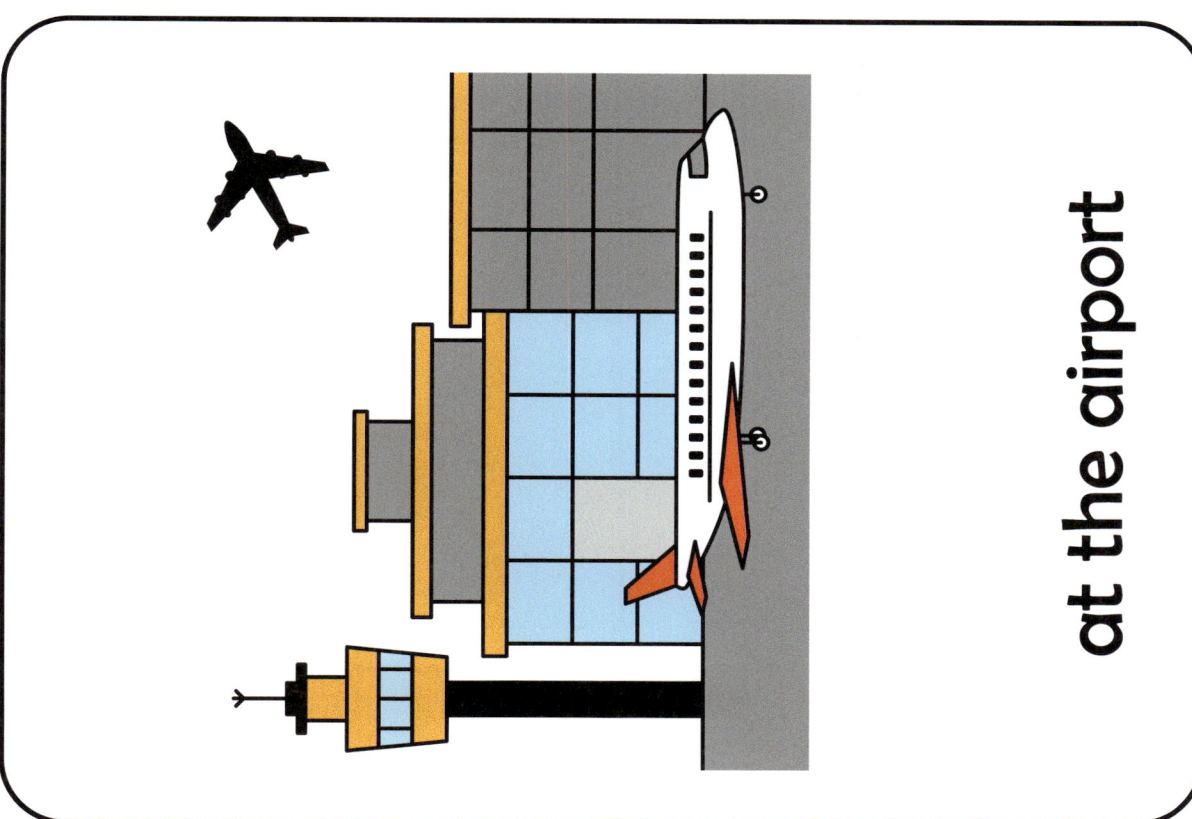

at the airport

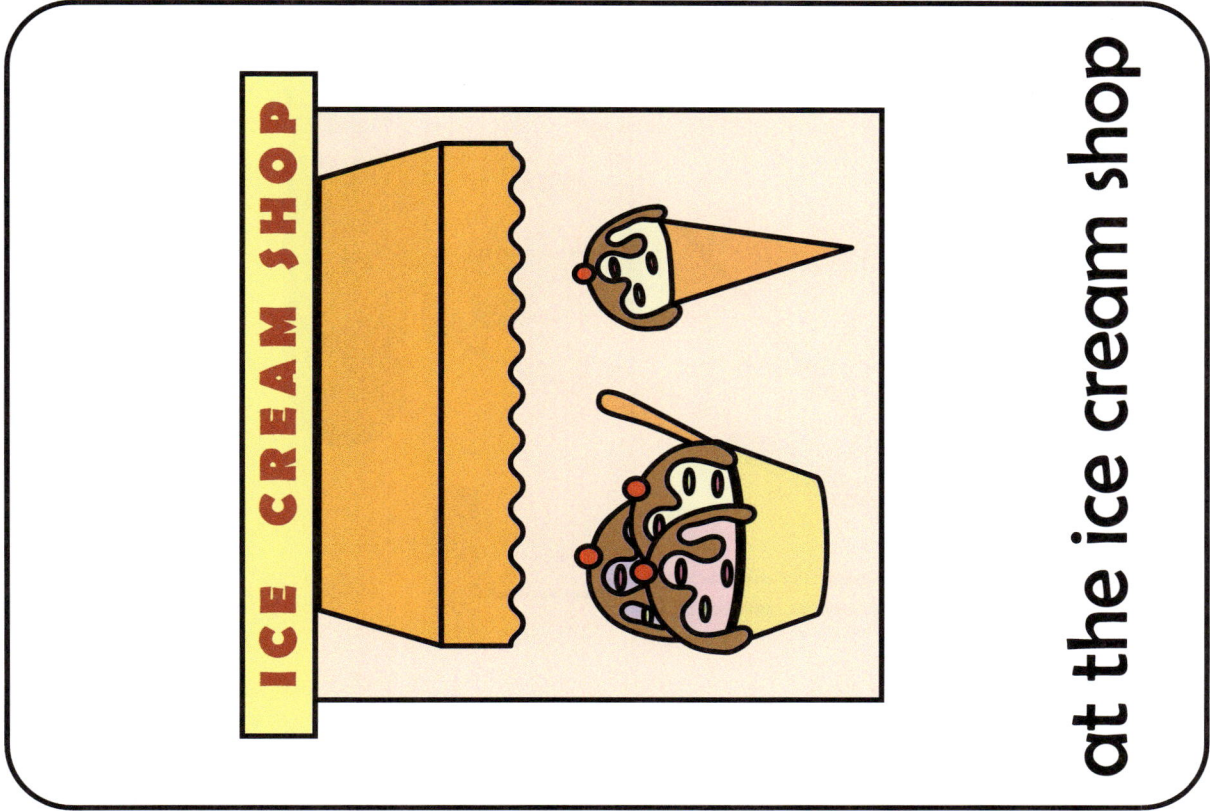

at the ice cream shop

Copyright material from NHS Forth Valley (2020), *Colourful Semantics*, Routledge

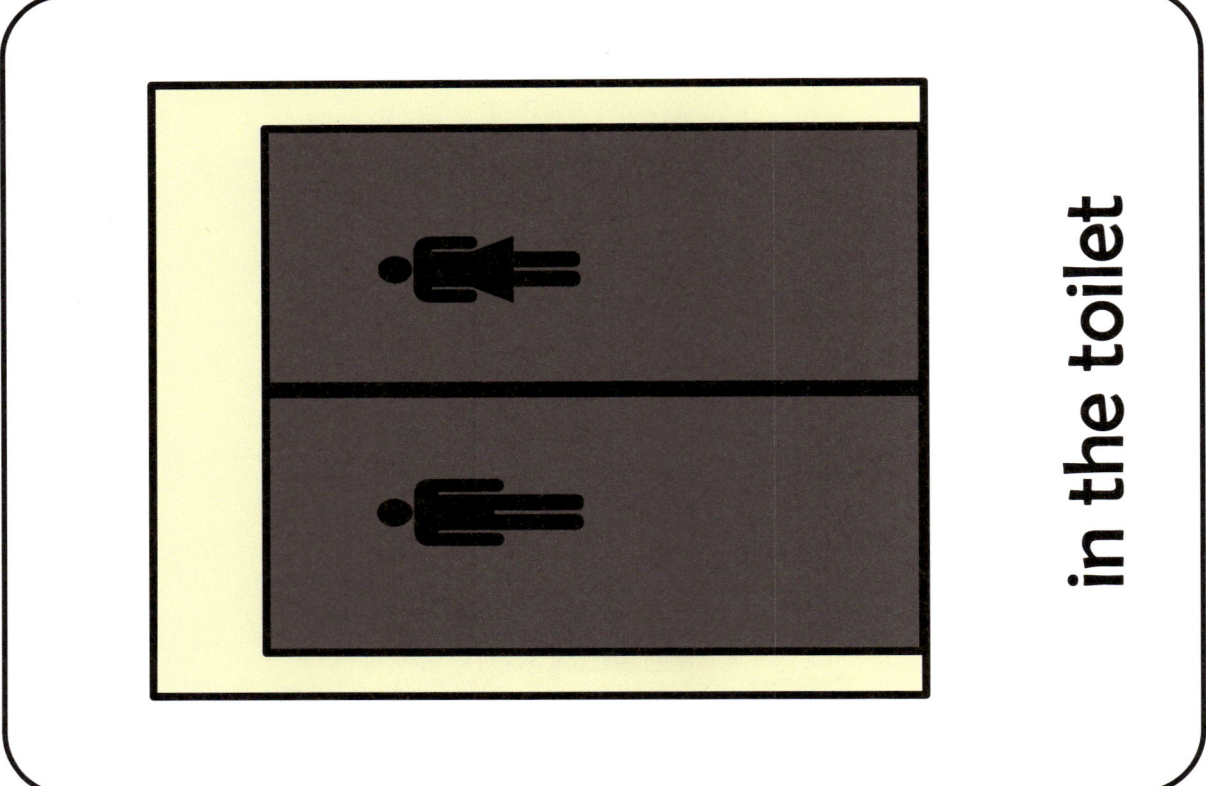

in the toilet

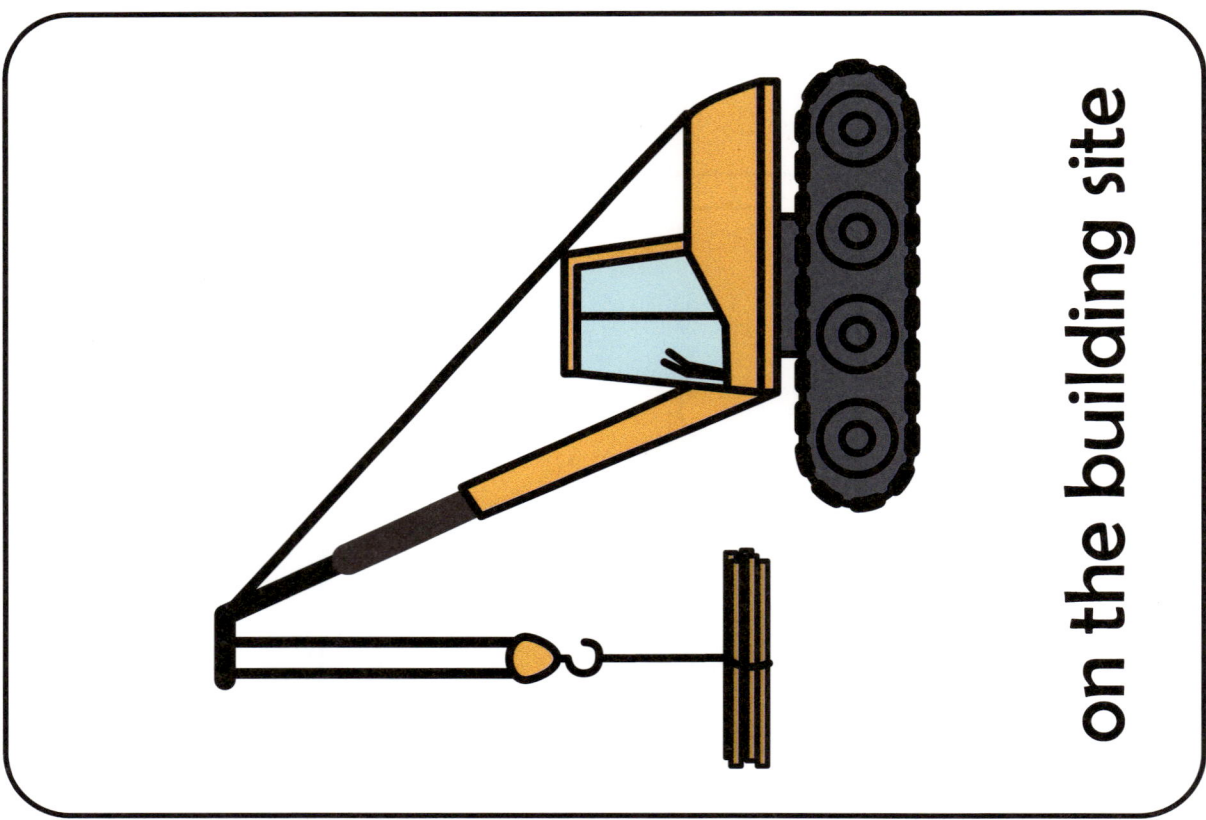

on the building site

Copyright material from NHS Forth Valley (2020), *Colourful Semantics*, Routledge

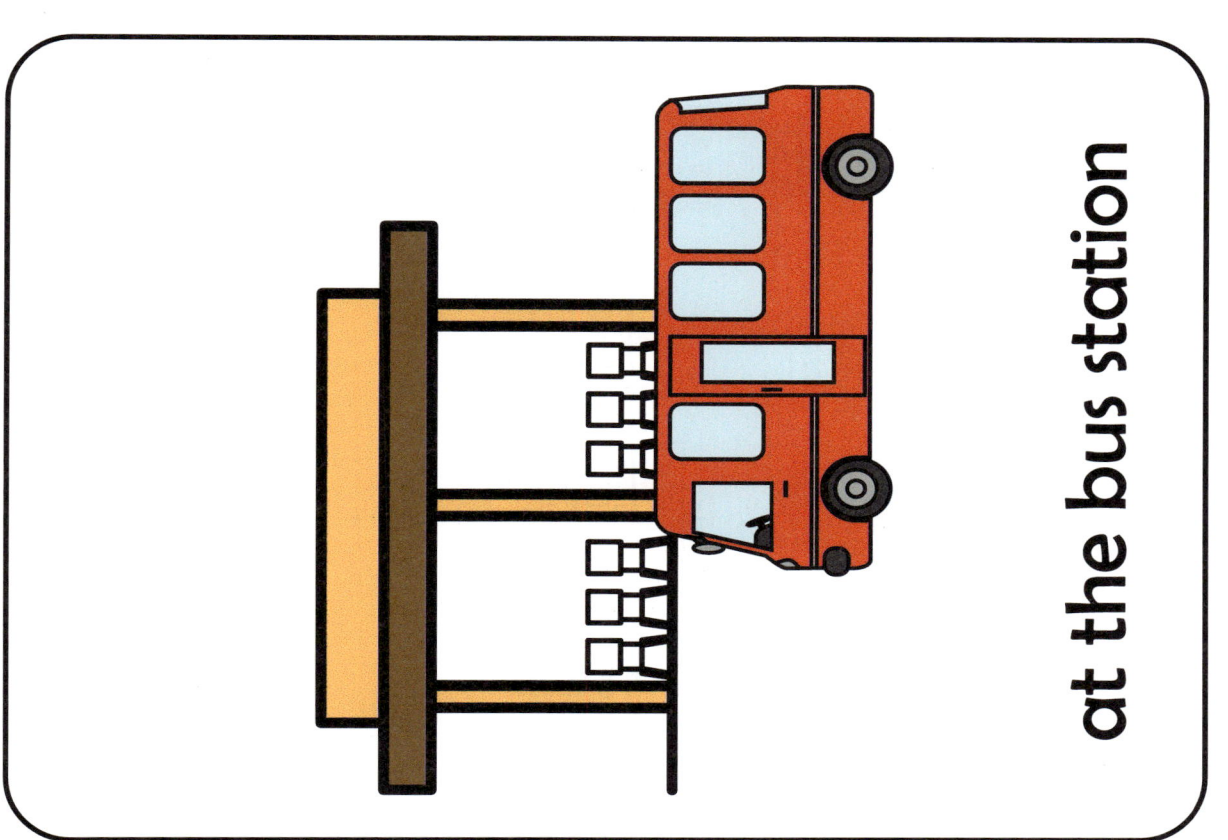

at the bus station

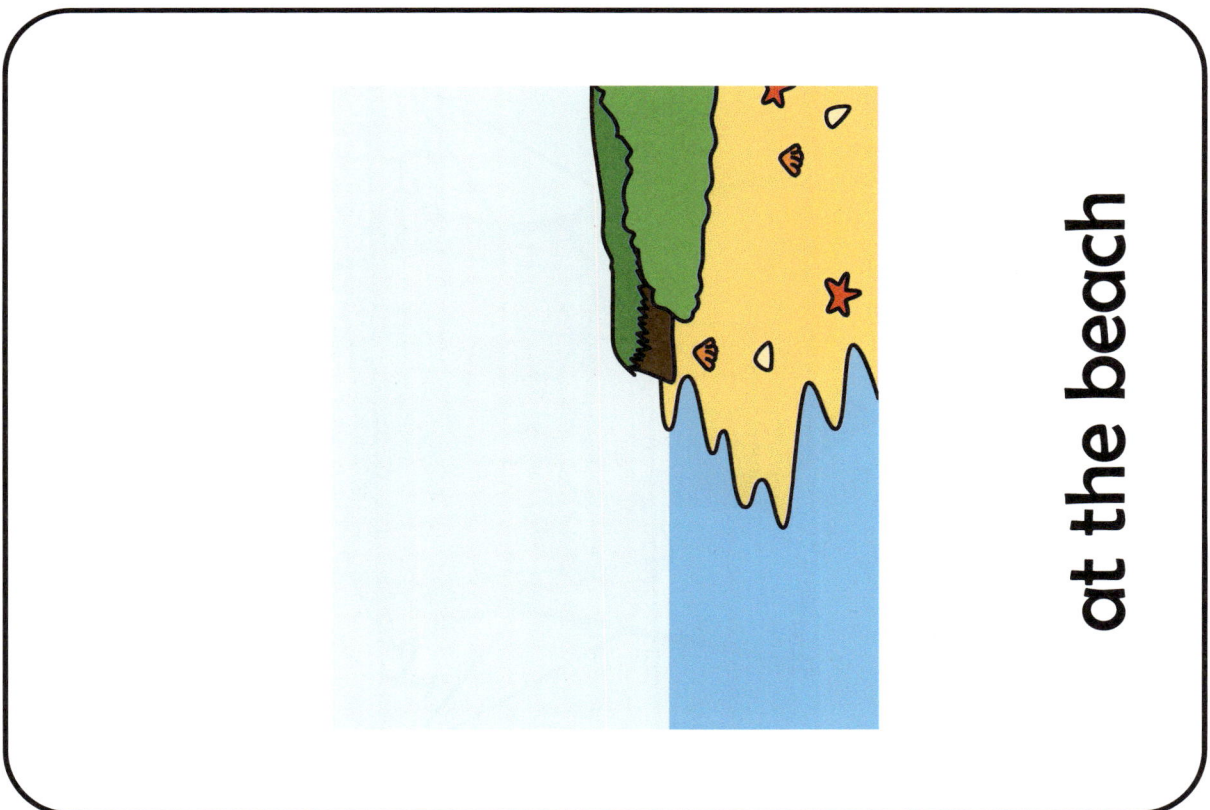

at the beach

Copyright material from NHS Forth Valley (2020), *Colourful Semantics*, Routledge

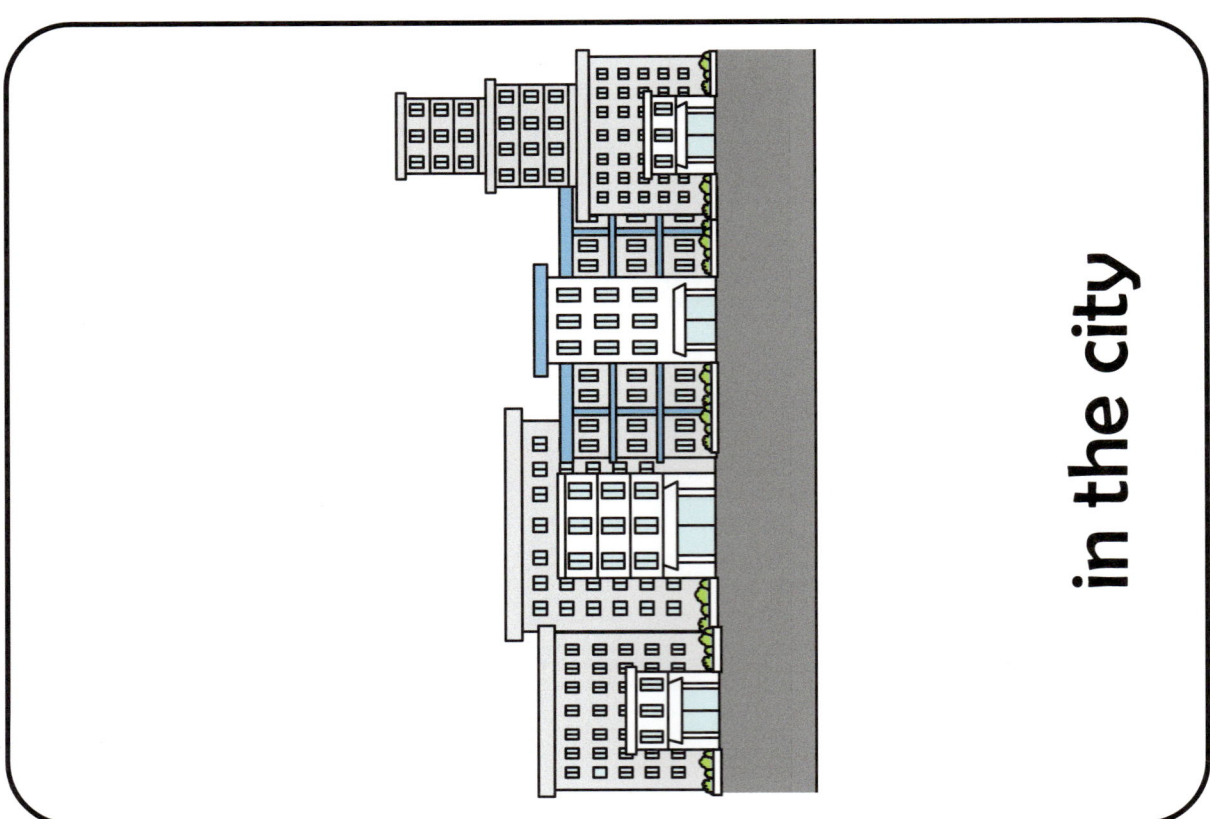

in the city

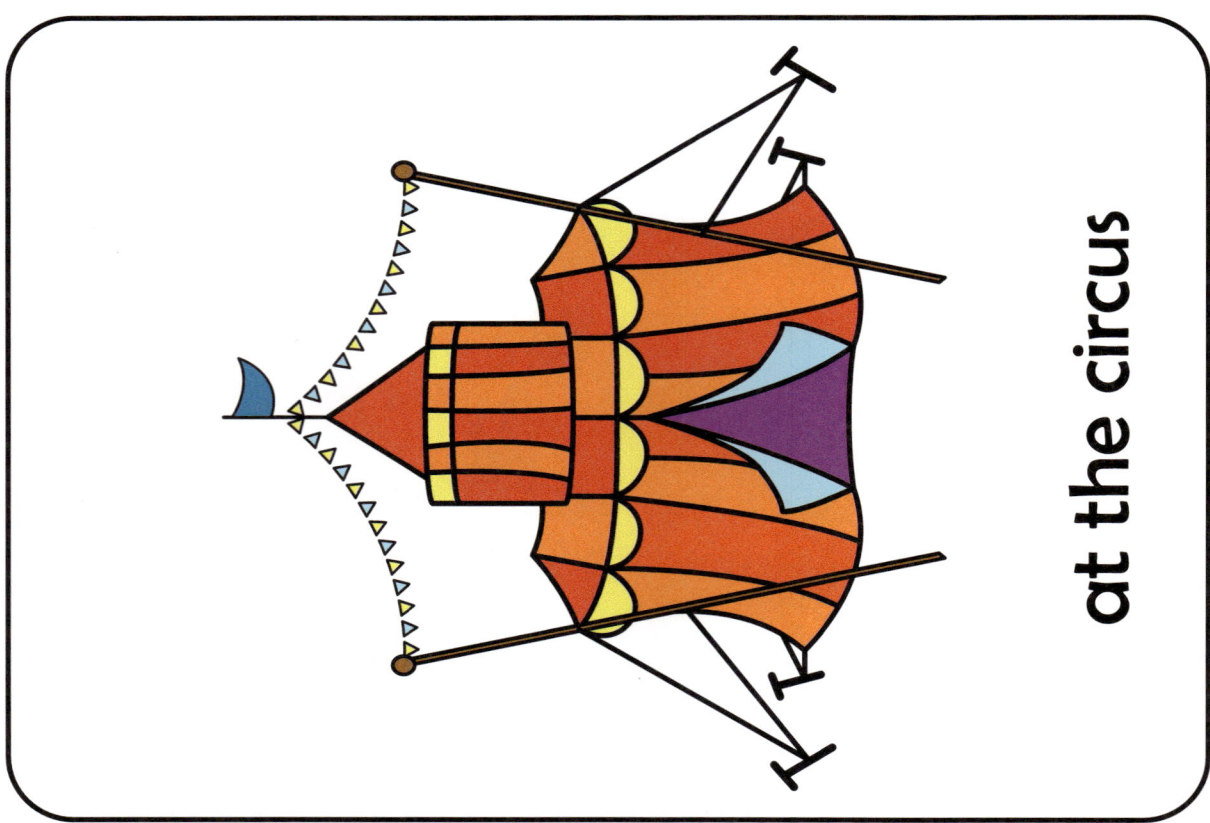

at the circus

Copyright material from NHS Forth Valley (2020), *Colourful Semantics*, Routledge

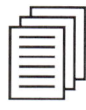

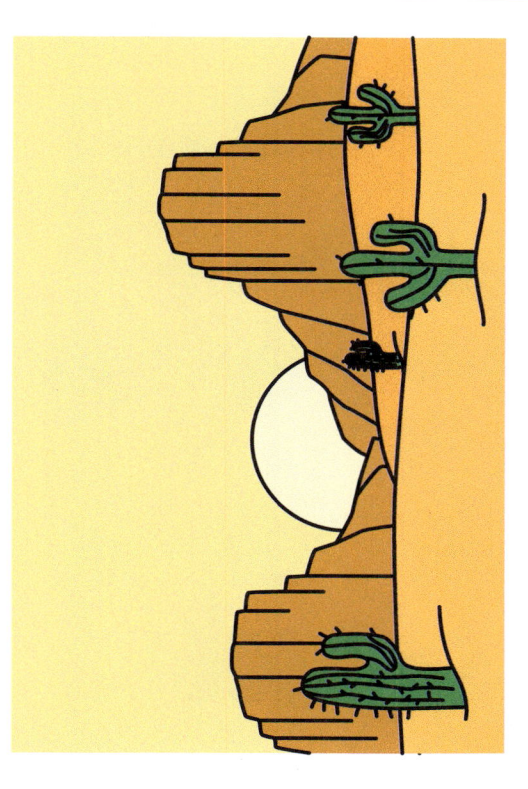

in the desert

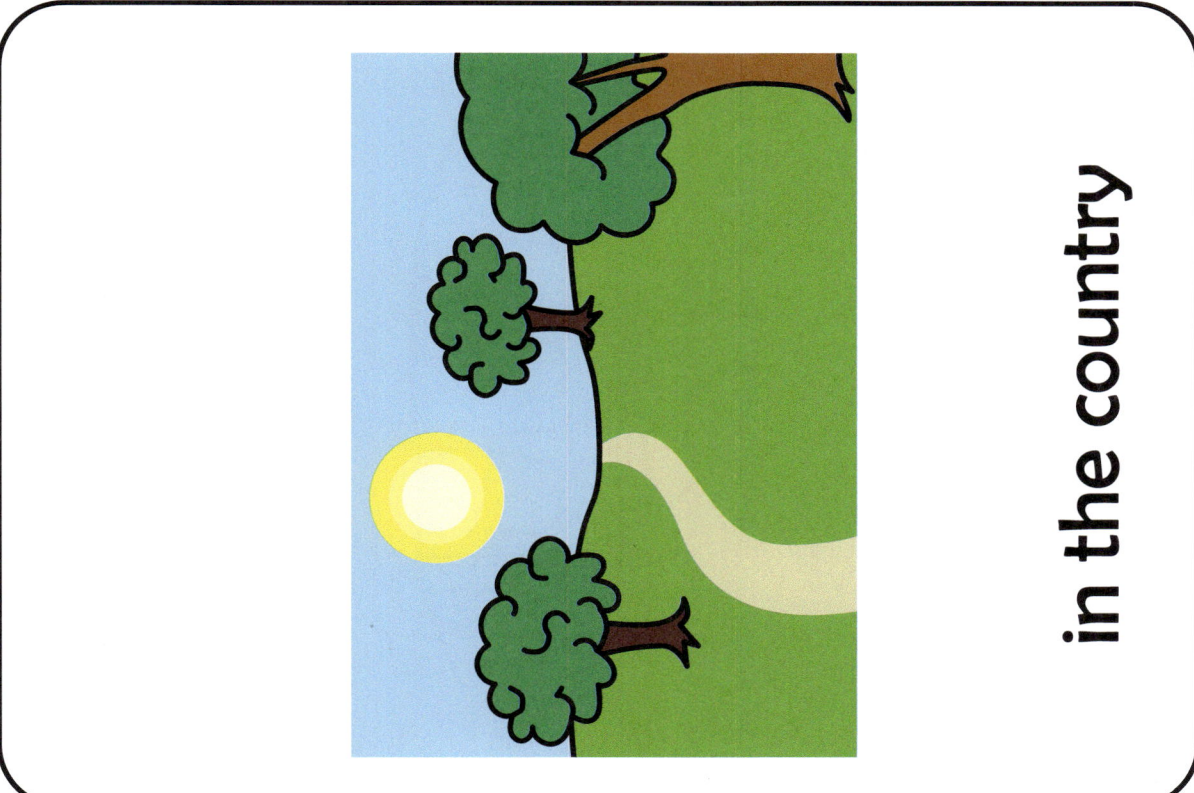

in the country

Copyright material from NHS Forth Valley (2020), *Colourful Semantics*, Routledge

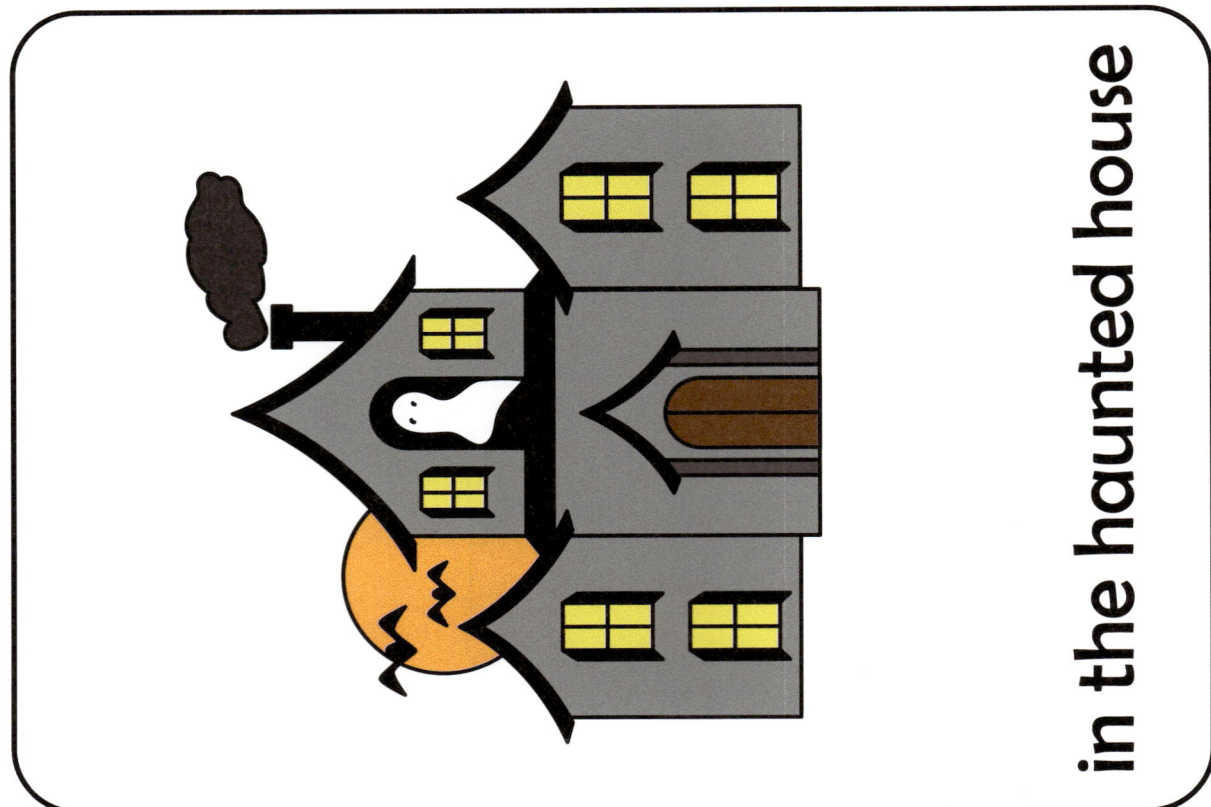

in the haunted house

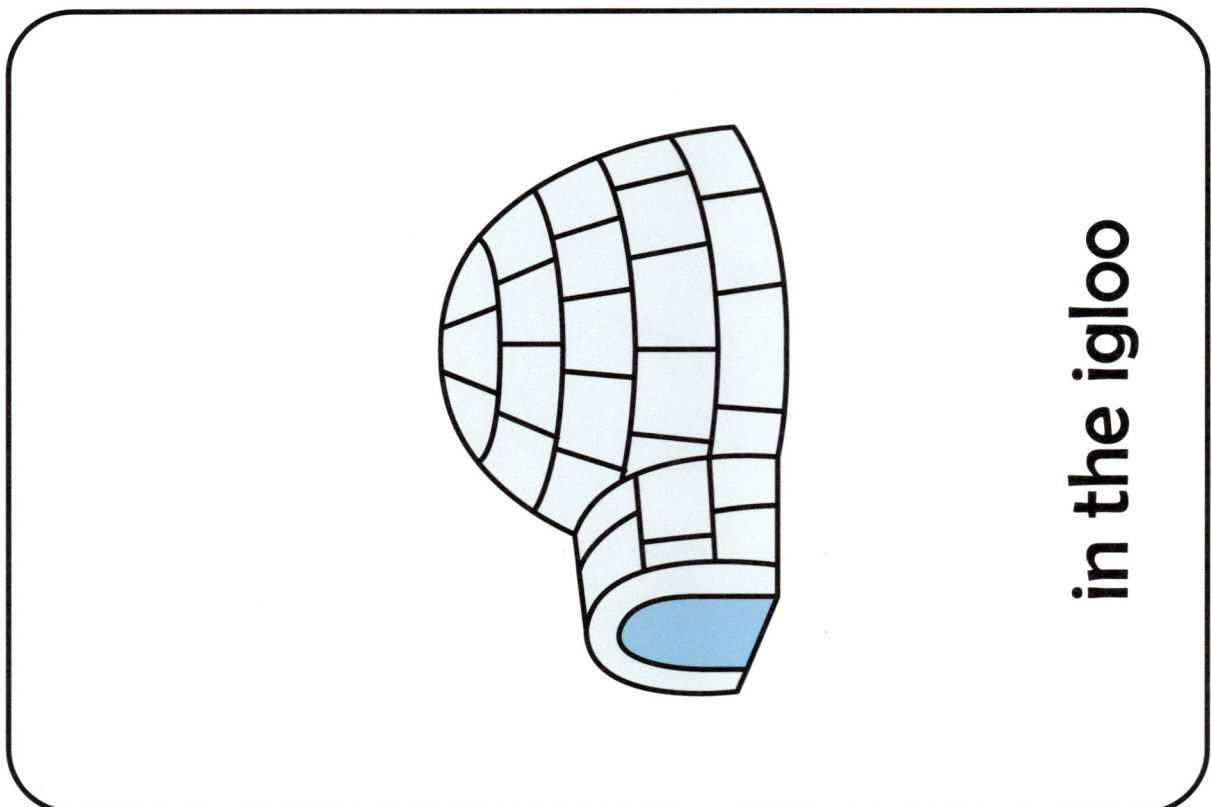

in the igloo

Copyright material from NHS Forth Valley (2020), *Colourful Semantics*, Routledge

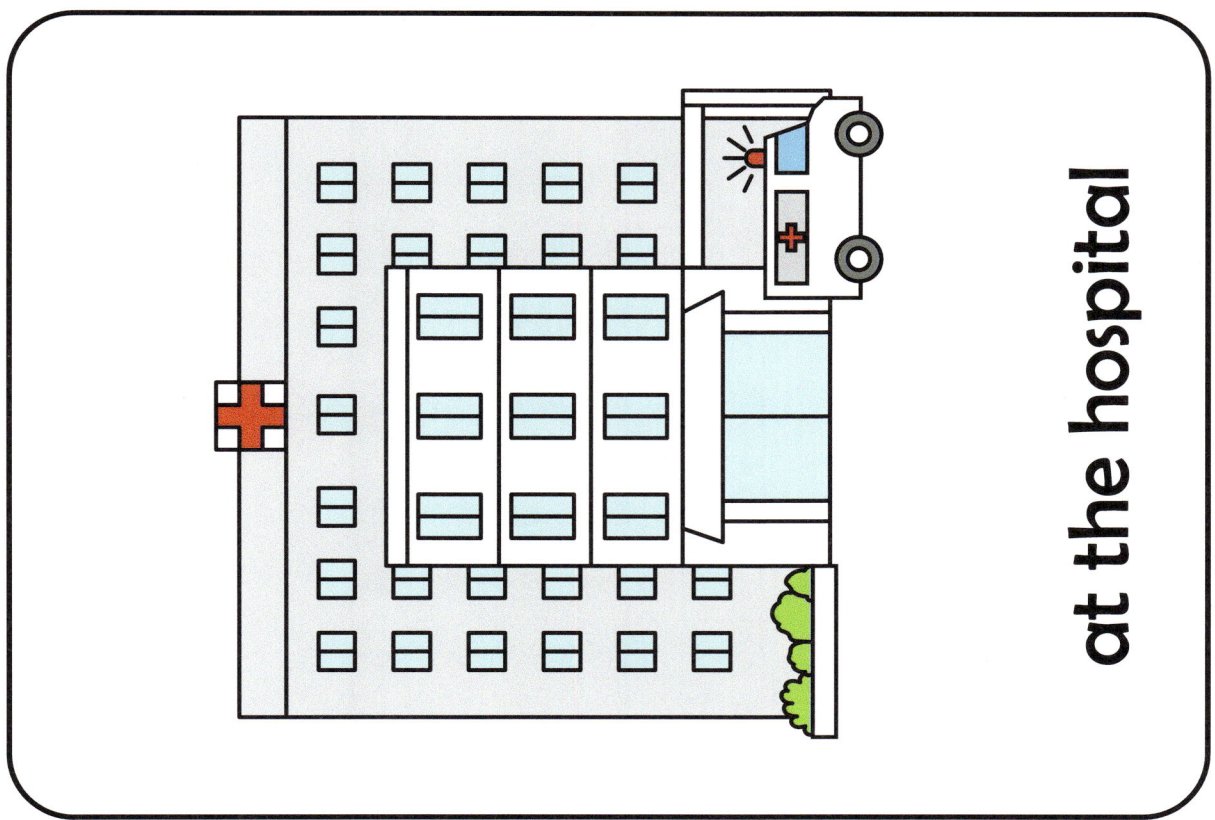

on a bridge

at the hospital

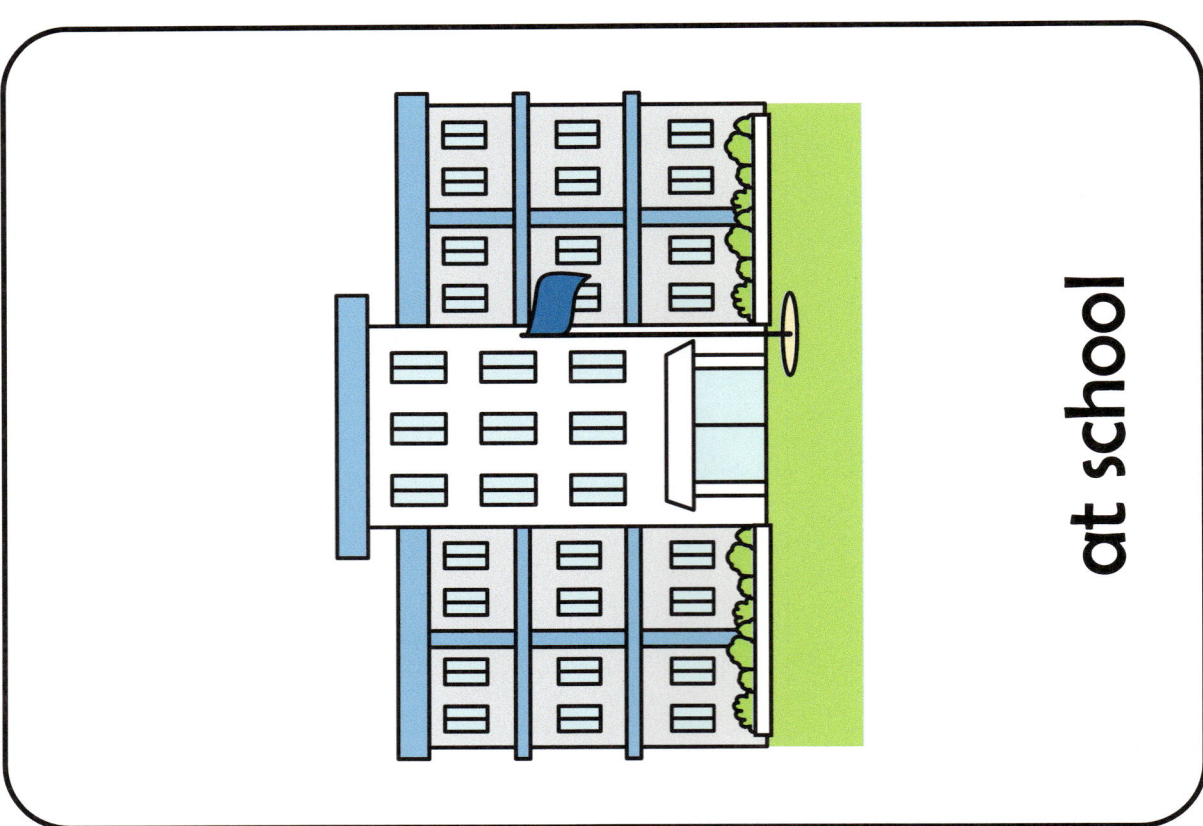

at school

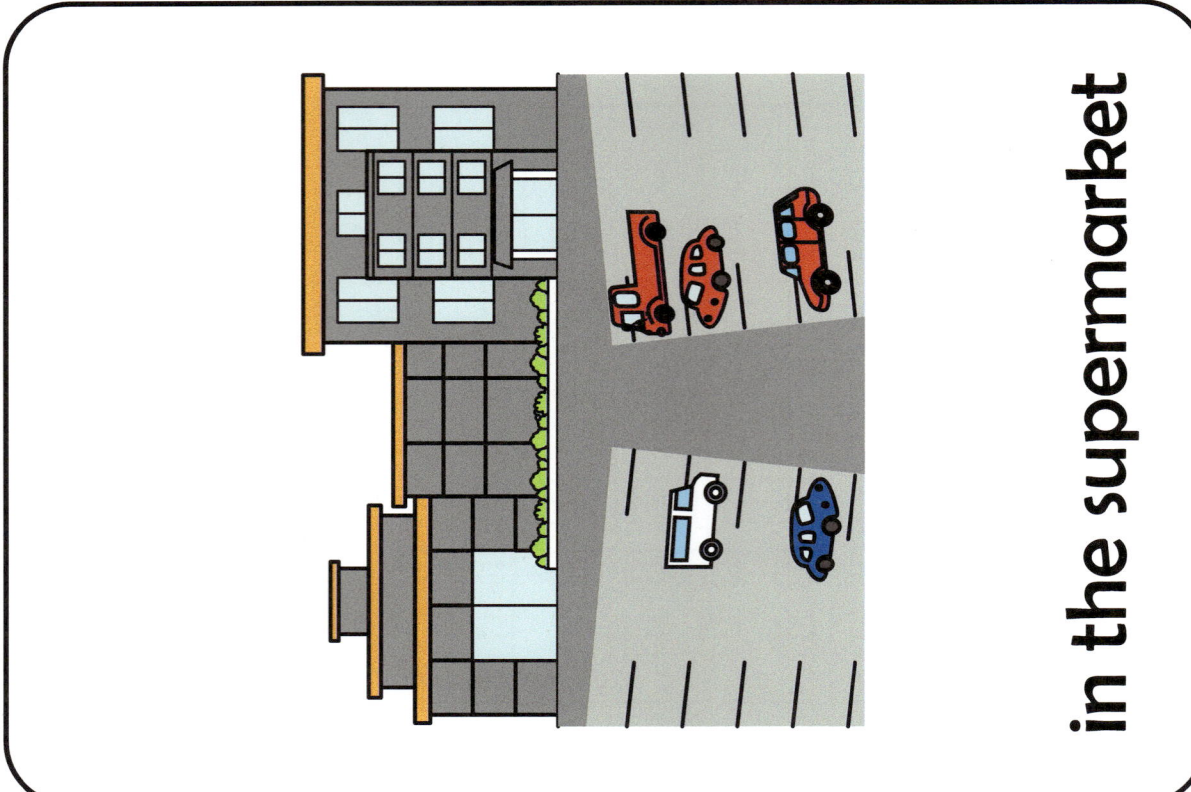

in the supermarket

Copyright material from NHS Forth Valley (2020), *Colourful Semantics*, Routledge

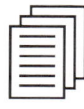

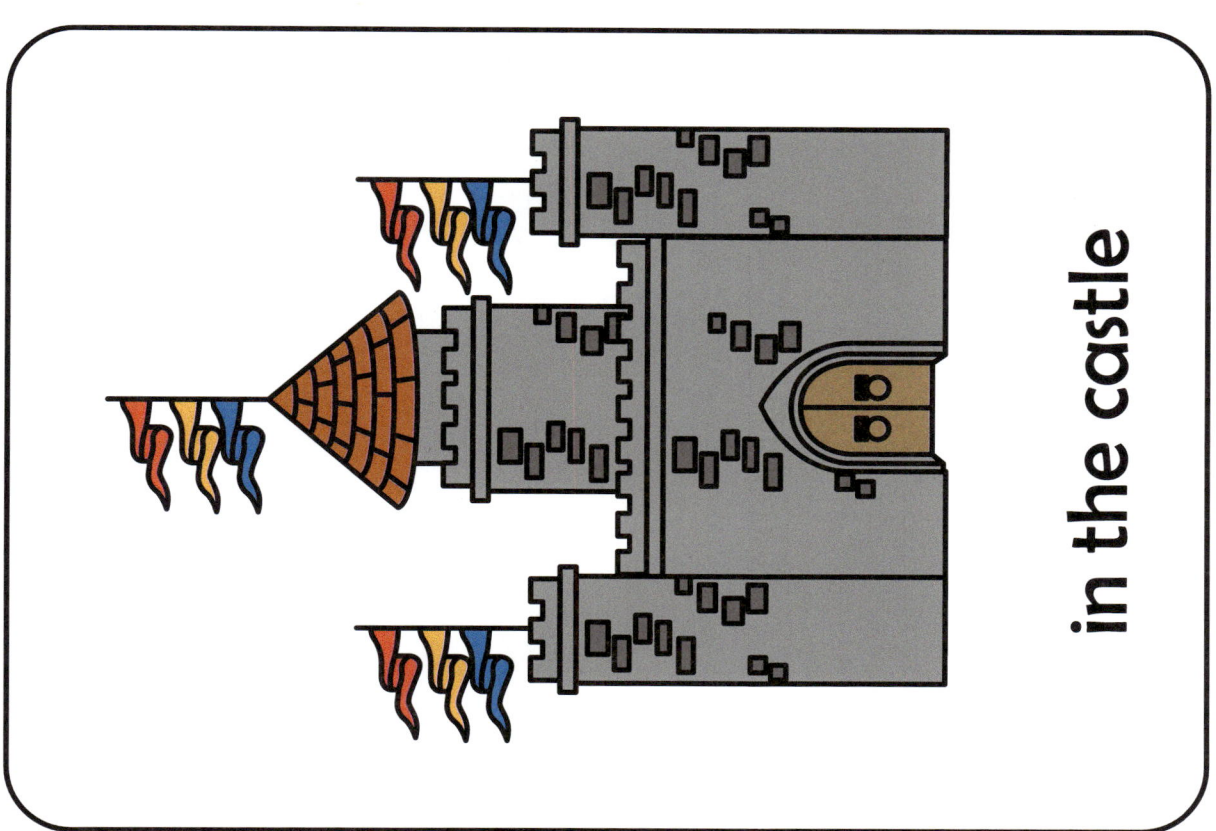

in the castle

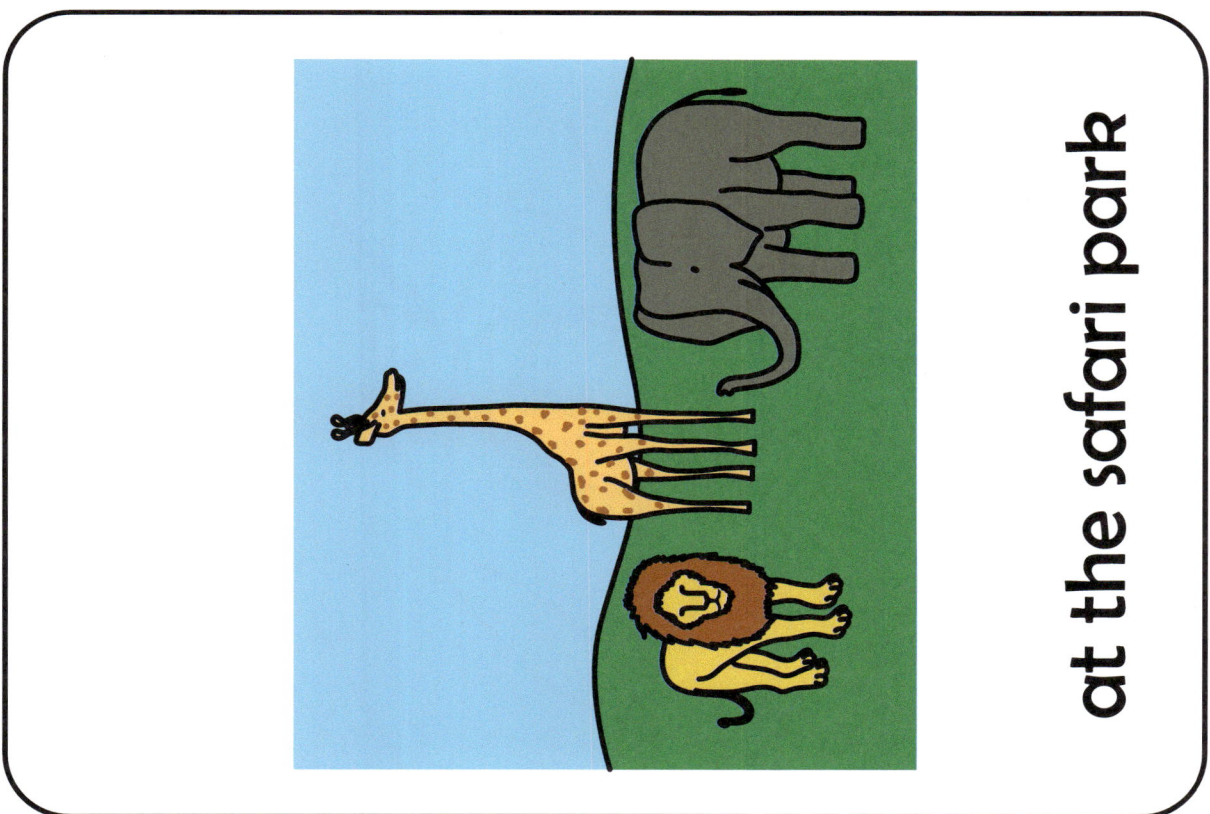

at the safari park

Copyright material from NHS Forth Valley (2020), *Colourful Semantics*, Routledge

'When' vocabulary

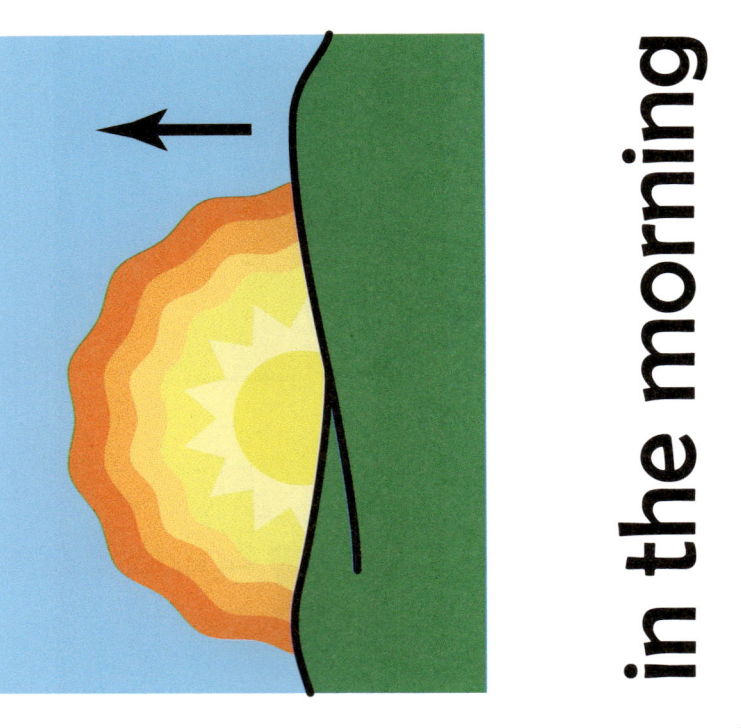

in the morning

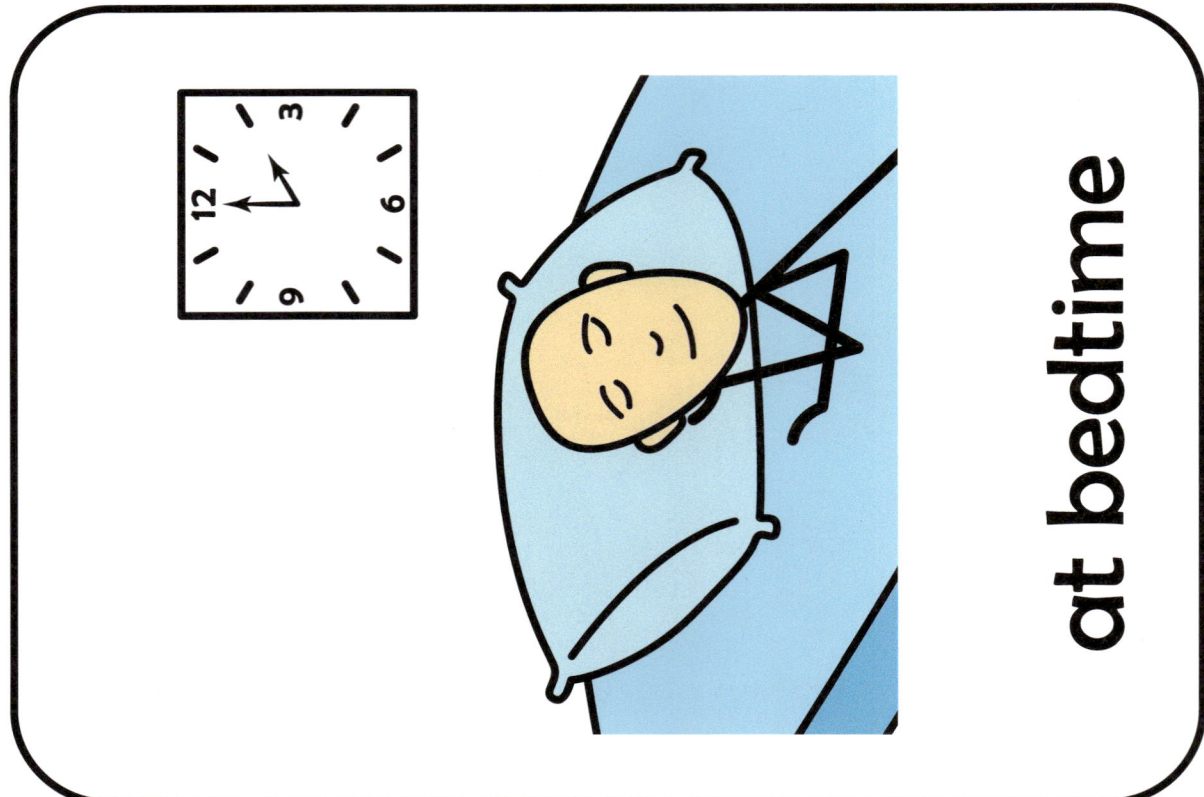

at bedtime

Copyright material from NHS Forth Valley (2020), *Colourful Semantics*, Routledge

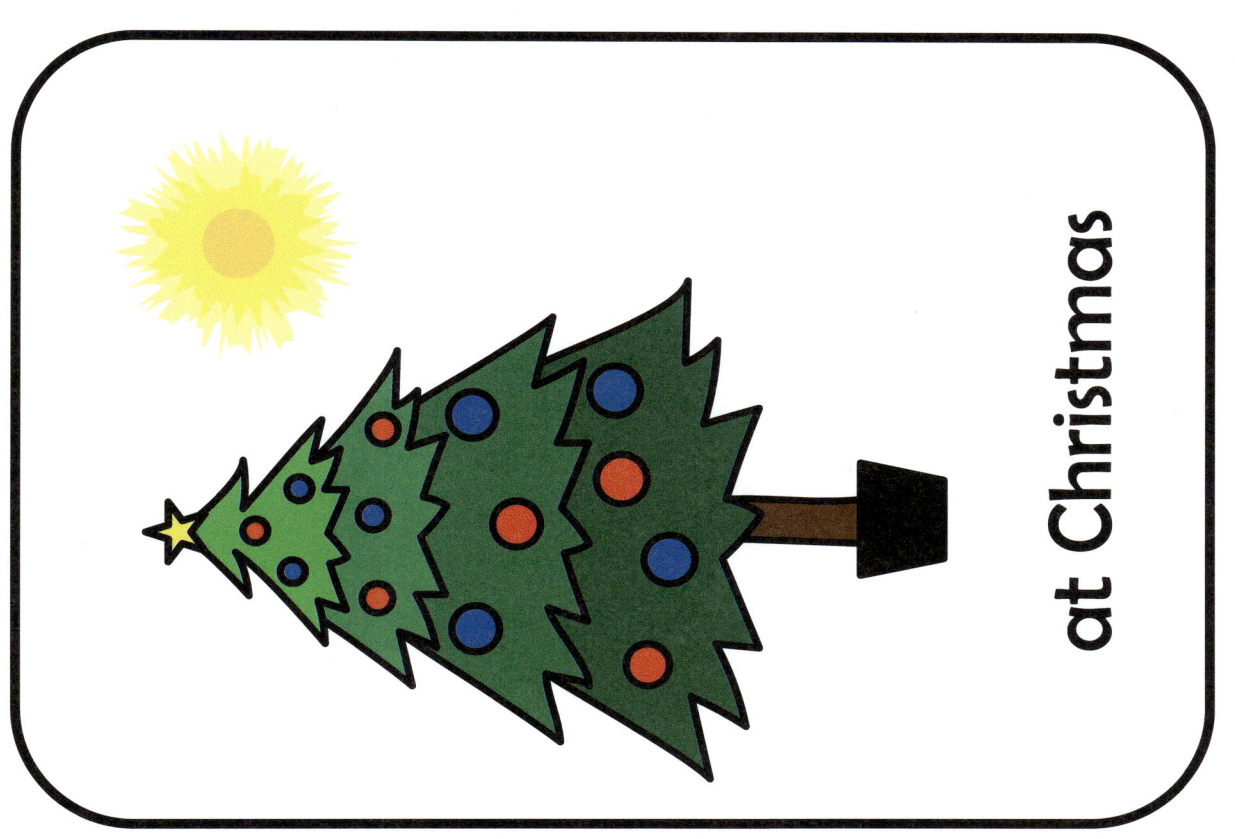

at Christmas

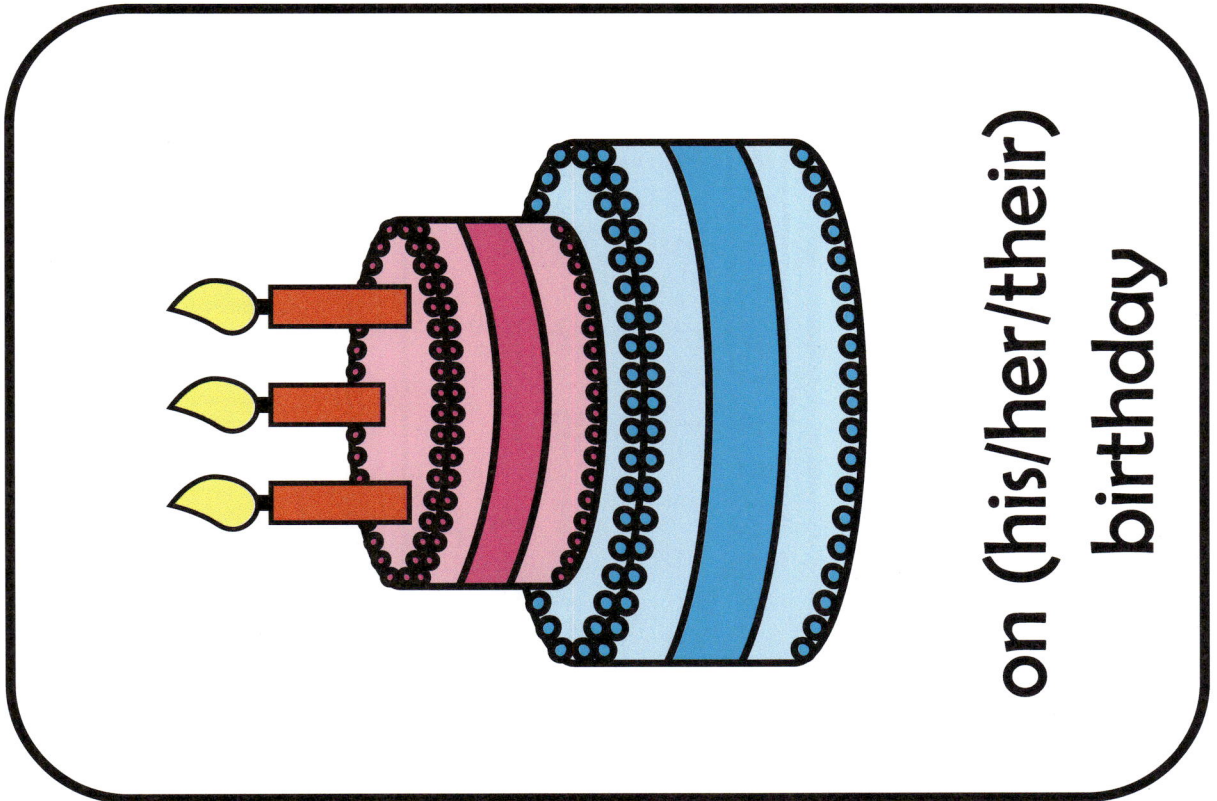

on (his/her/their) birthday

Copyright material from NHS Forth Valley (2020), *Colourful Semantics*, Routledge

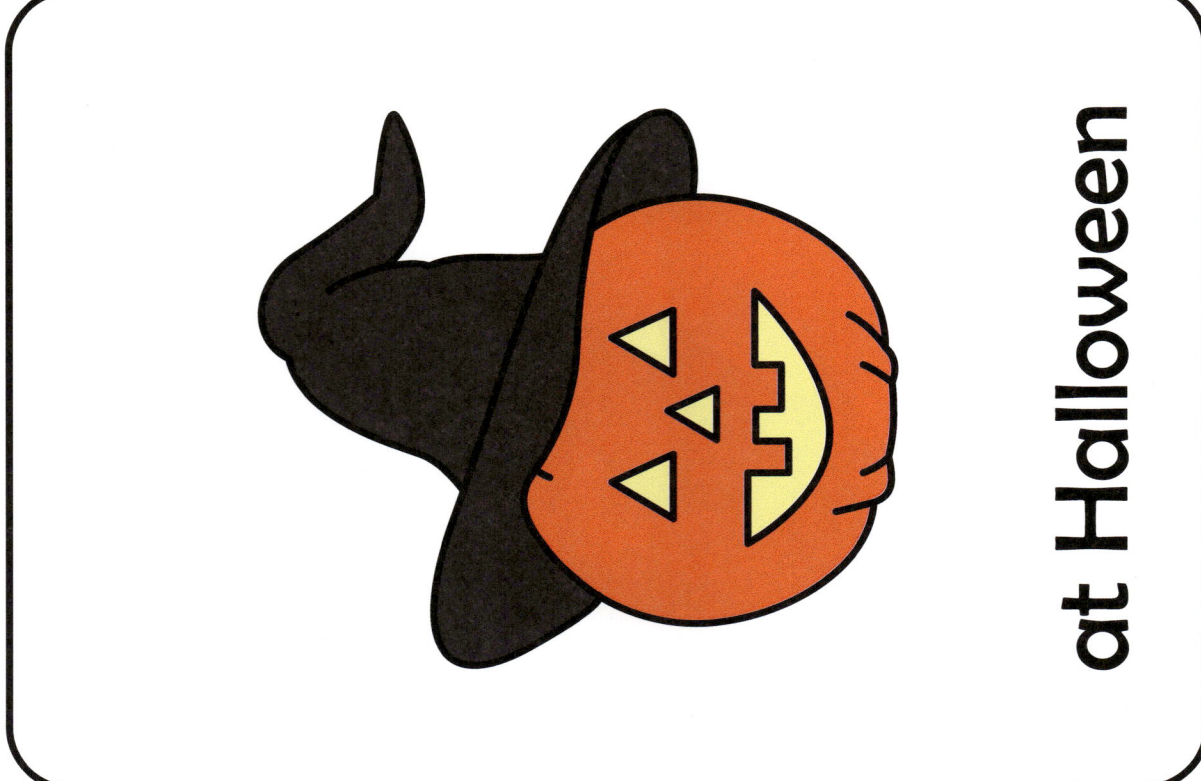

at Halloween

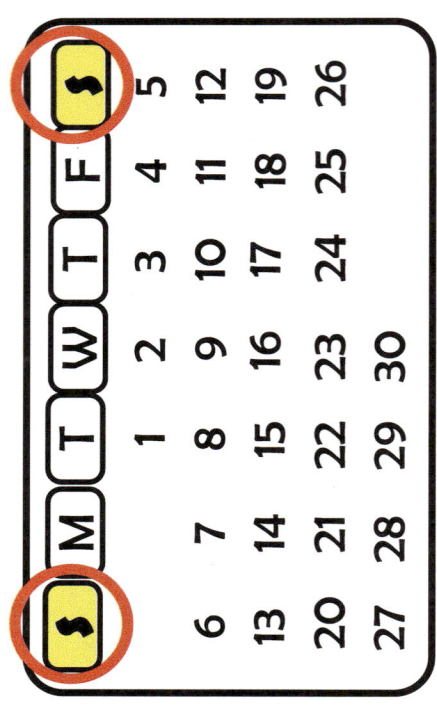

at the
weekend

Copyright material from NHS Forth Valley (2020), *Colourful Semantics*, Routledge

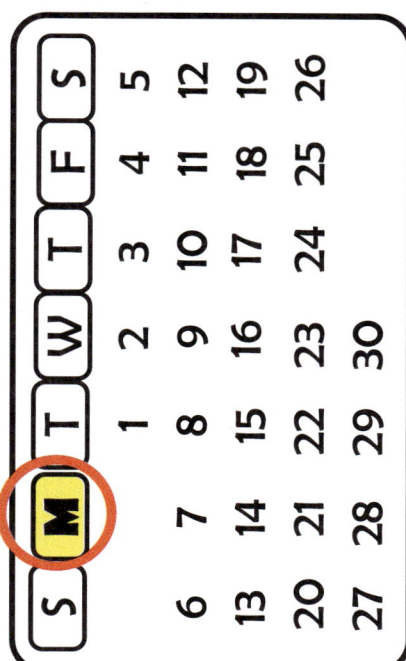

on Monday

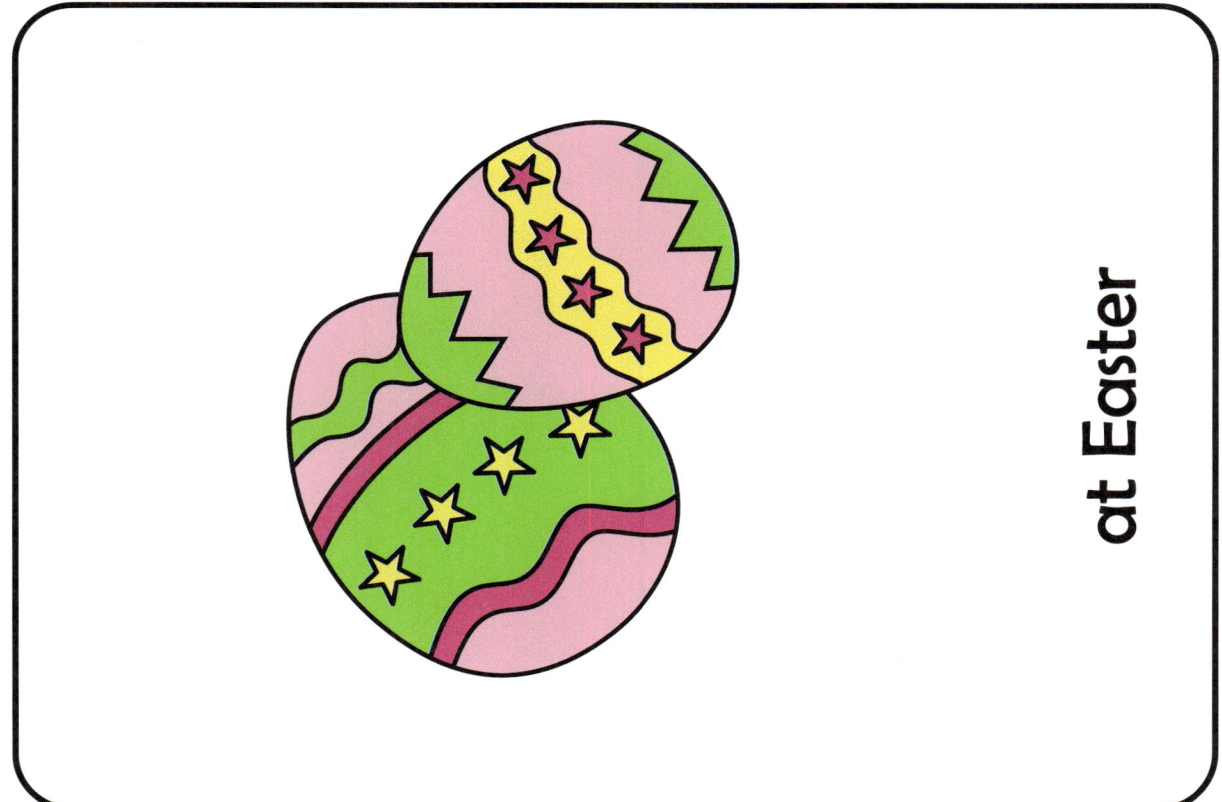

at Easter

Copyright material from NHS Forth Valley (2020), *Colourful Semantics*, Routledge

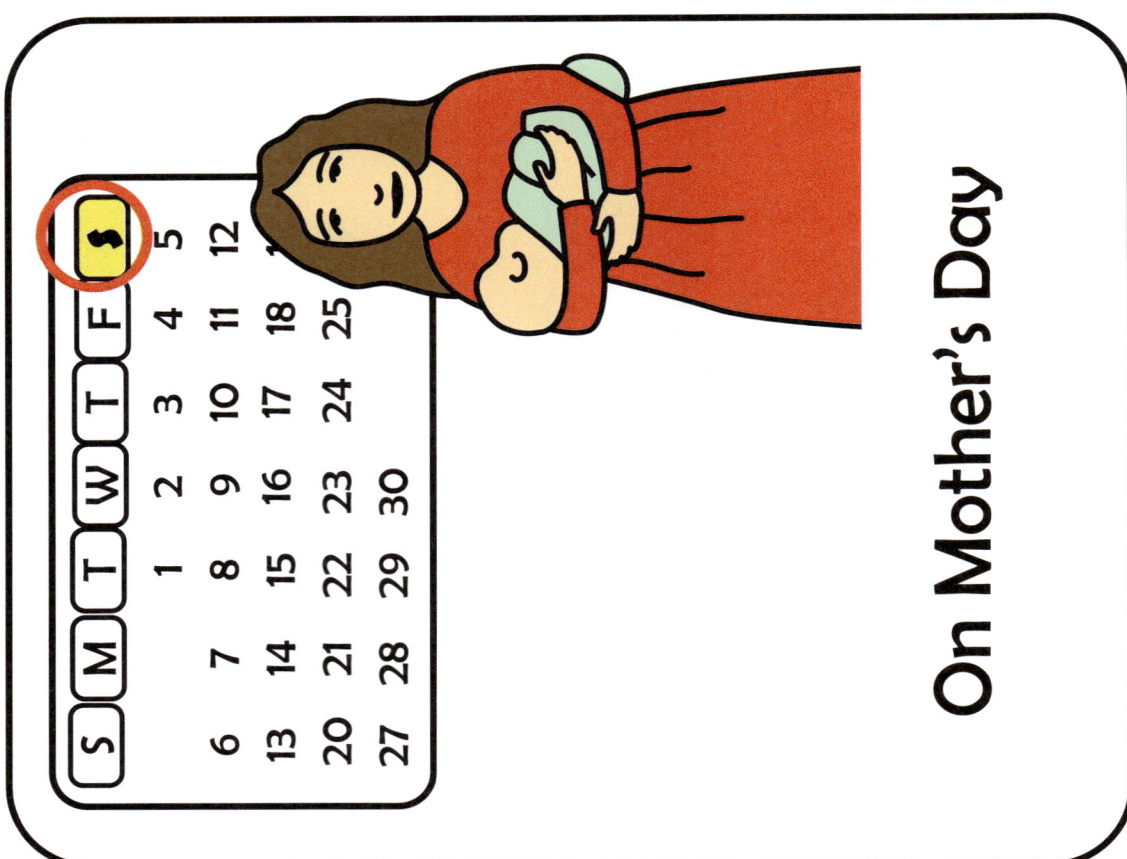

On Mother's Day

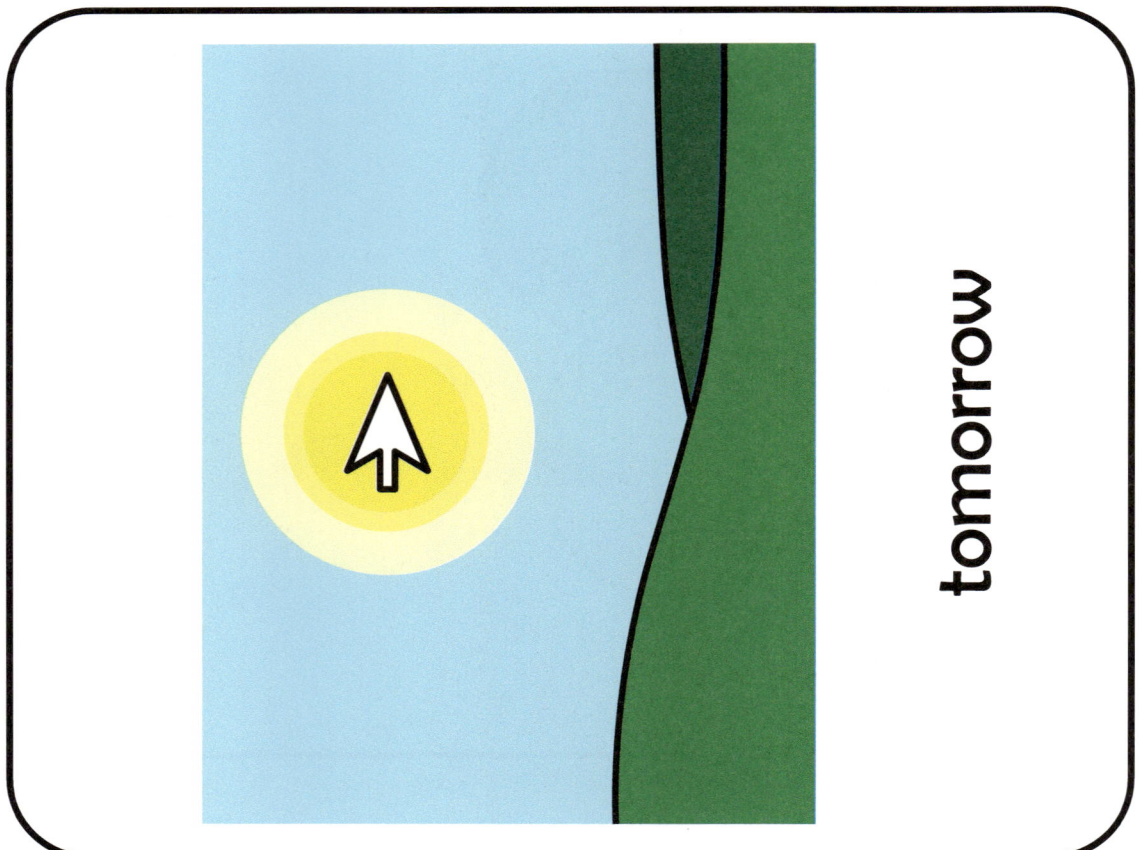

tomorrow

Copyright material from NHS Forth Valley (2020), *Colourful Semantics*, Routledge

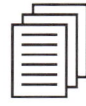

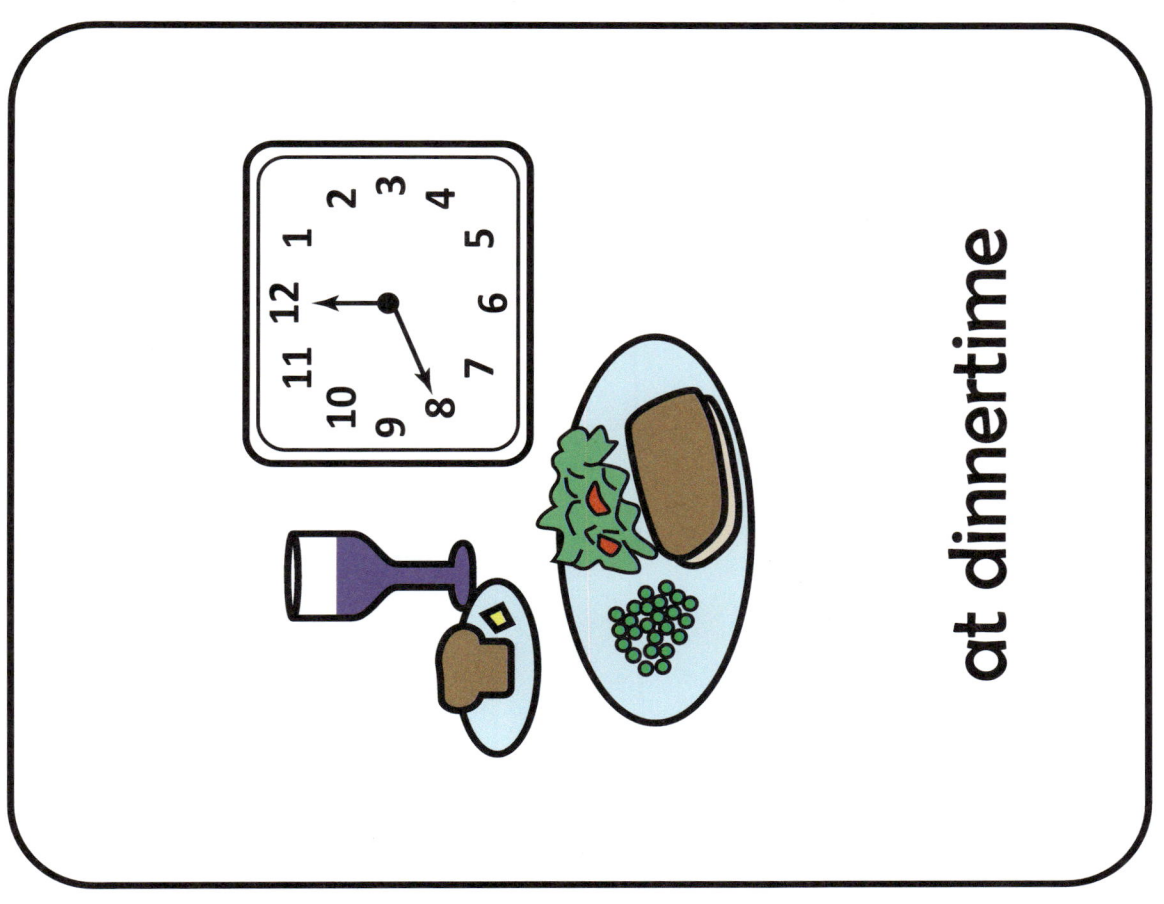

at dinnertime

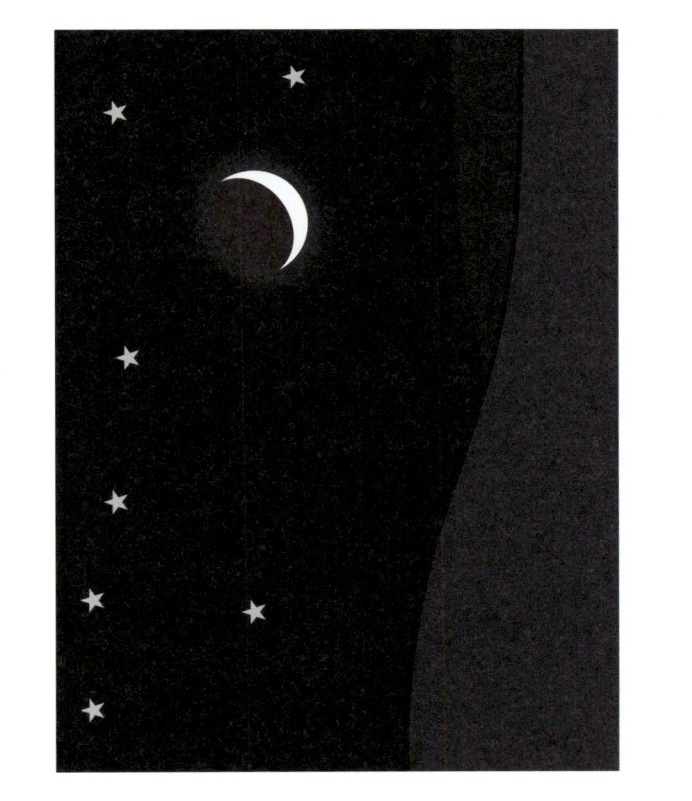

at night time

Copyright material from NHS Forth Valley (2020), *Colourful Semantics*, Routledge

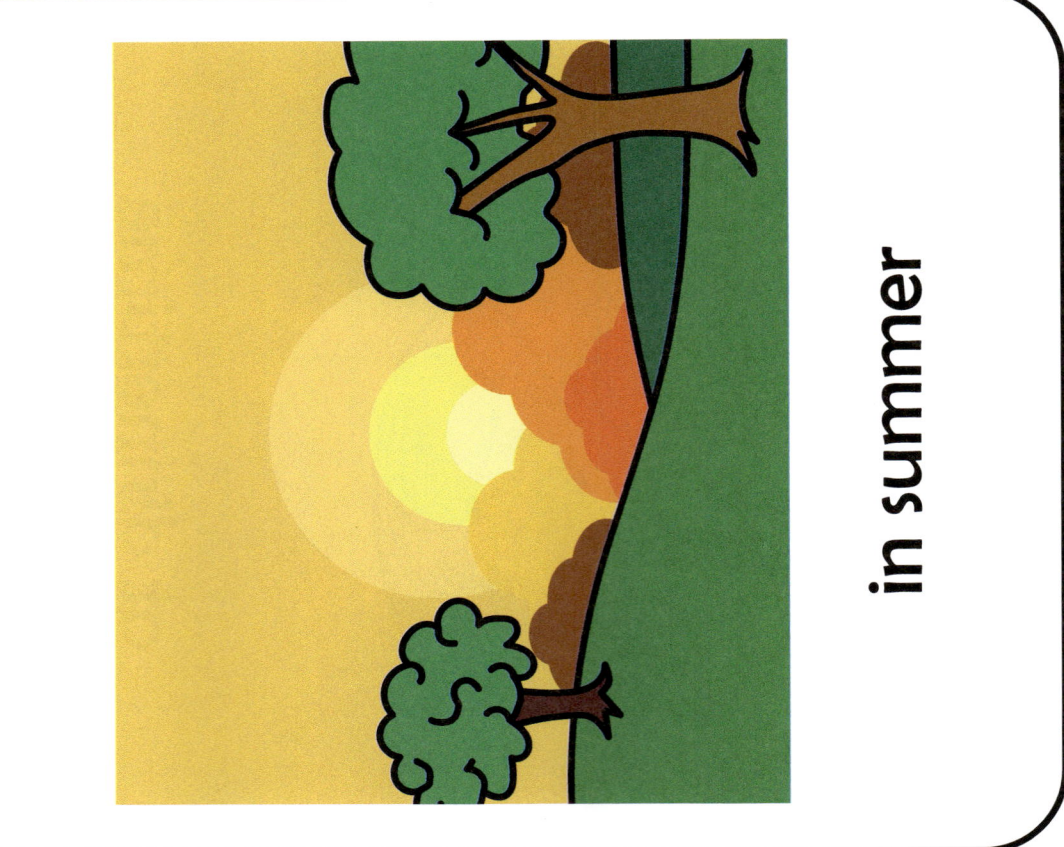

in summer

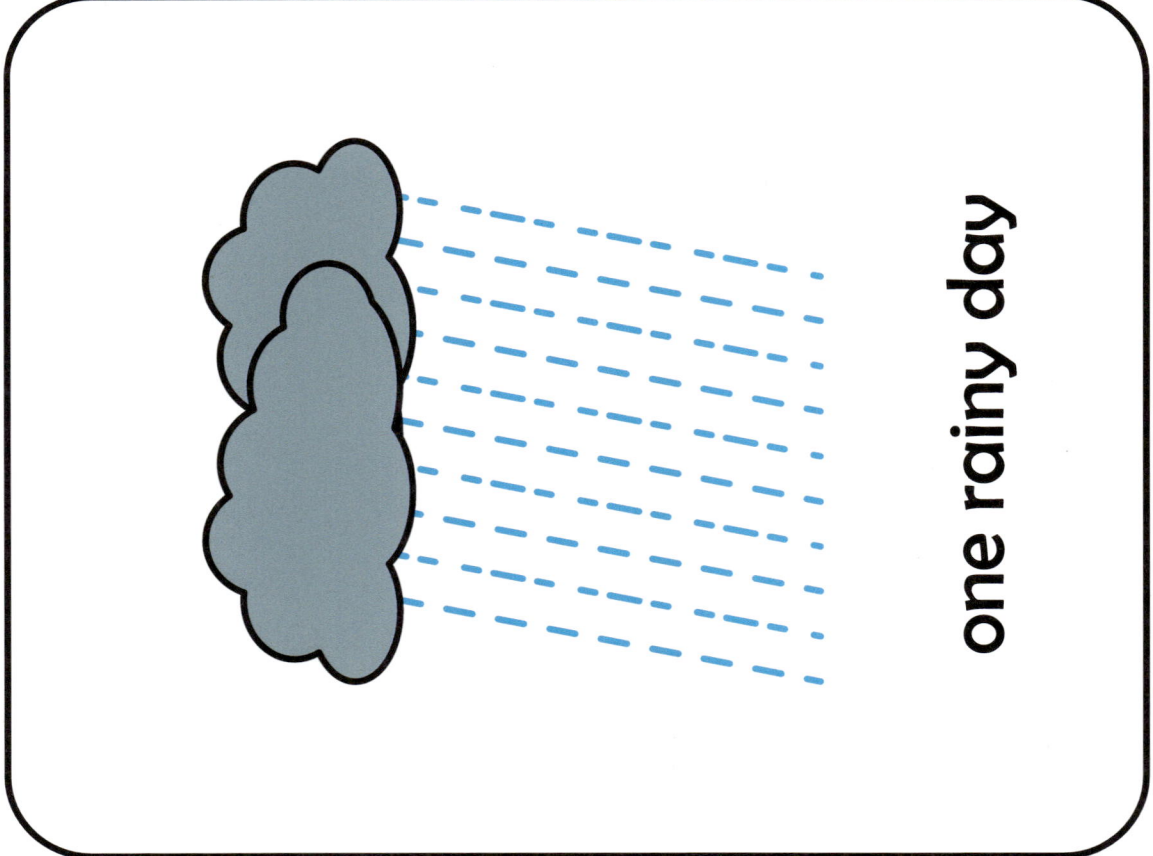

one rainy day

Copyright material from NHS Forth Valley (2020), *Colourful Semantics*, Routledge

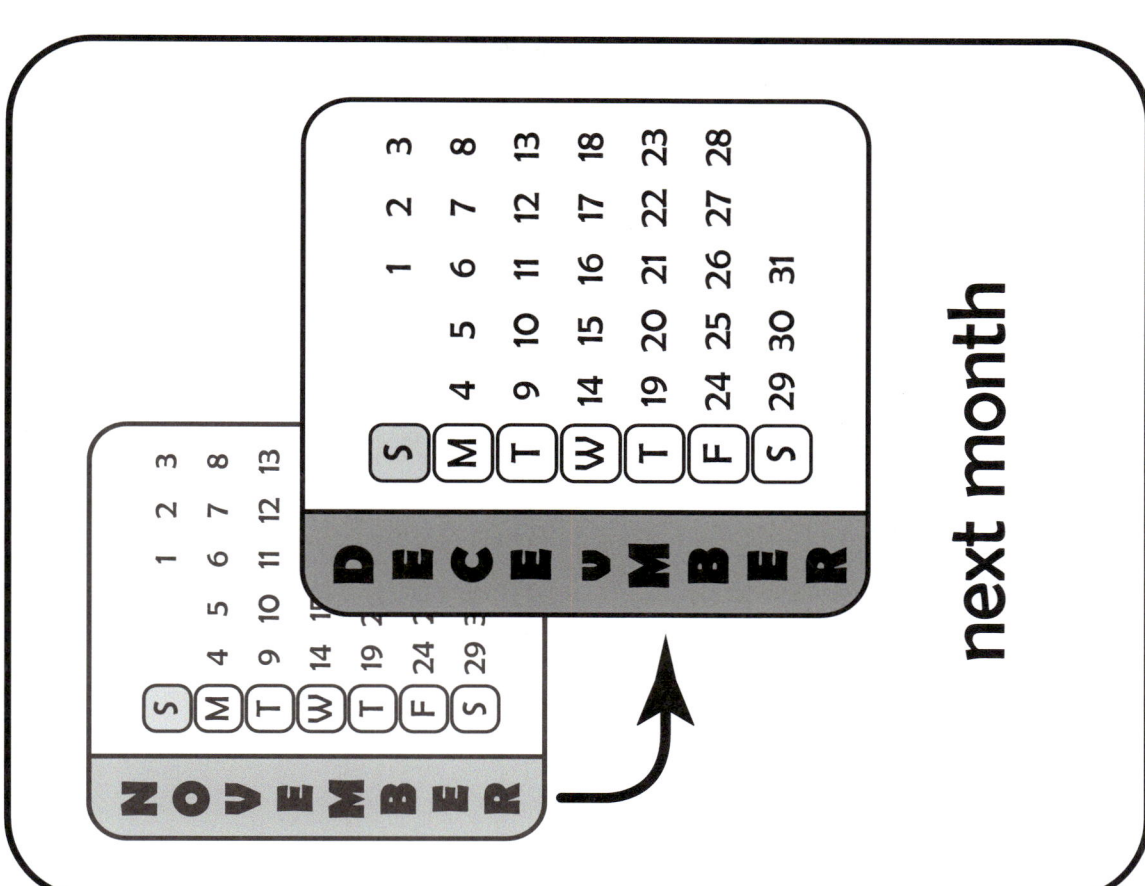

next month

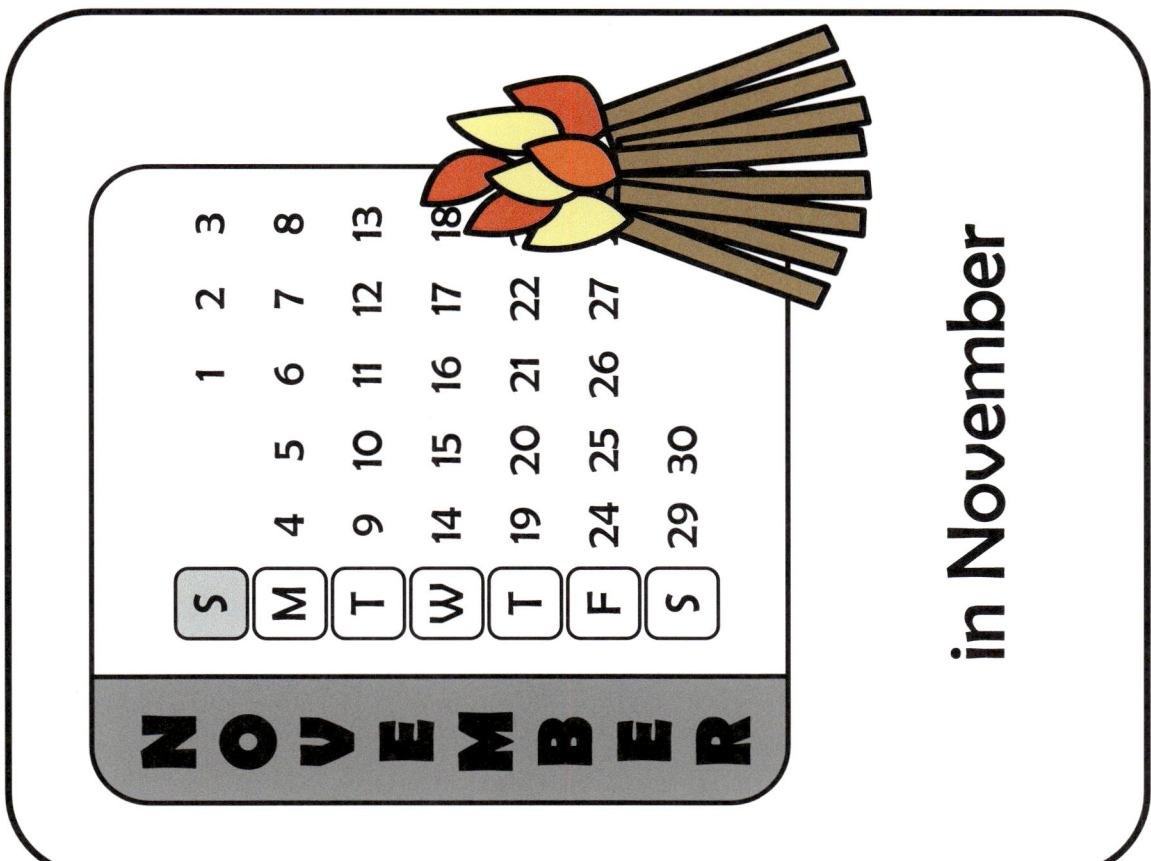

in November

Copyright material from NHS Forth Valley (2020), *Colourful Semantics*, Routledge

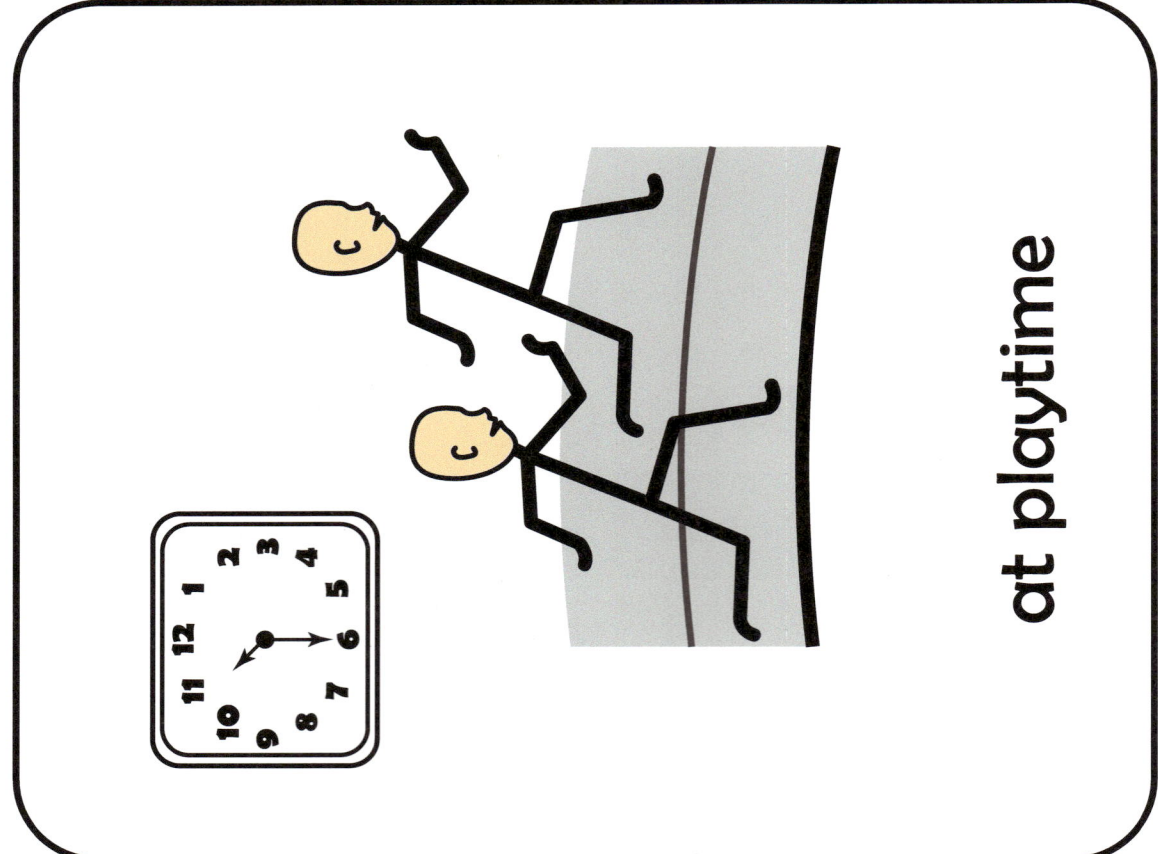

at playtime

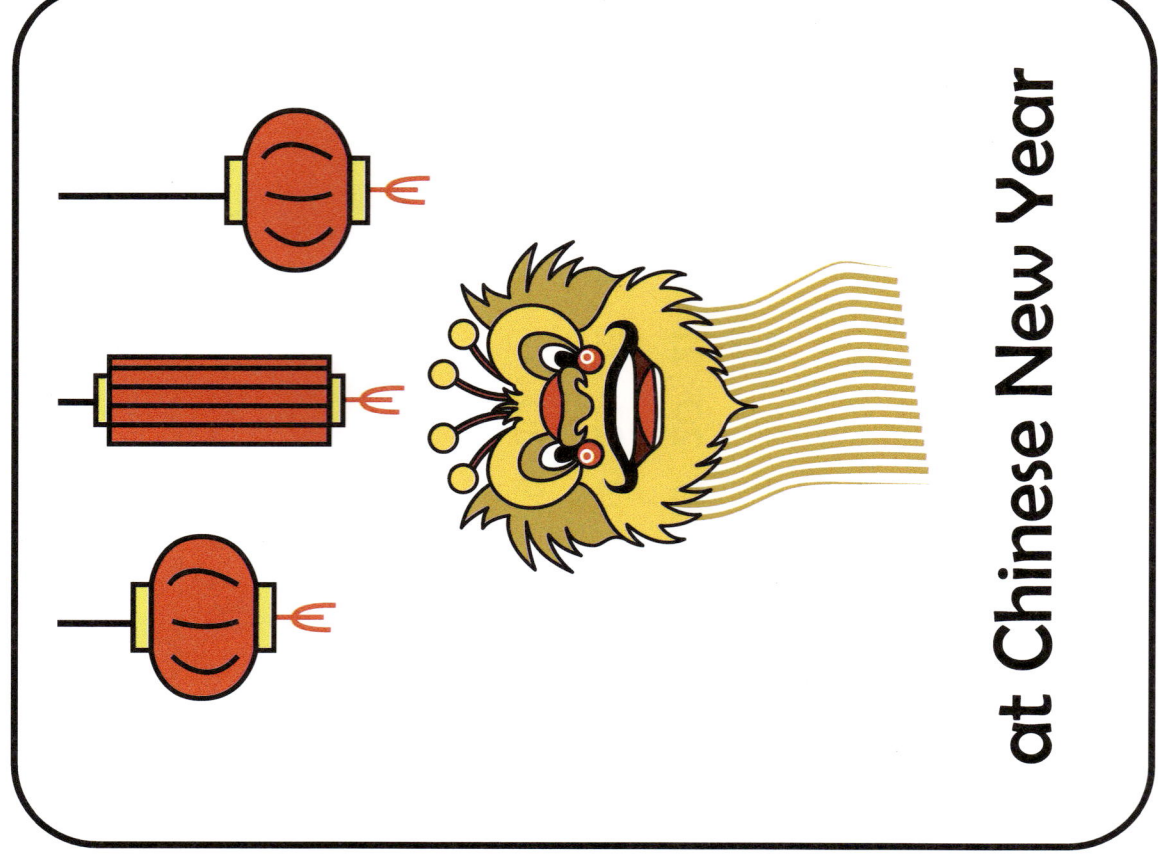

at Chinese New Year

Copyright material from NHS Forth Valley (2020), *Colourful Semantics*, Routledge

Appendix 5
Small vocabulary cards

Copyright material from NHS Forth Valley (2020), *Colourful Semantics*, Routledge

'Who' vocabulary
General people and family

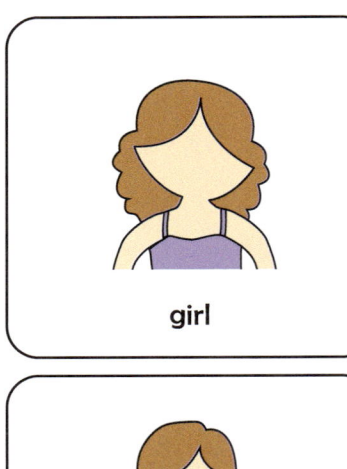

girl

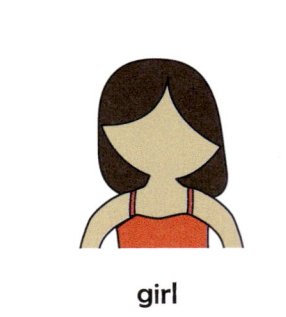

girl

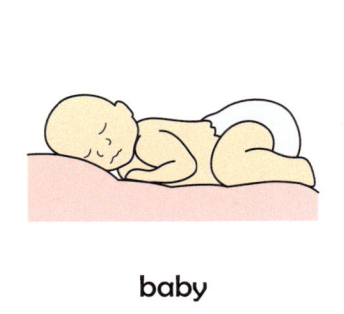

baby

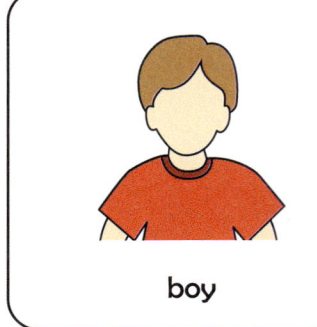

boy

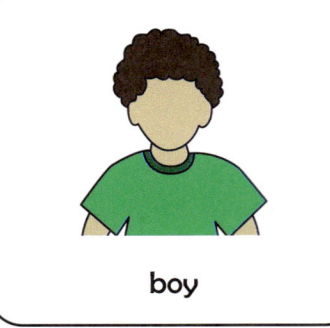

boy

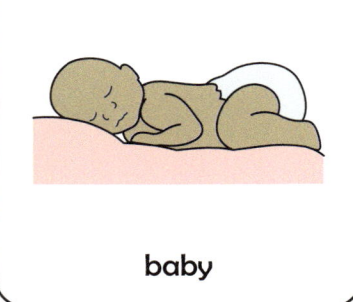

baby

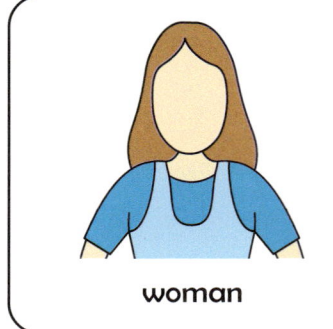

woman

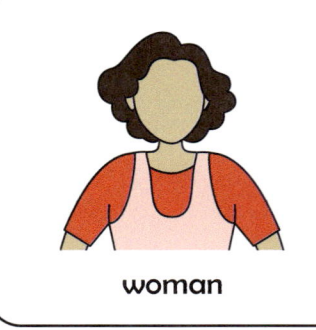

woman

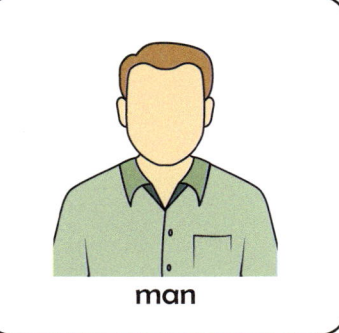

man

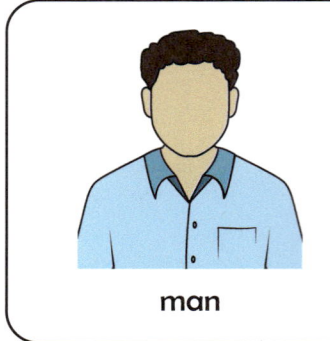

man

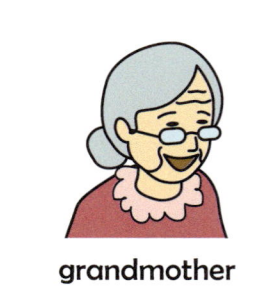

grandmother

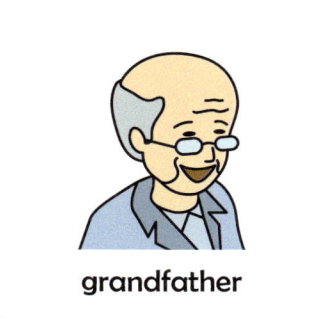

grandfather

Copyright material from NHS Forth Valley (2020), *Colourful Semantics*, Routledge

Family and occupations

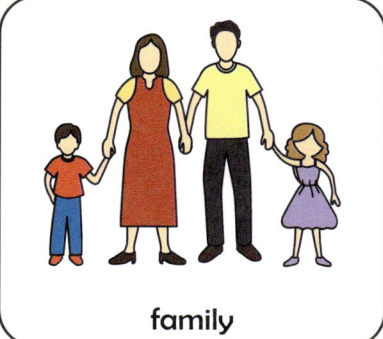
family

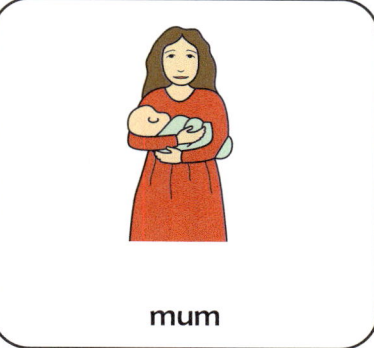
mum

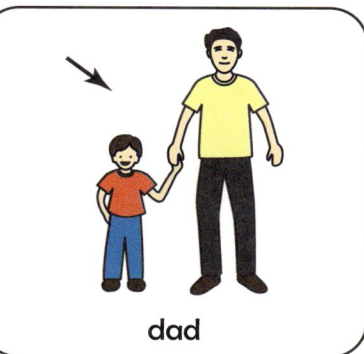
dad

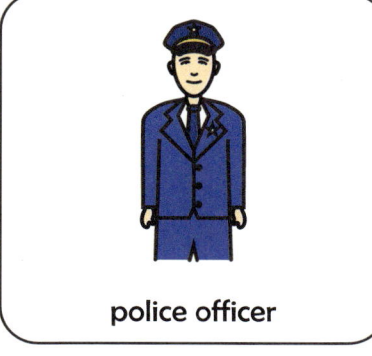
police officer

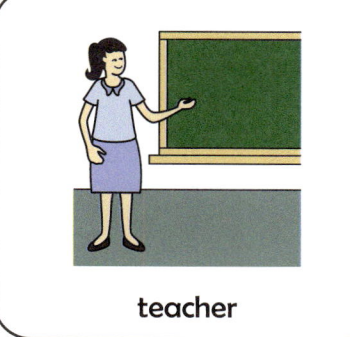
teacher

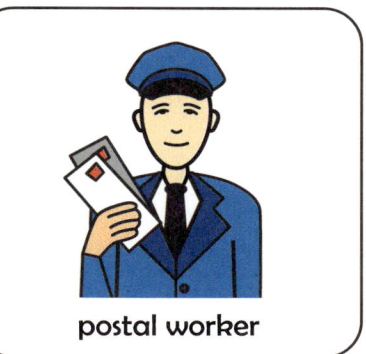
postal worker

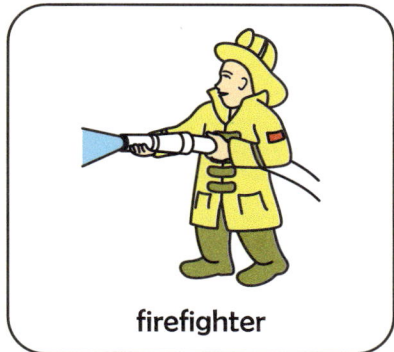
firefighter

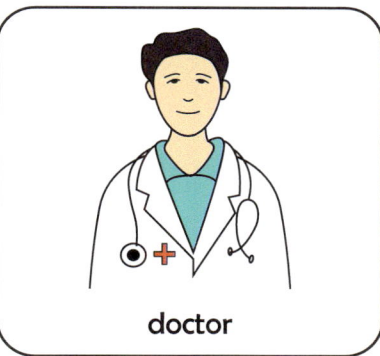
doctor

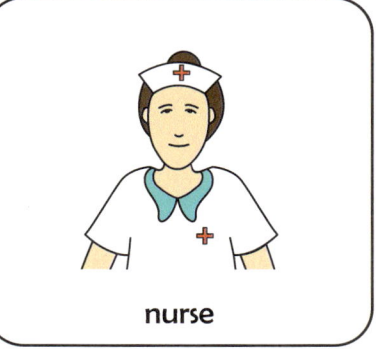
nurse

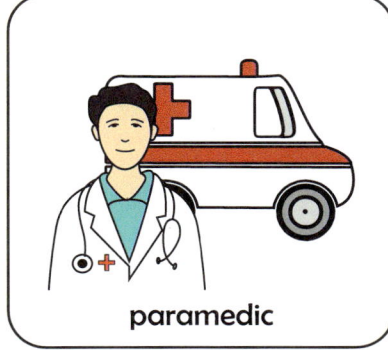
paramedic

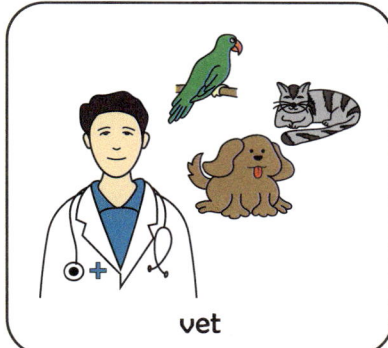
vet

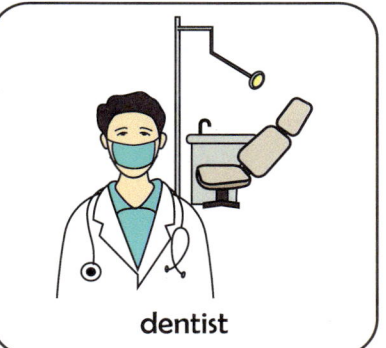
dentist

Copyright material from NHS Forth Valley (2020), *Colourful Semantics*, Routledge

Occupations

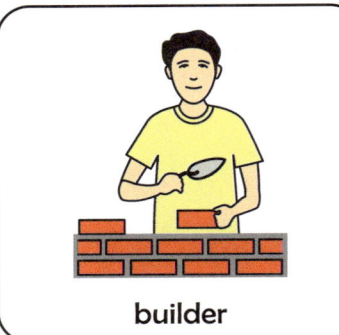

builder

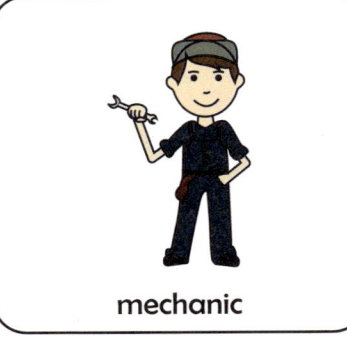

mechanic

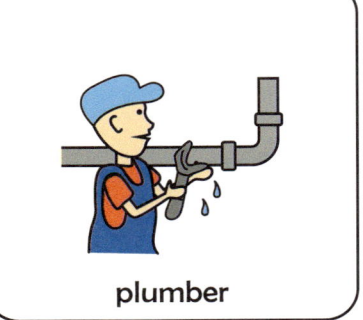

plumber

painter

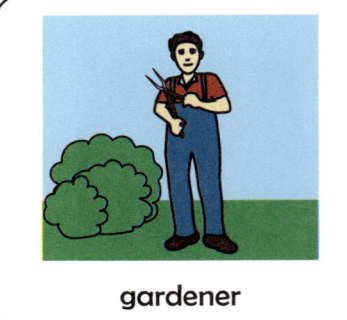

gardener

cleaner

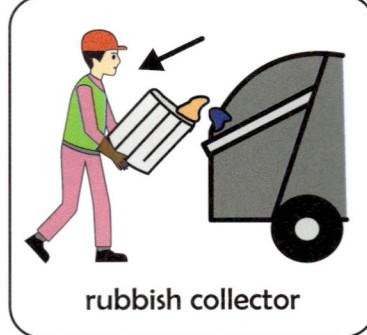

rubbish collector

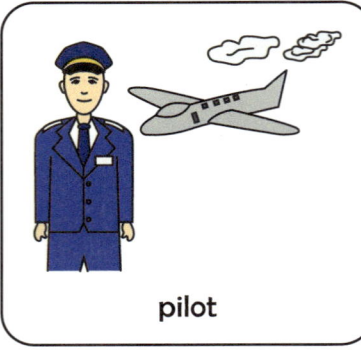

pilot

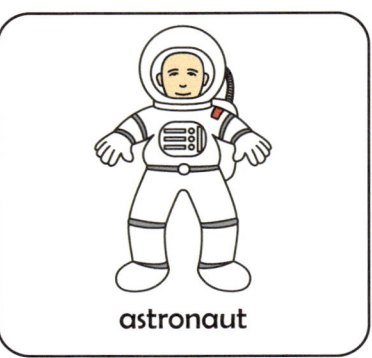

astronaut

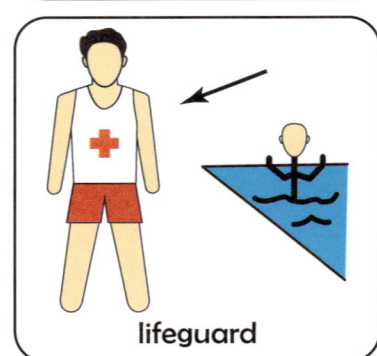

lifeguard

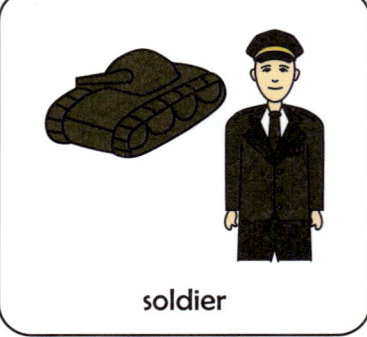

soldier

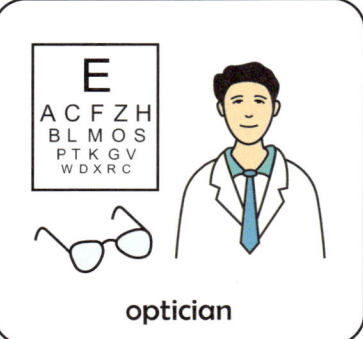

optician

Copyright material from NHS Forth Valley (2020), *Colourful Semantics*, Routledge

Additional occupations

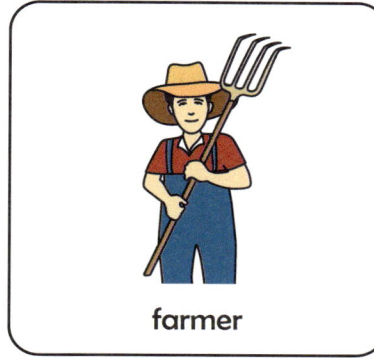

farmer

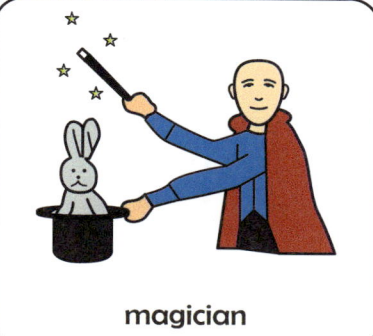

magician

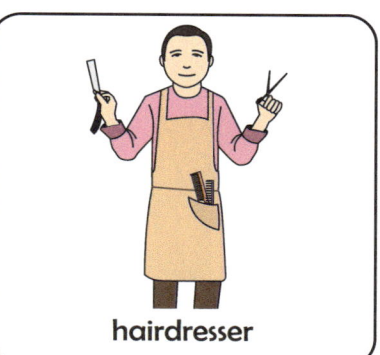

hairdresser

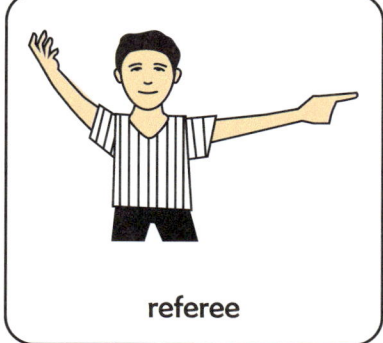

referee

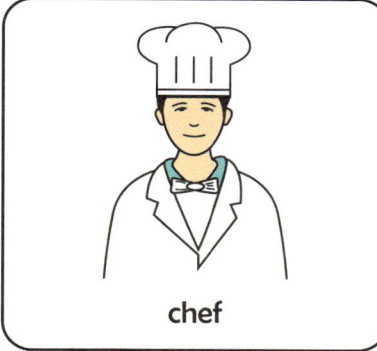

chef

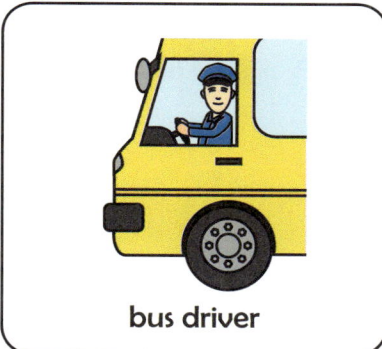

bus driver

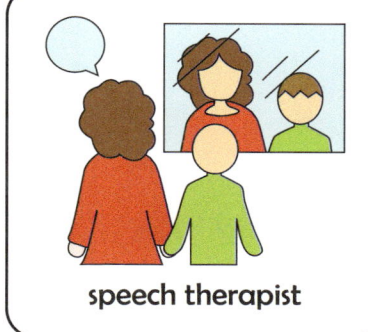

speech therapist

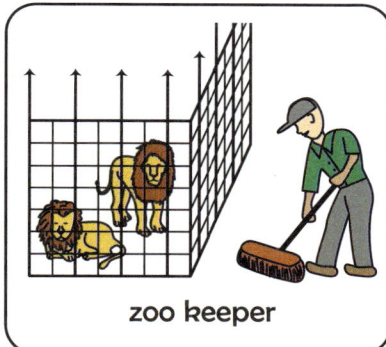

zoo keeper

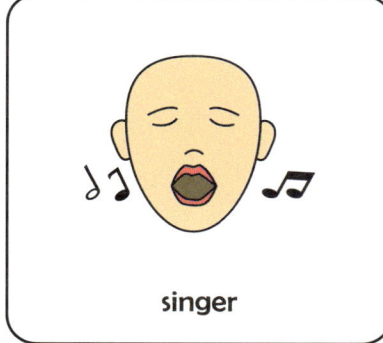

singer

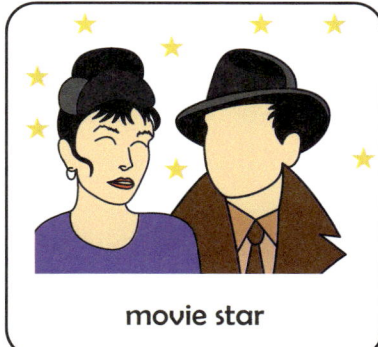

movie star

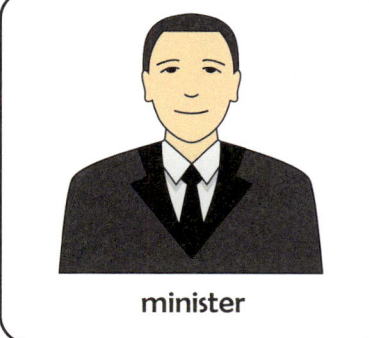

minister

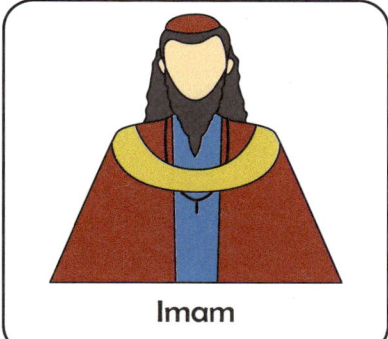

Imam

Copyright material from NHS Forth Valley (2020), *Colourful Semantics*, Routledge

Characters

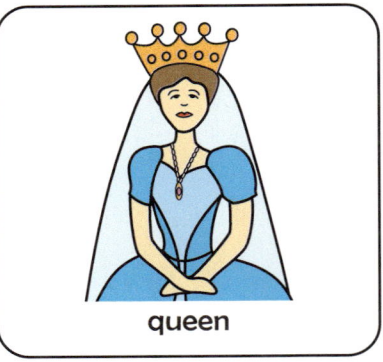
queen

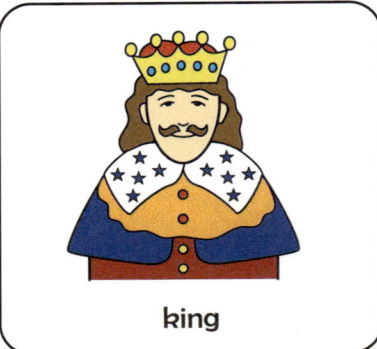
king

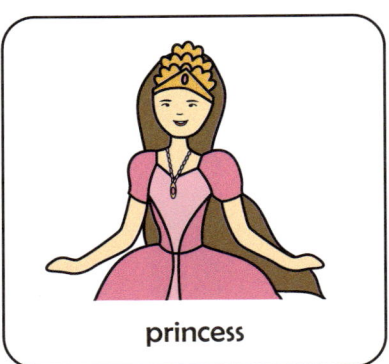
princess

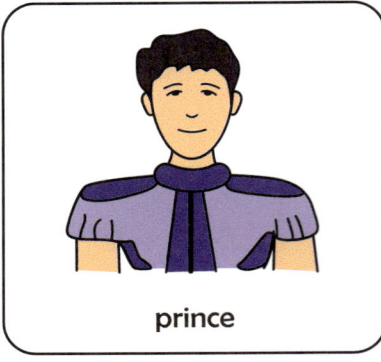
prince

clown

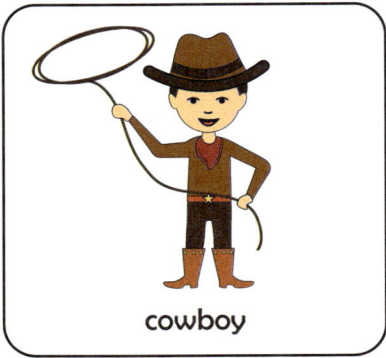
cowboy

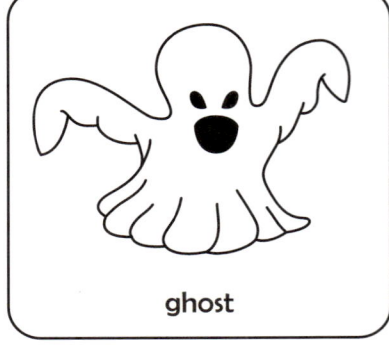
ghost

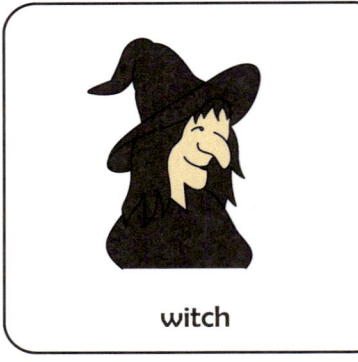
witch

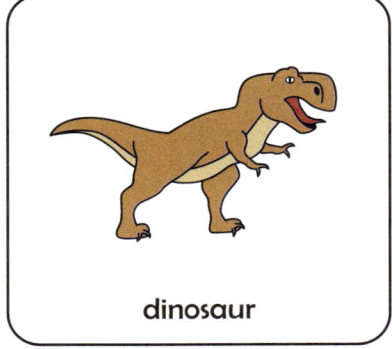
dinosaur

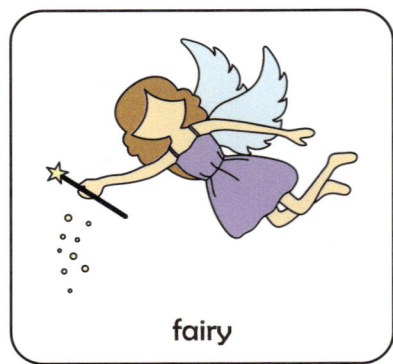
fairy

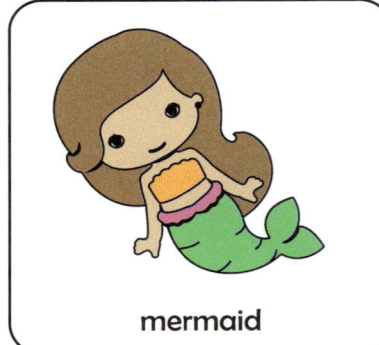
mermaid

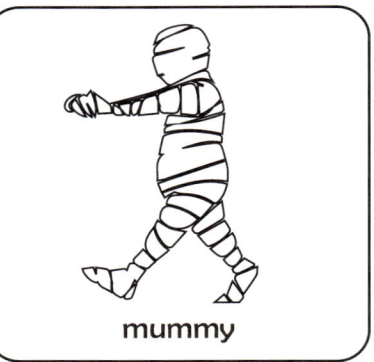
mummy

Copyright material from NHS Forth Valley (2020), *Colourful Semantics*, Routledge

Additional characters

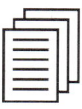

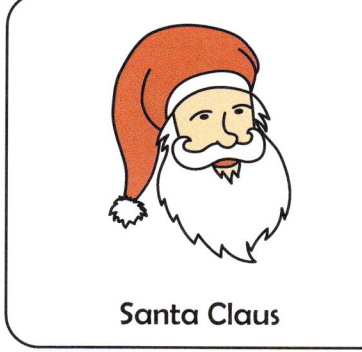	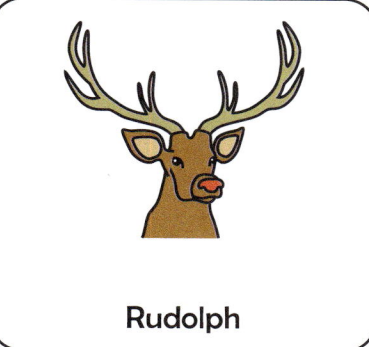	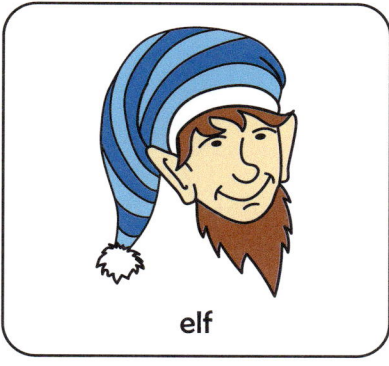
Santa Claus	Rudolph	elf
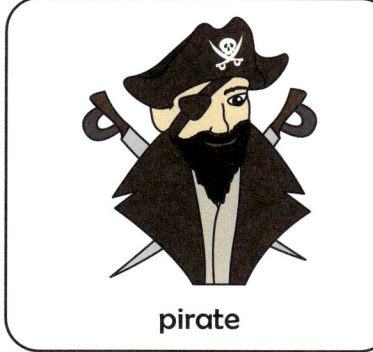	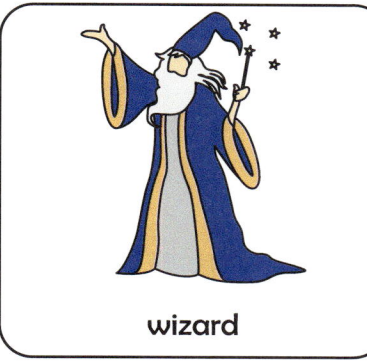	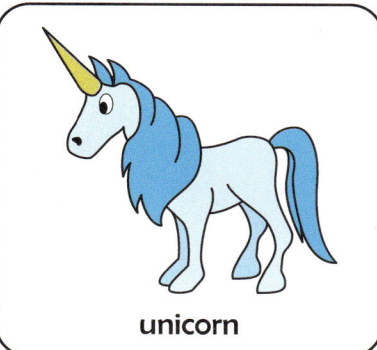
pirate	wizard	unicorn
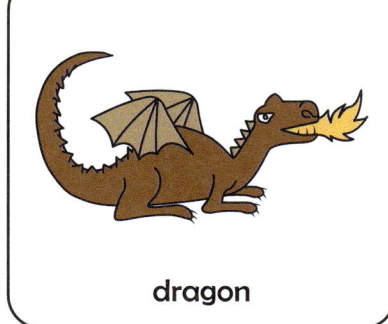	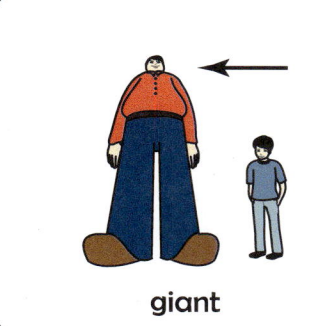	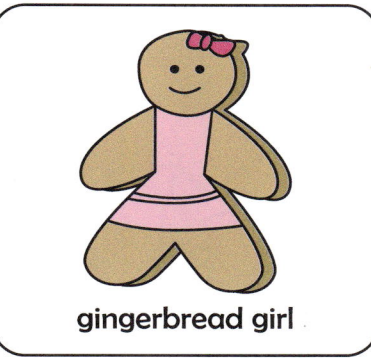
dragon	giant	gingerbread girl
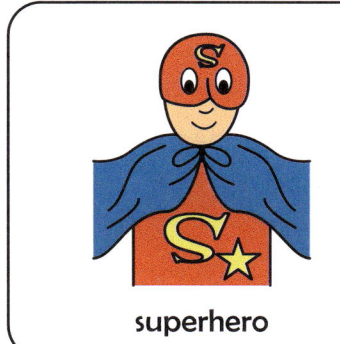	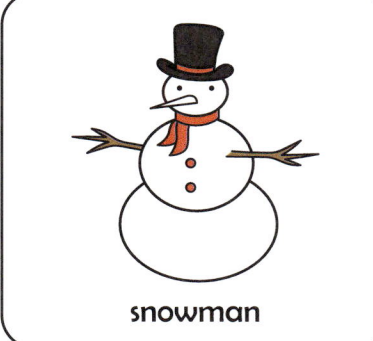	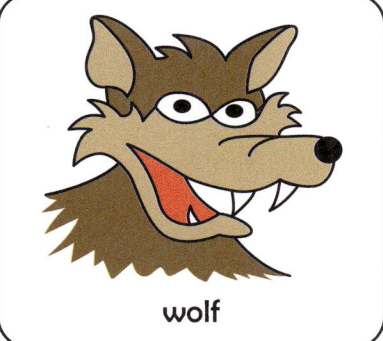
superhero	snowman	wolf

Copyright material from NHS Forth Valley (2020), *Colourful Semantics*, Routledge

'Doing' vocabulary
Early verbs

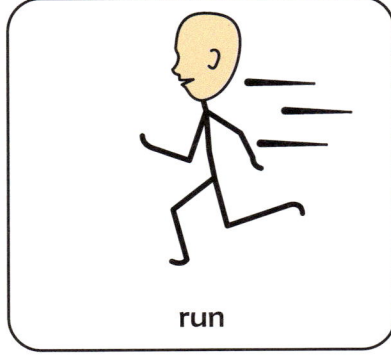

run

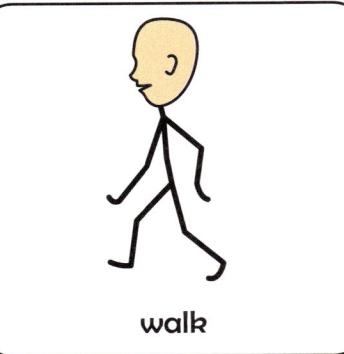

walk

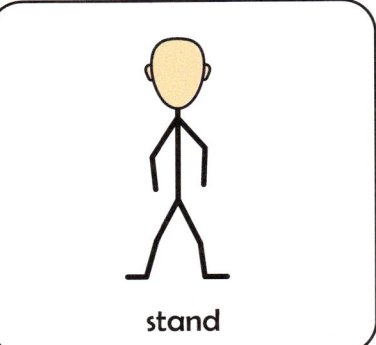

stand

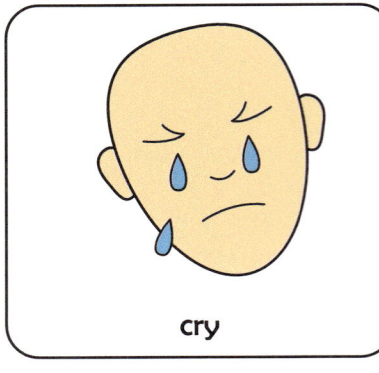

cry

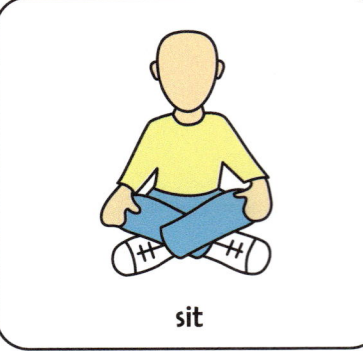

sit

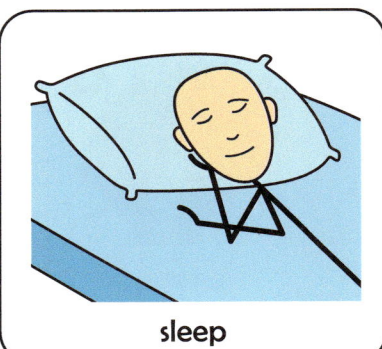

sleep

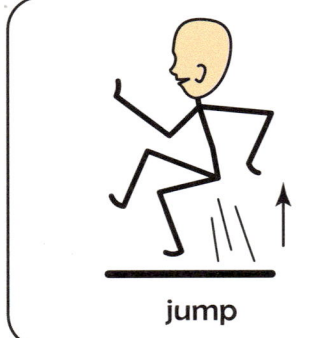

jump

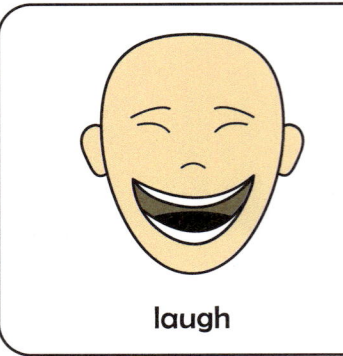

laugh

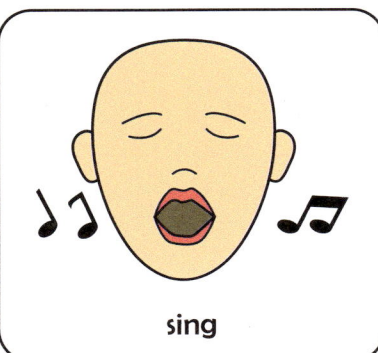

sing

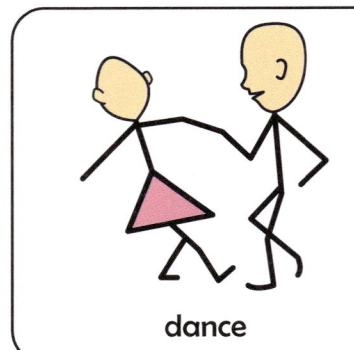

dance

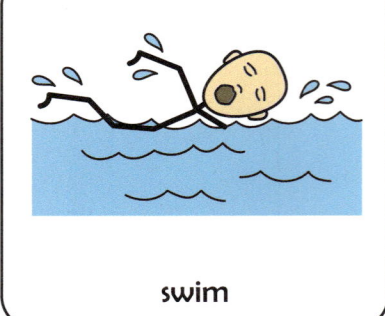

swim

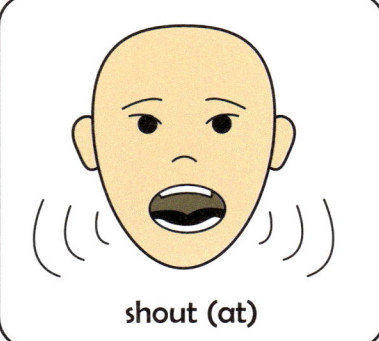

shout (at)

Copyright material from NHS Forth Valley (2020), *Colourful Semantics*, Routledge

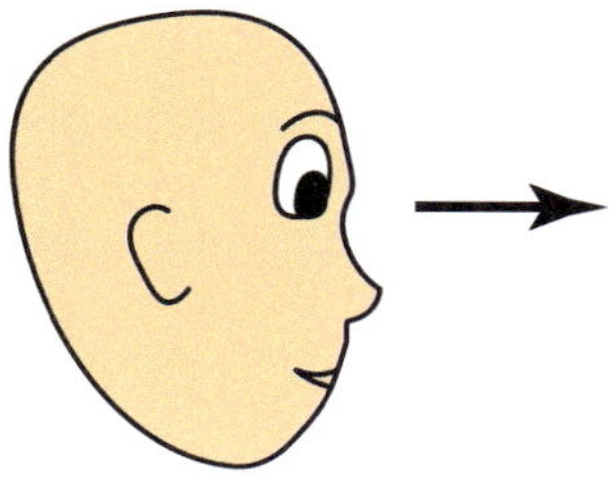

look (at)	eat	play (with)
drink	read	throw
brush	wash	kick
paint	cut	climb

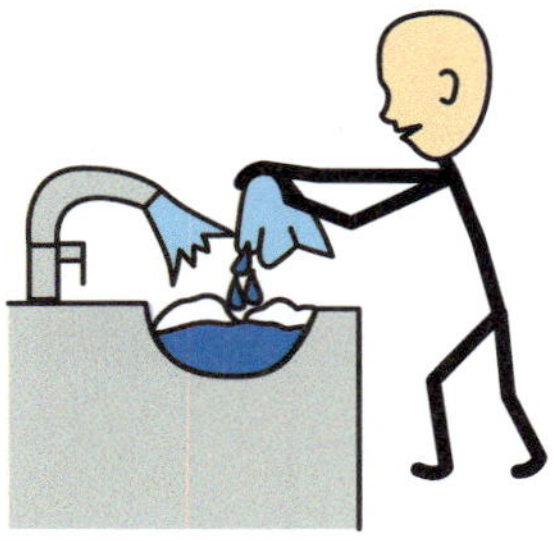

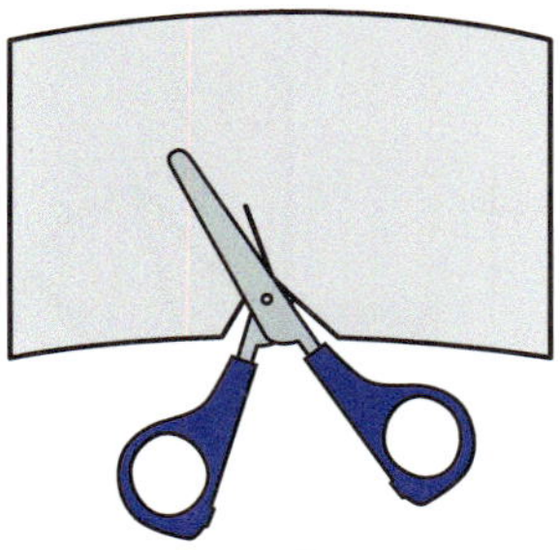

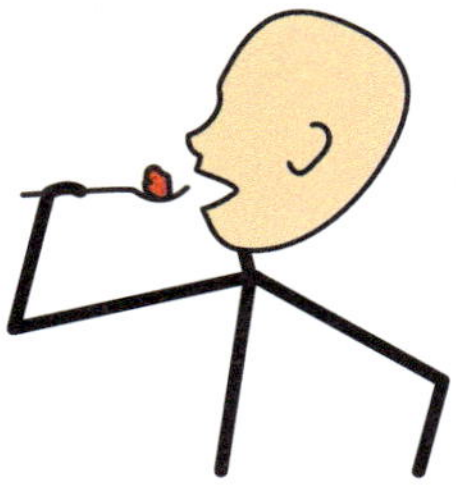

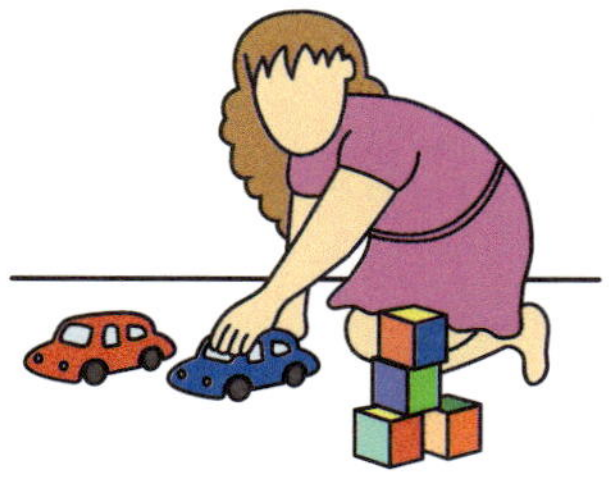

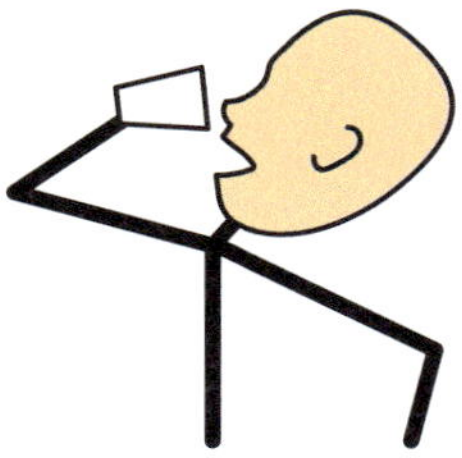

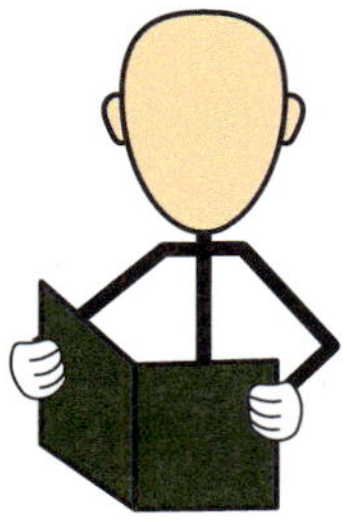

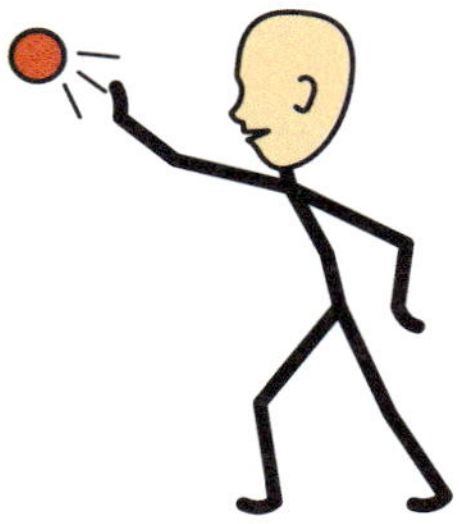

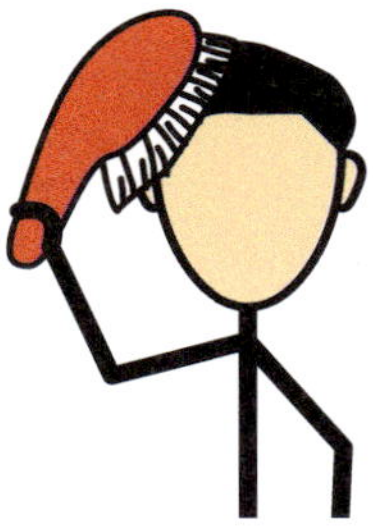

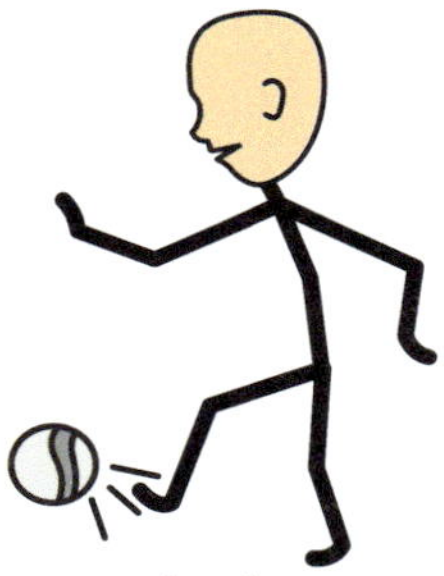

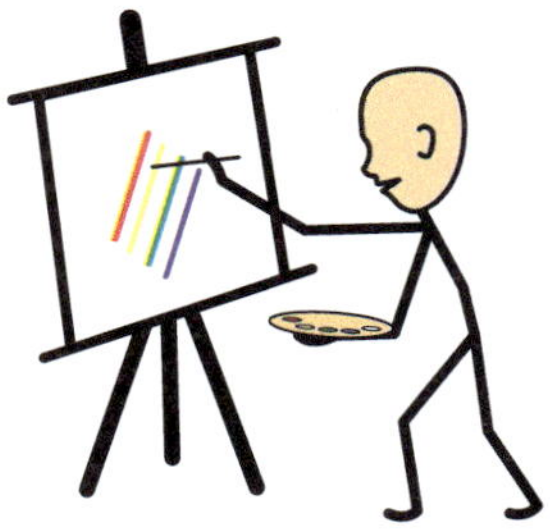

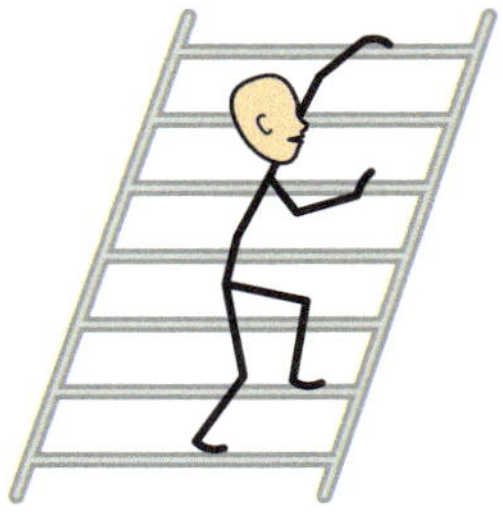

General verb selection

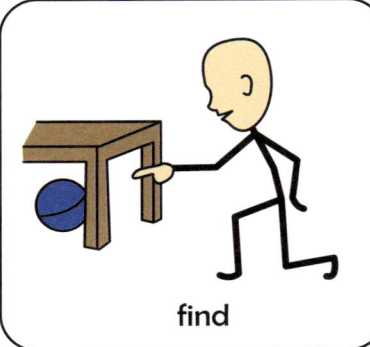

find

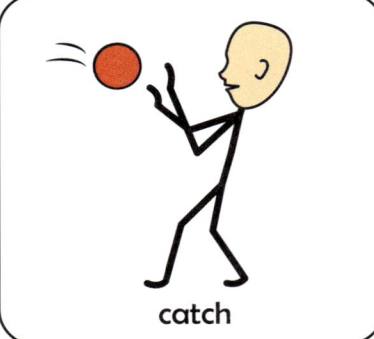

catch

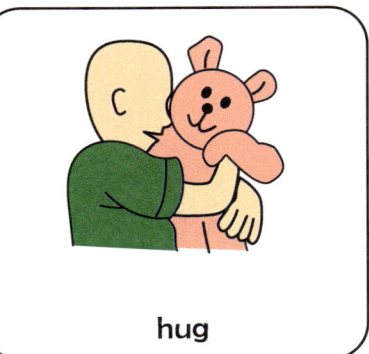

hug

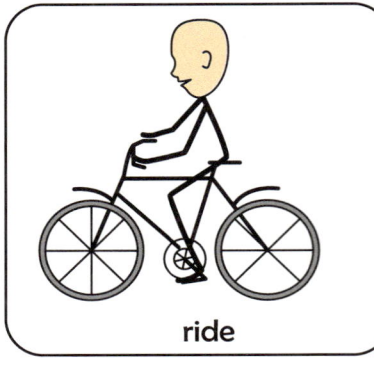

ride

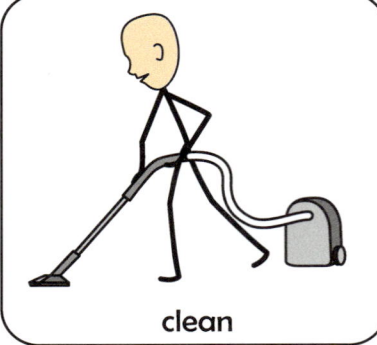

clean

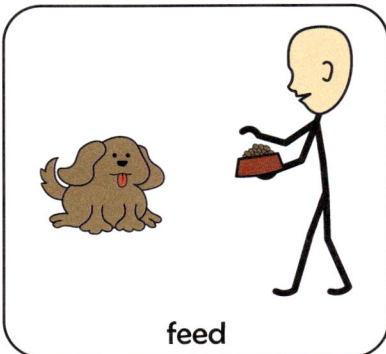

feed

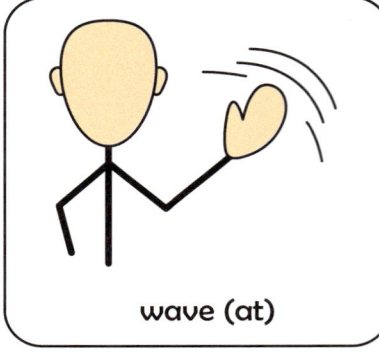

wave (at)

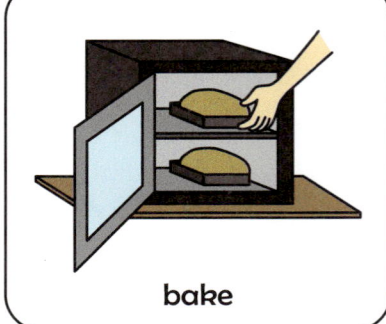

bake

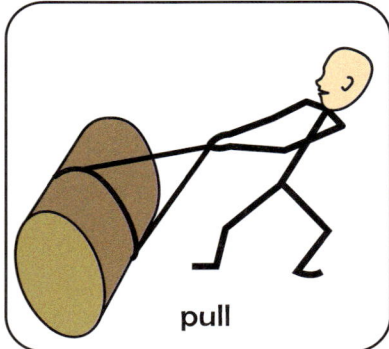

pull

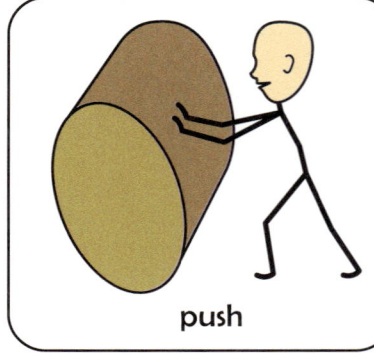

push

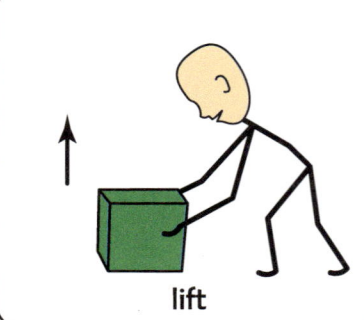

lift

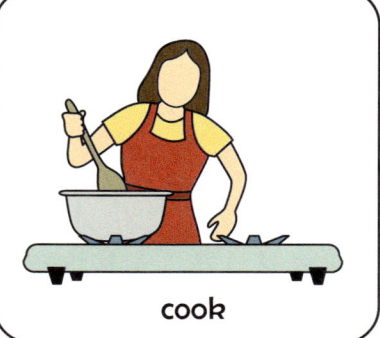

cook

Copyright material from NHS Forth Valley (2020), *Colourful Semantics*, Routledge

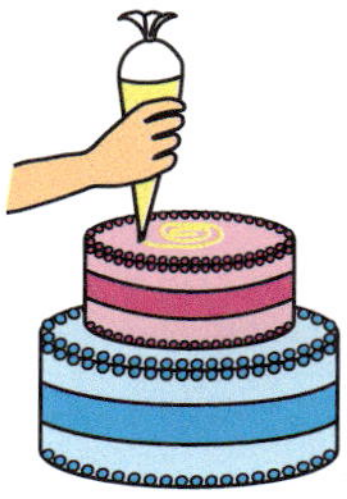

decorate	pack	drive
row	draw	choose
write	carry	build
put on	kiss	listen to

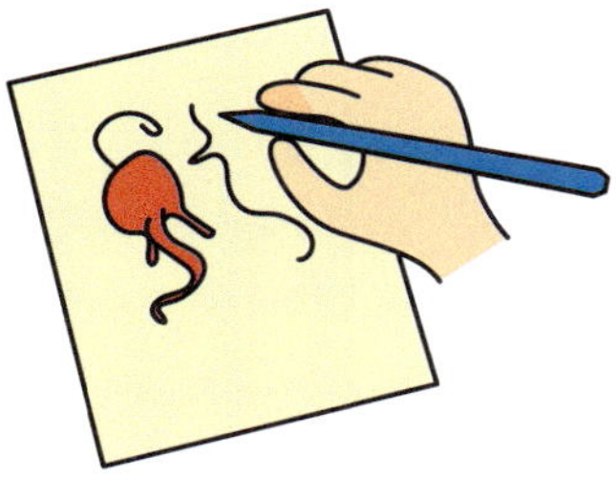

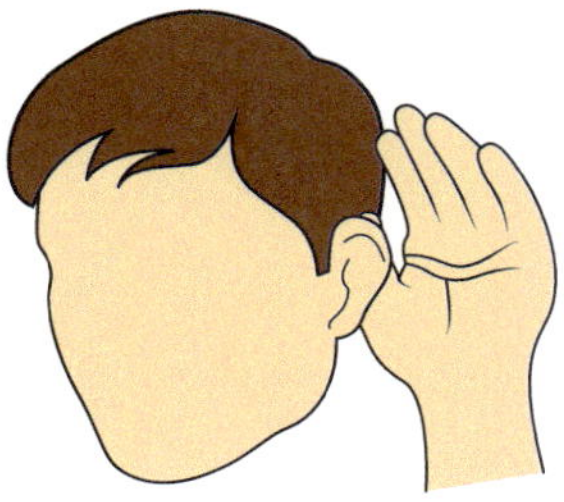

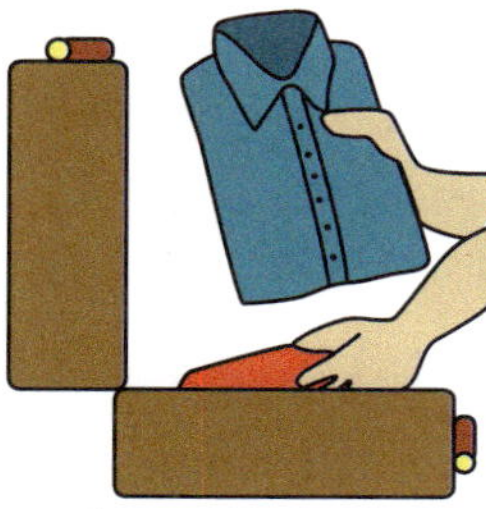

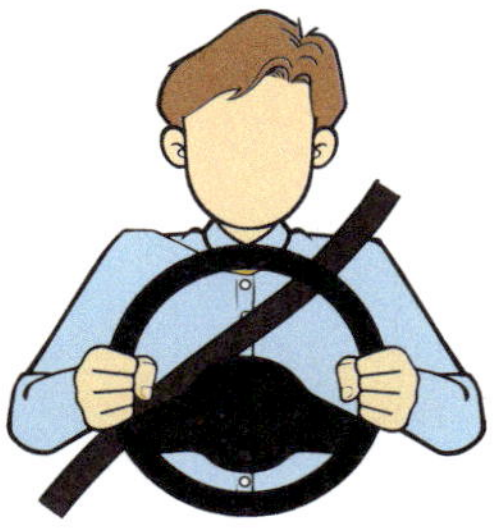

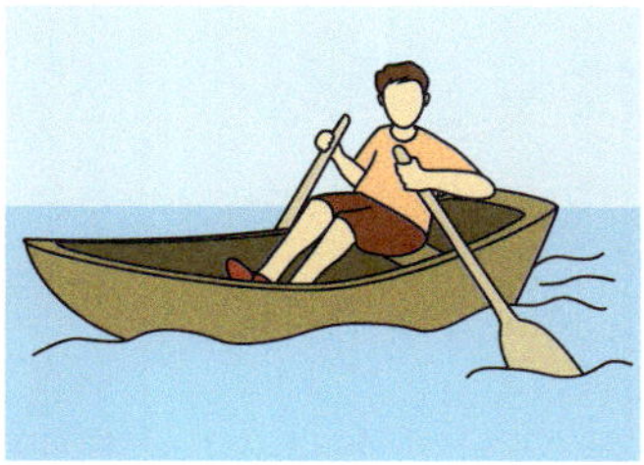

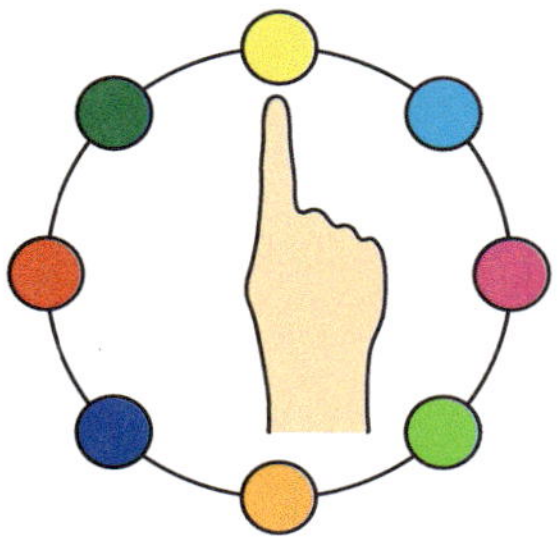

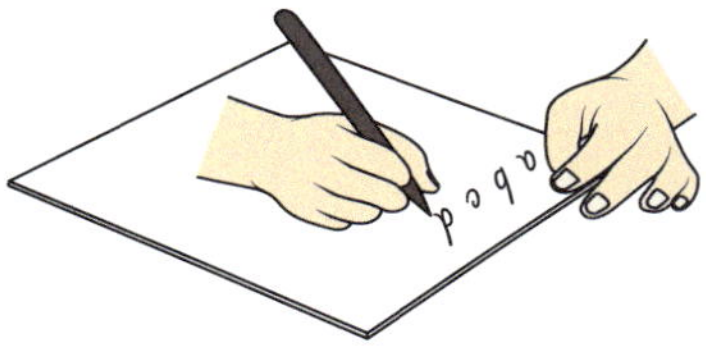

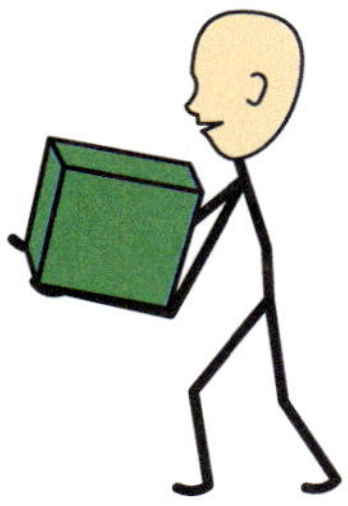

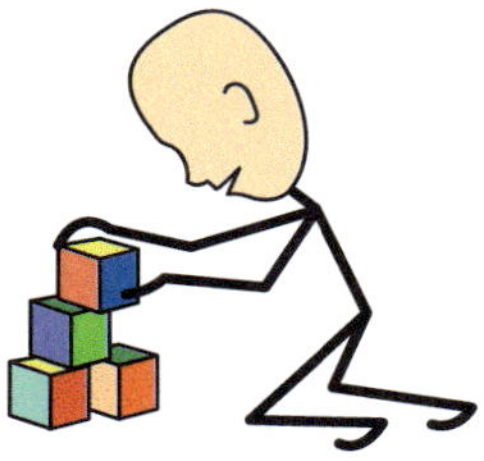

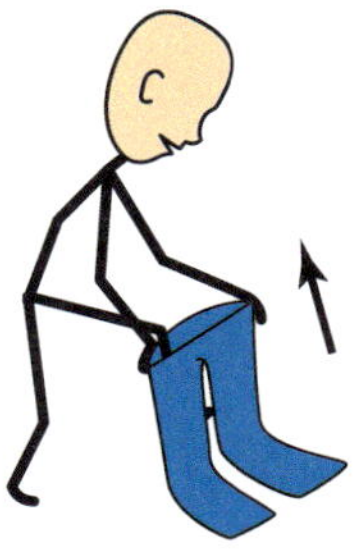

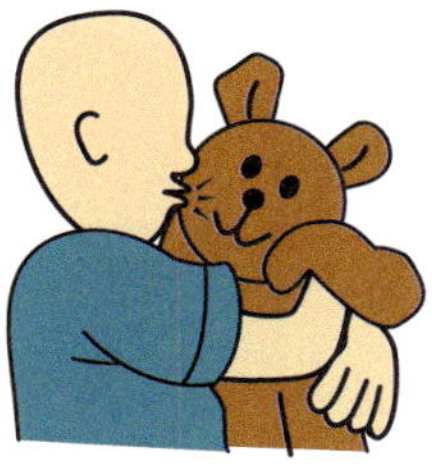

Copyright material from NHS Forth Valley (2020), *Colourful Semantics*, Routledge

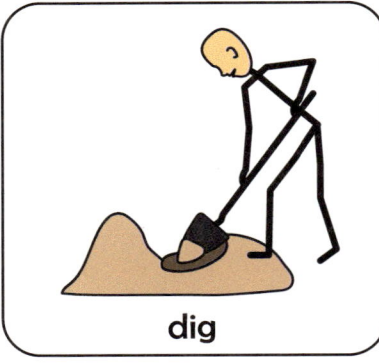

dig

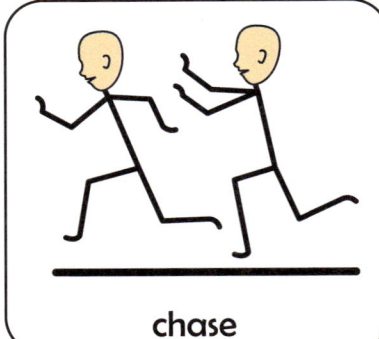

chase

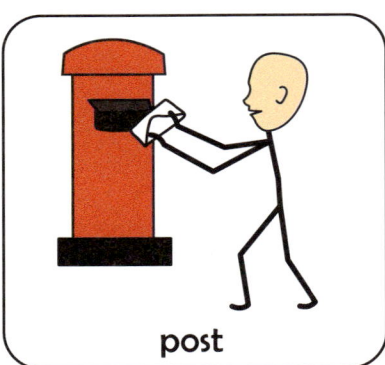

post

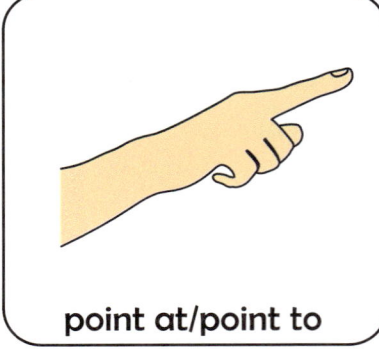

point at/point to

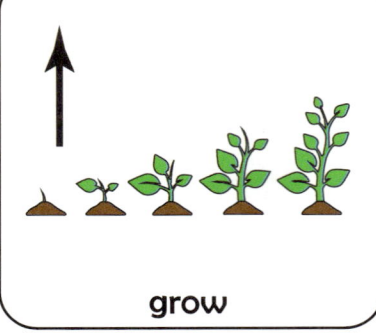

grow

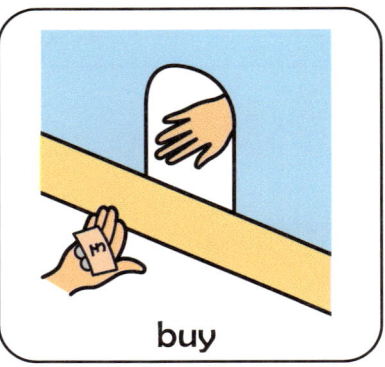

buy

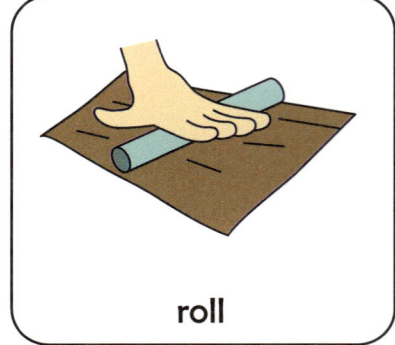

roll

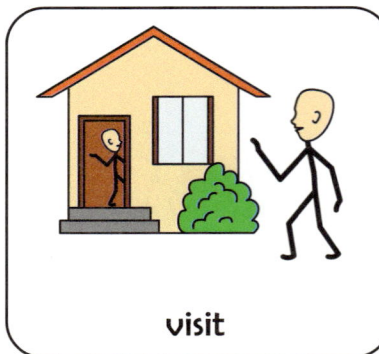

visit

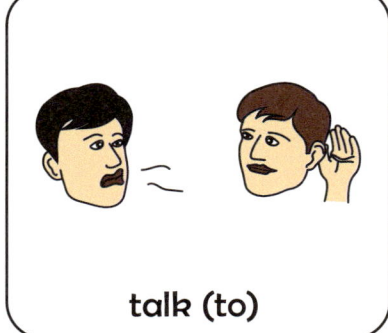

talk (to)

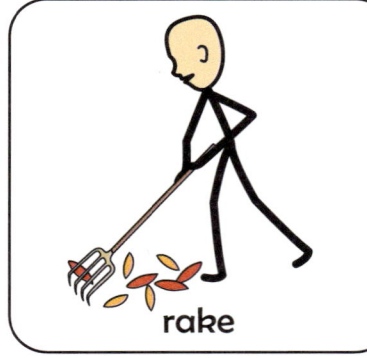

rake

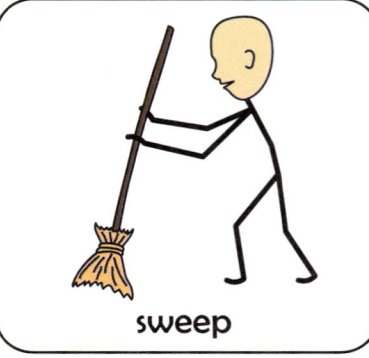

sweep

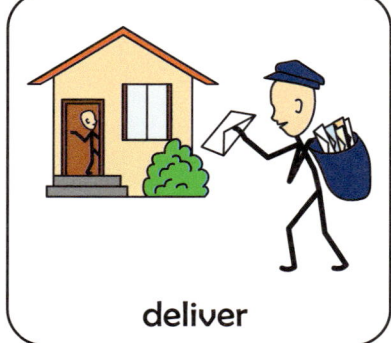

deliver

Copyright material from NHS Forth Valley (2020), *Colourful Semantics*, Routledge

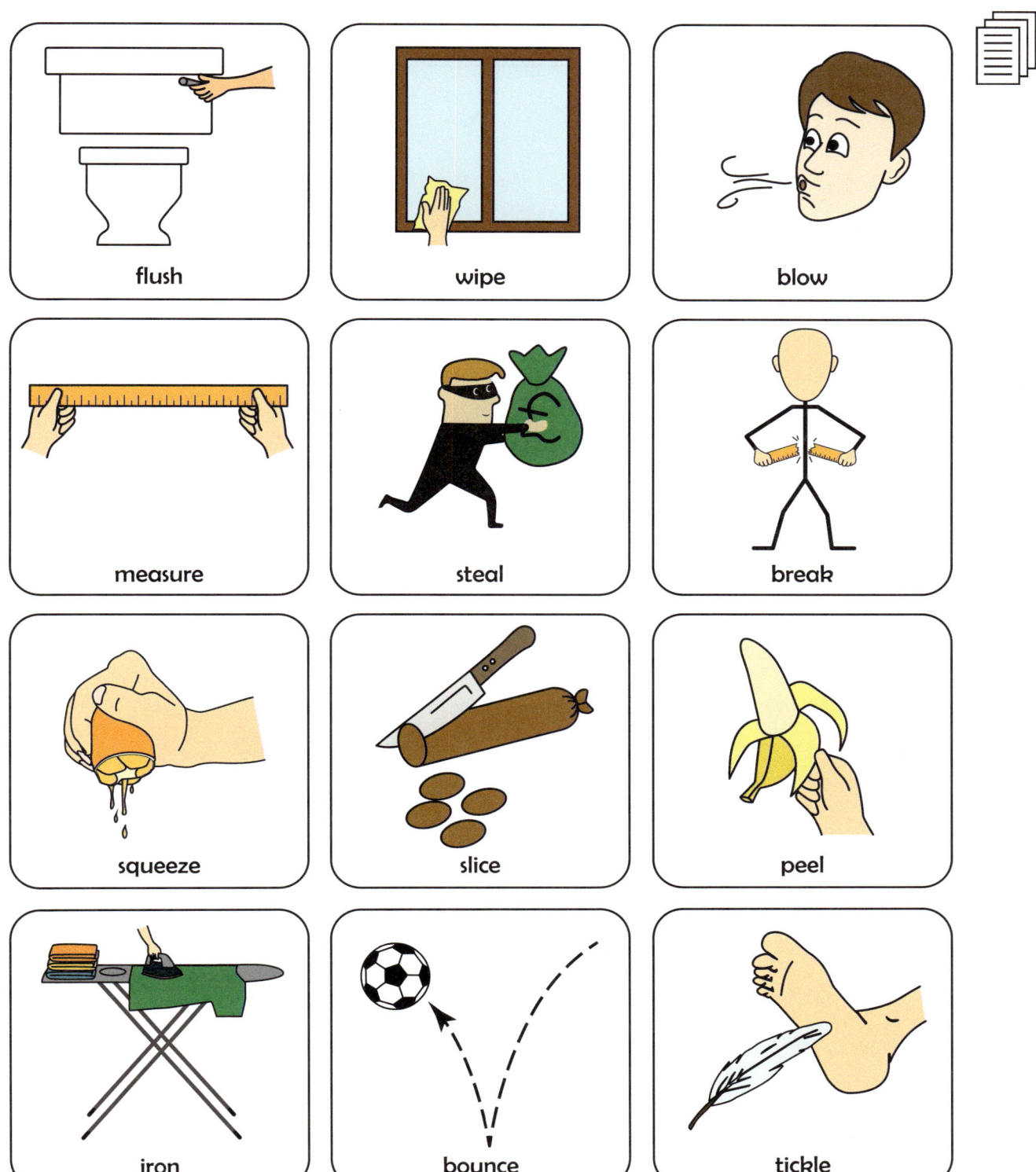

flush

wipe

blow

measure

steal

break

squeeze

slice

peel

iron

bounce

tickle

Copyright material from NHS Forth Valley (2020), *Colourful Semantics*, Routledge

'What' vocabulary

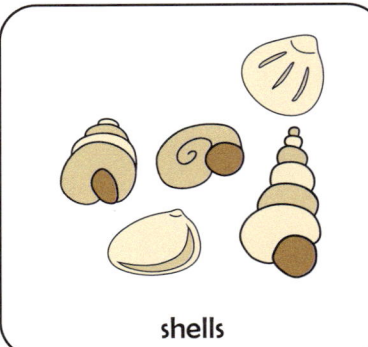

shells

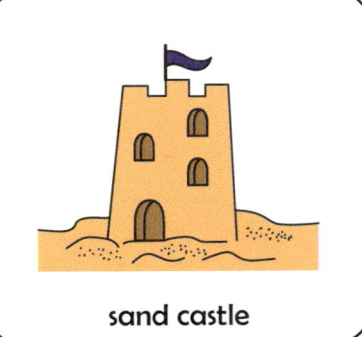

sand castle

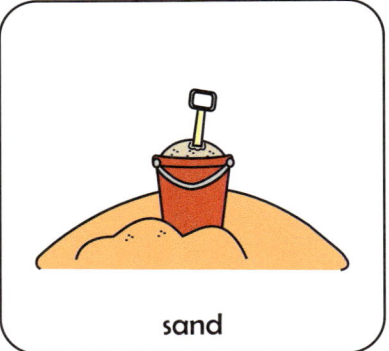

sand

hat

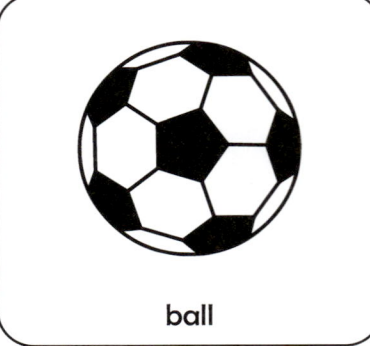

ball

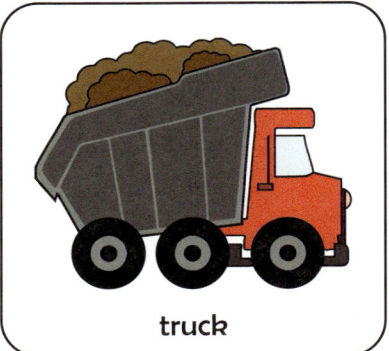

truck

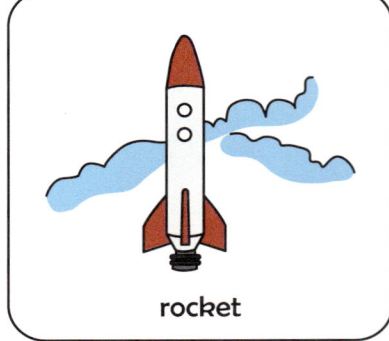

rocket

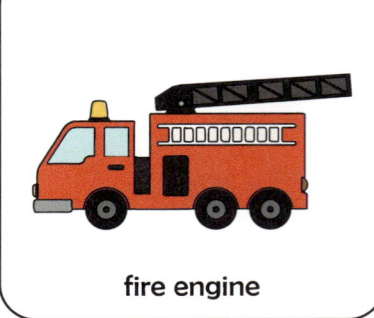

fire engine

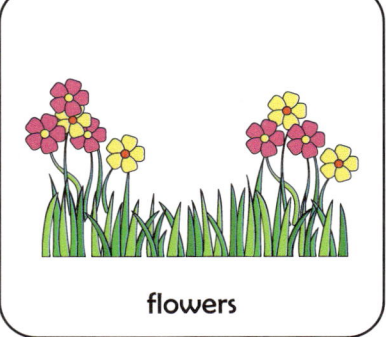

flowers

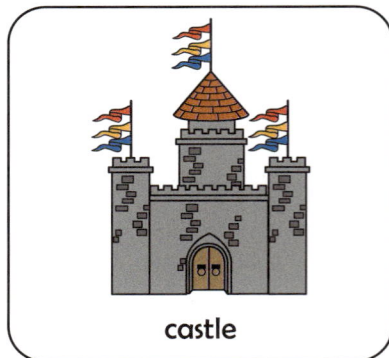

castle

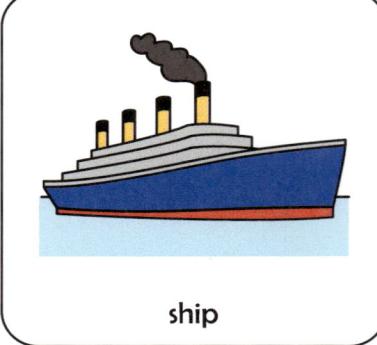

ship

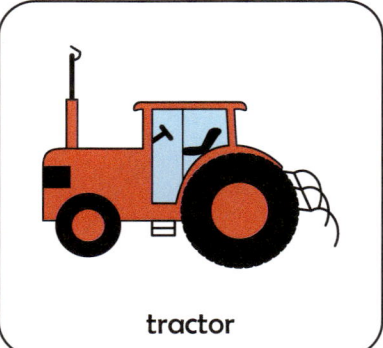

tractor

Copyright material from NHS Forth Valley (2020), *Colourful Semantics*, Routledge

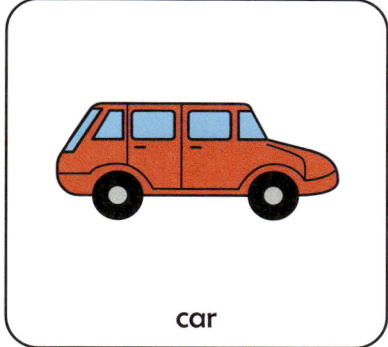

car

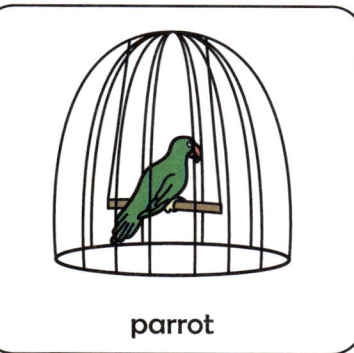

parrot

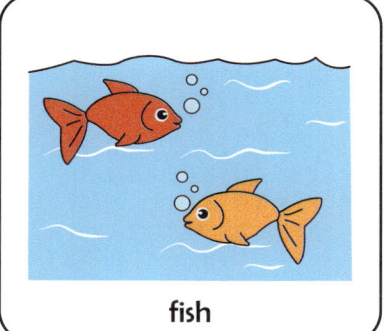

fish

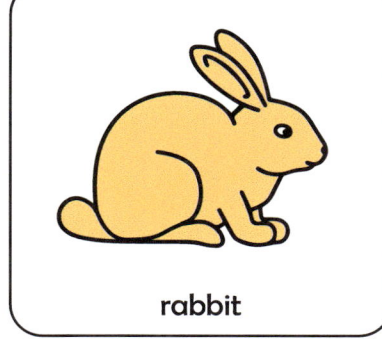

rabbit

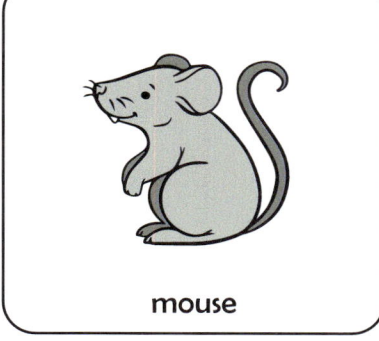

mouse

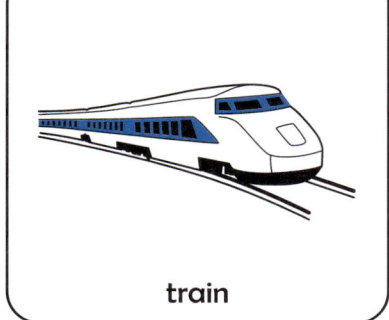

train

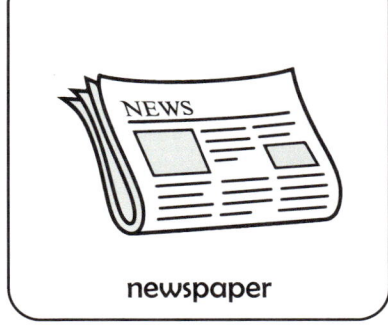

newspaper

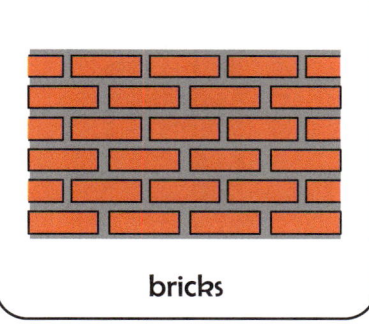

bricks

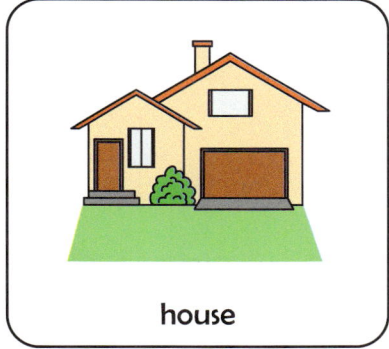

house

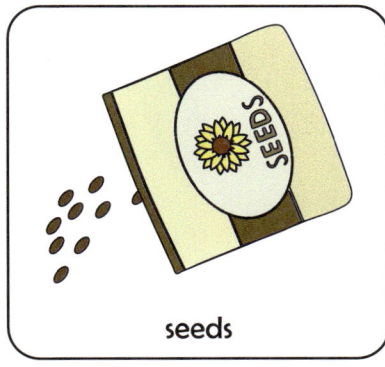

seeds

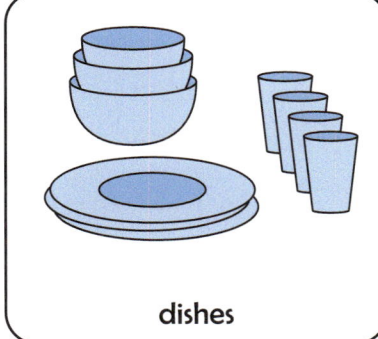

dishes

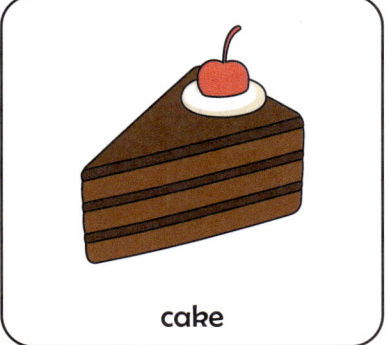

cake

Copyright material from NHS Forth Valley (2020), *Colourful Semantics*, Routledge

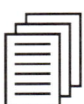

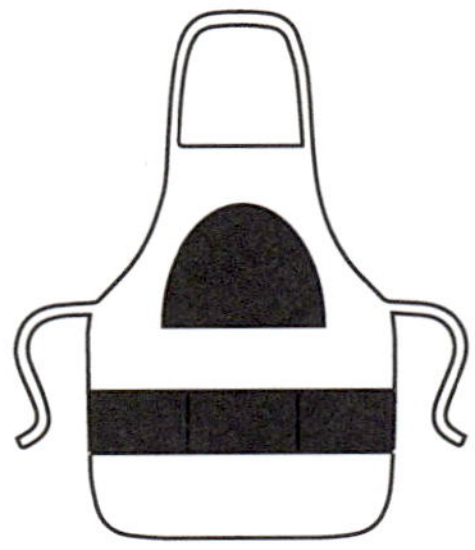

apron	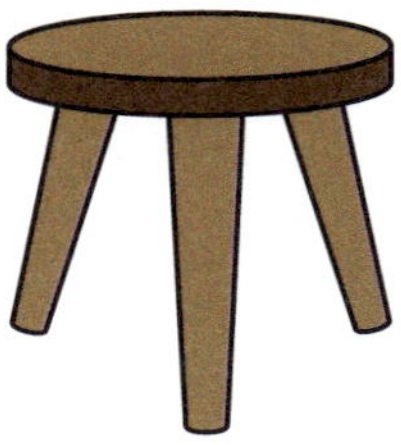 stool	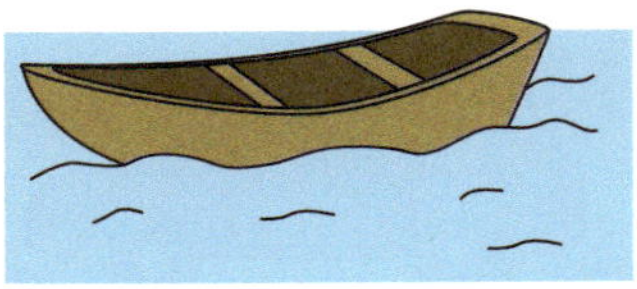 boat
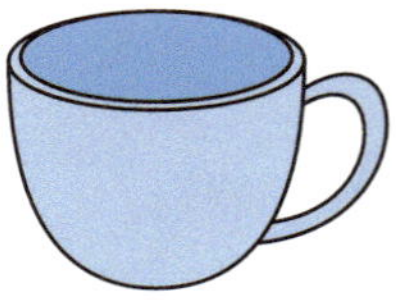 cup	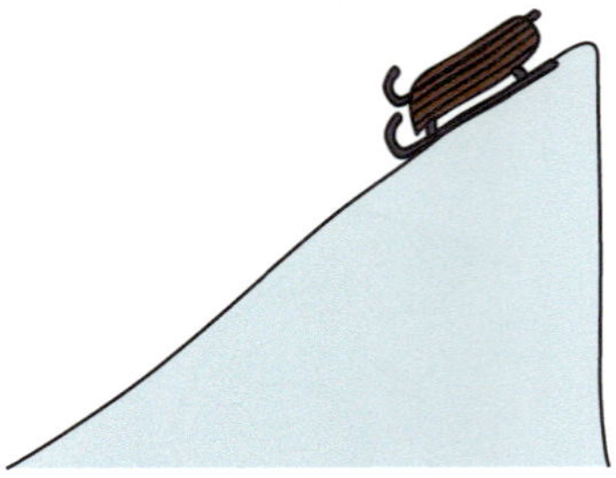 sledge	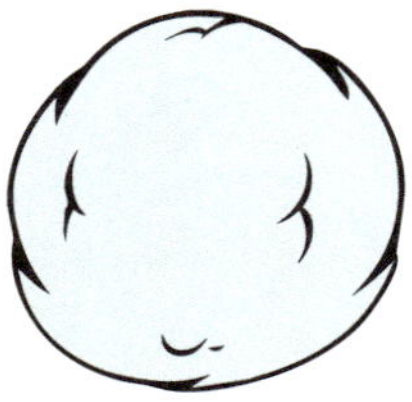 snowball
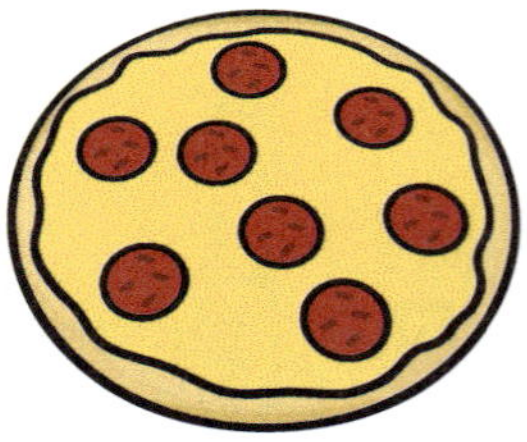 pizza	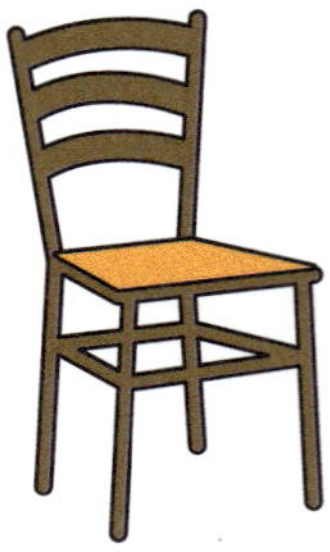 chair	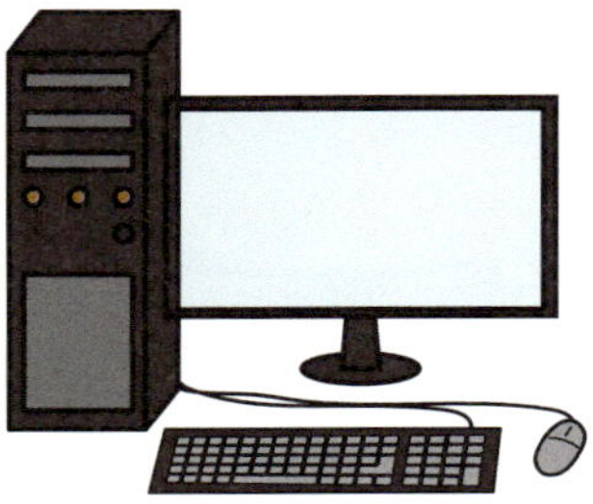 computer
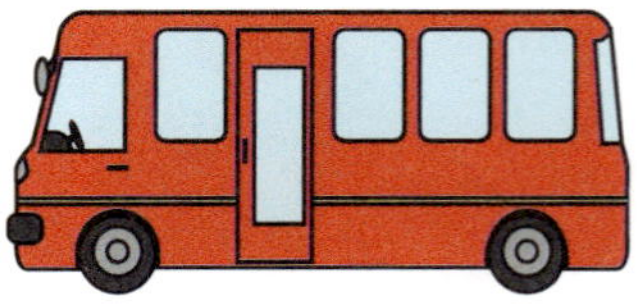 bus	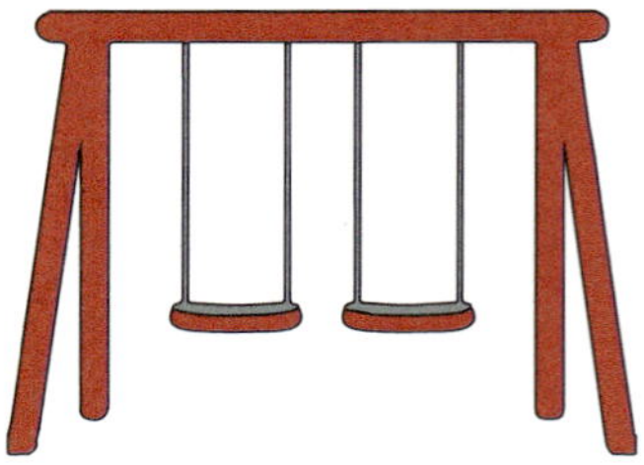 swings	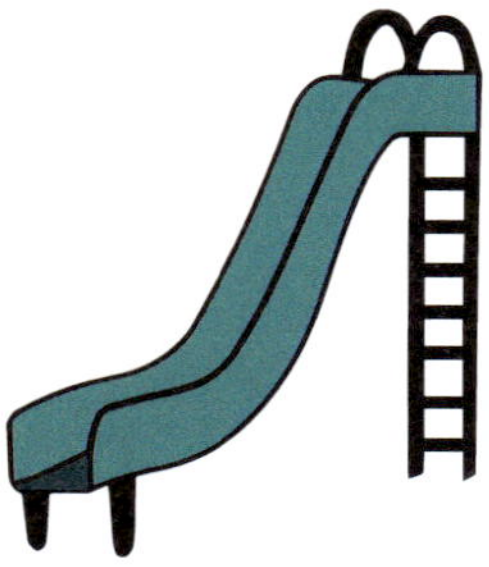 slide

Copyright material from NHS Forth Valley (2020), *Colourful Semantics*, Routledge
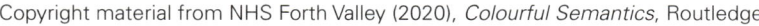

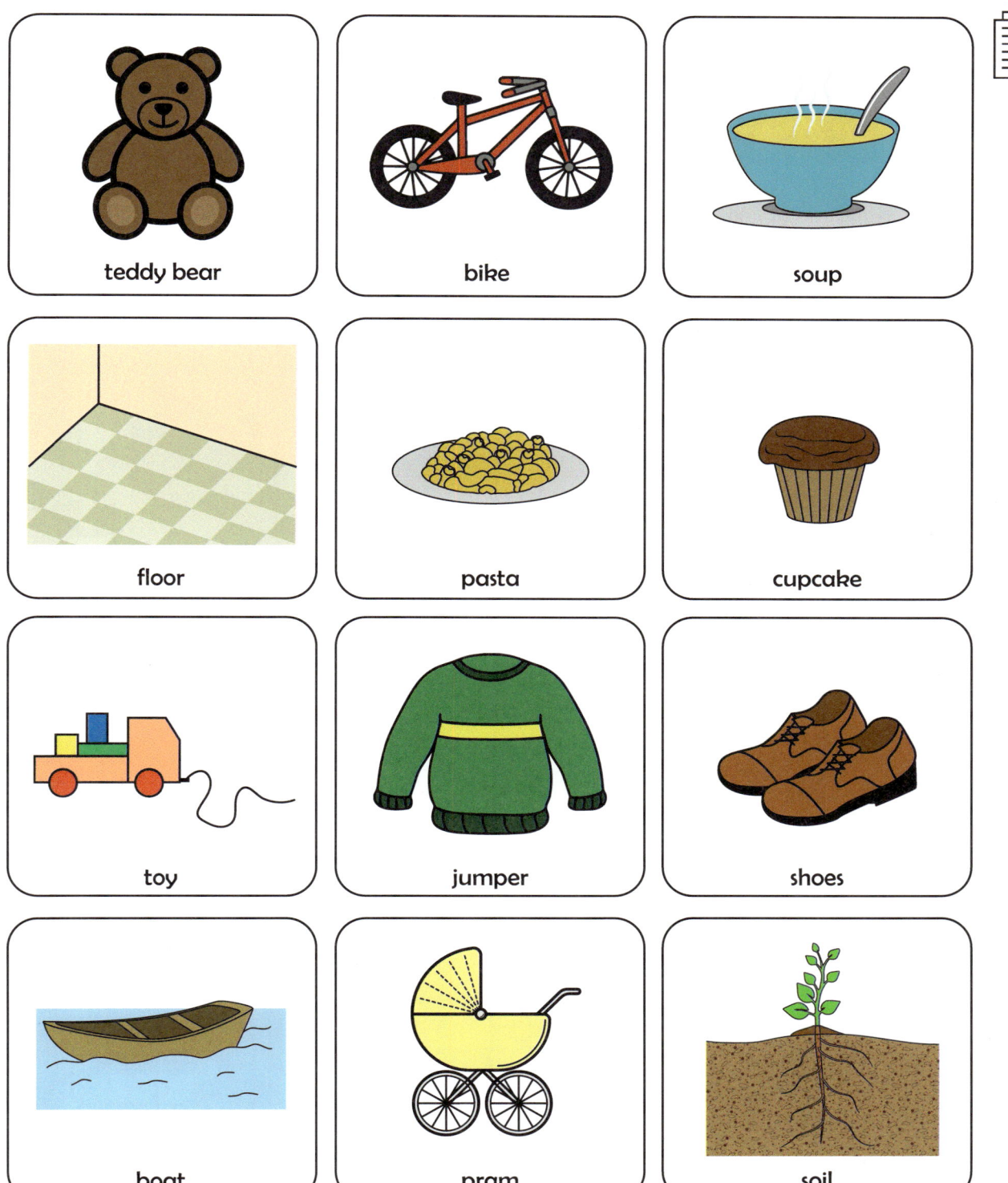

teddy bear

bike

soup

floor

pasta

cupcake

toy

jumper

shoes

boat

pram

soil

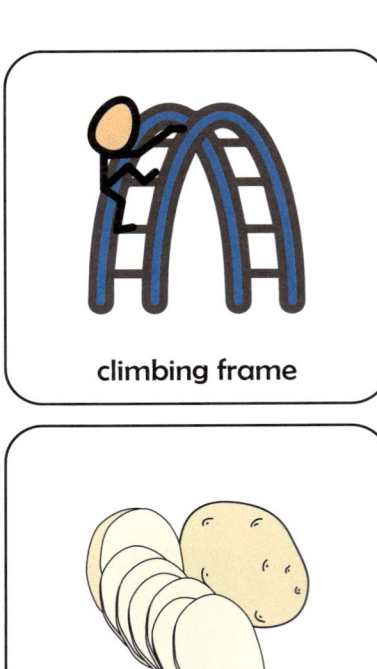

climbing frame

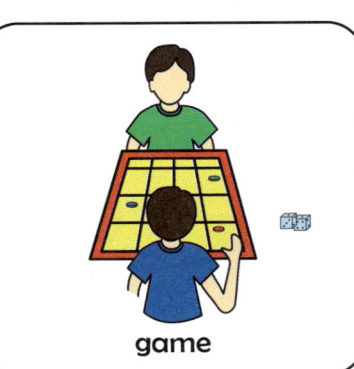

game

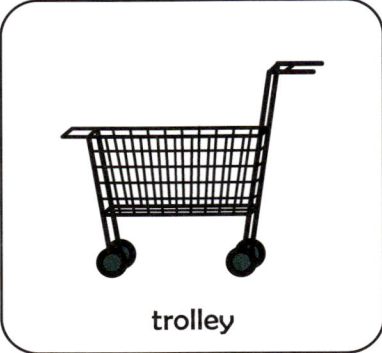

trolley

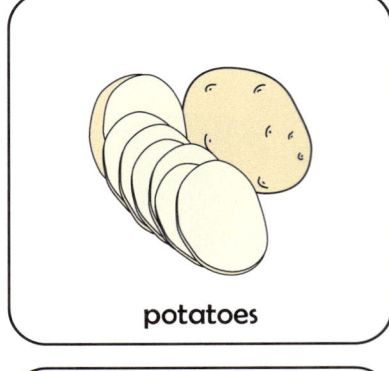

potatoes

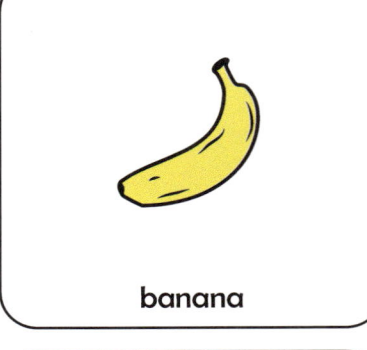

banana

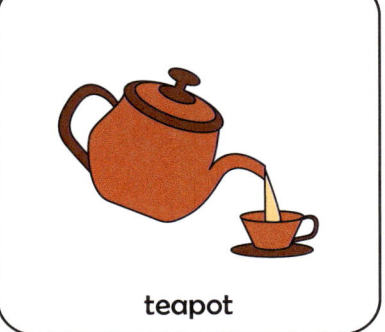

teapot

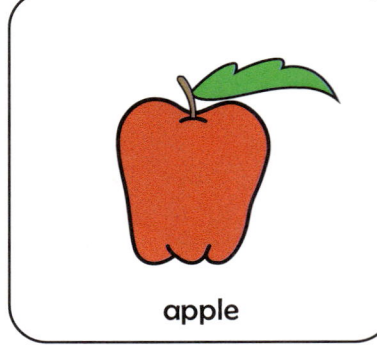

apple

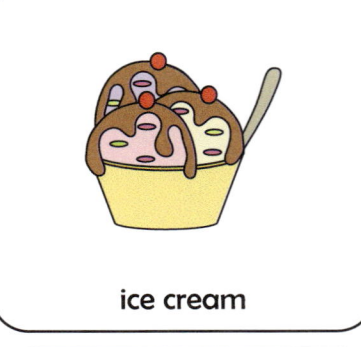

ice cream

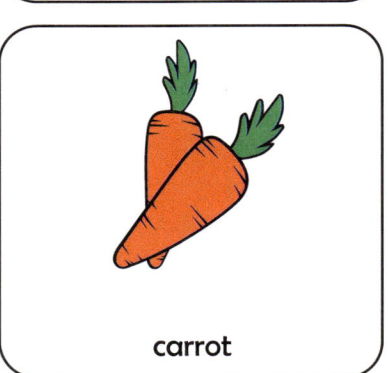

carrot

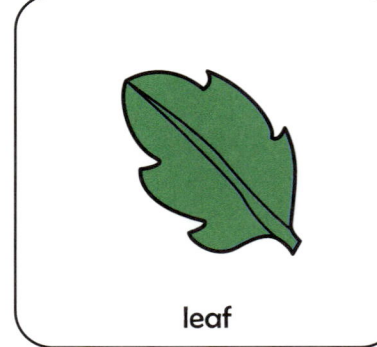

leaf

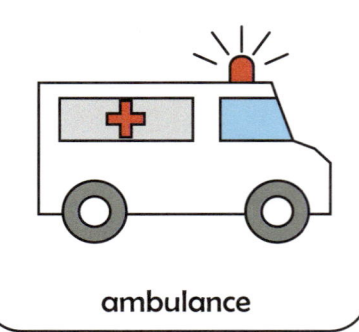

ambulance

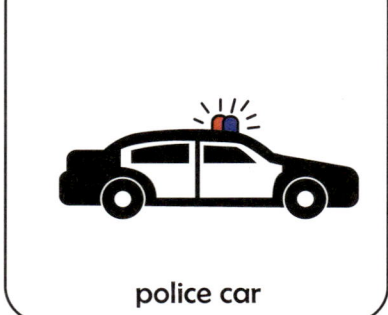

police car

Copyright material from NHS Forth Valley (2020), *Colourful Semantics*, Routledge

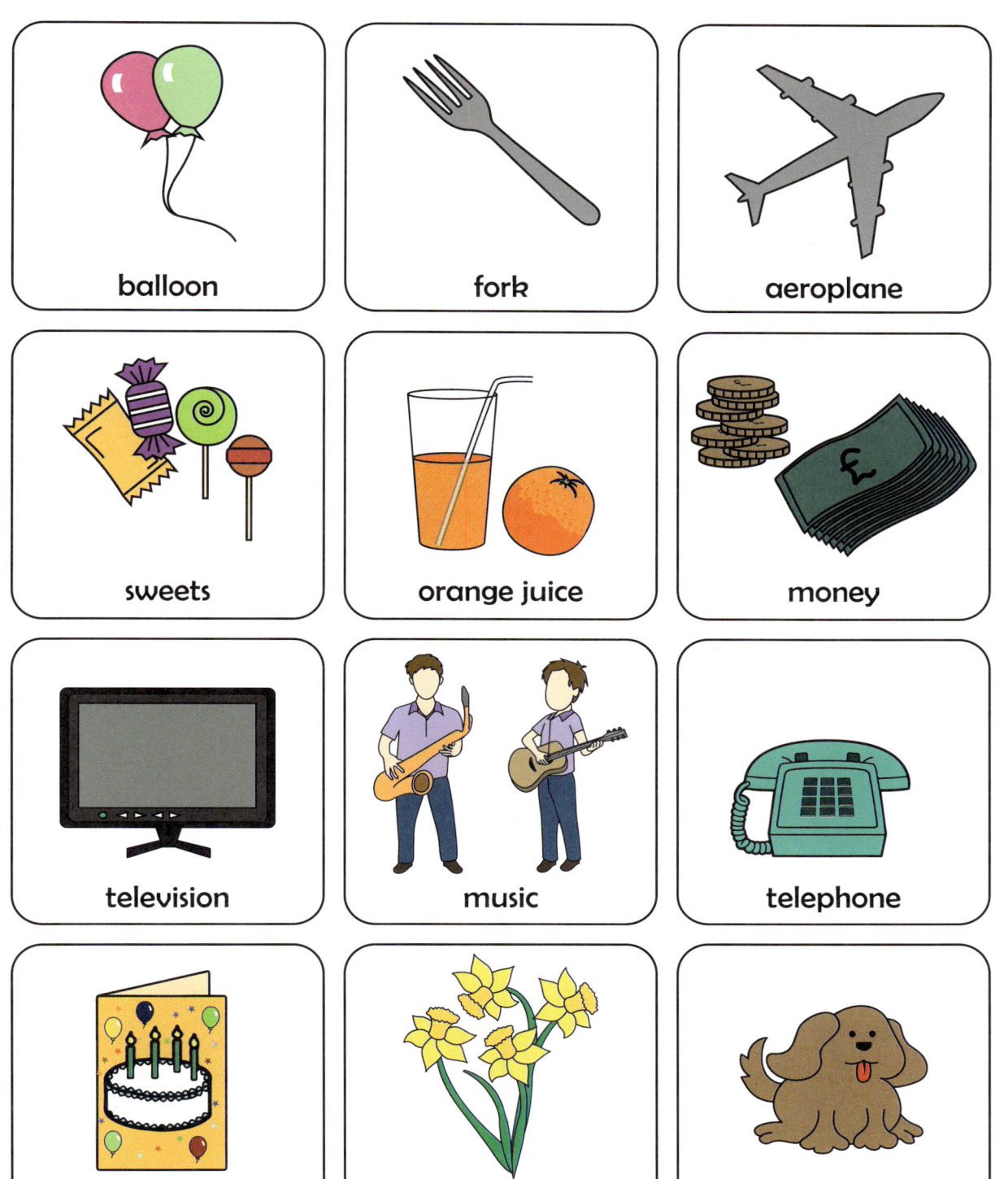

balloon

fork

aeroplane

sweets

orange juice

money

television

music

telephone

card

daffodil

dog

Copyright material from NHS Forth Valley (2020), *Colourful Semantics*, Routledge

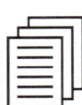

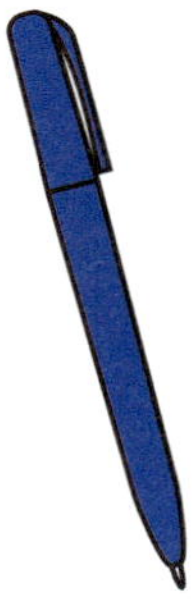

pen	letter	scissors
doll	bee	milk
book	hair	hands
picture	ladder	tree

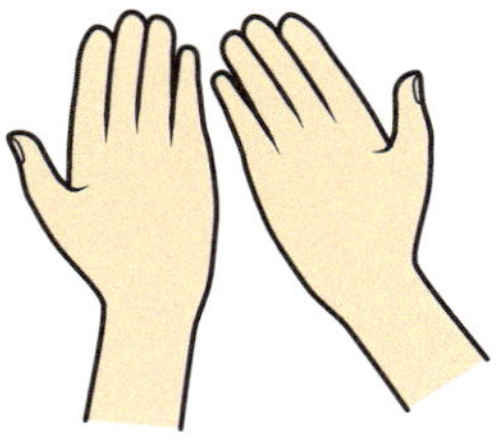

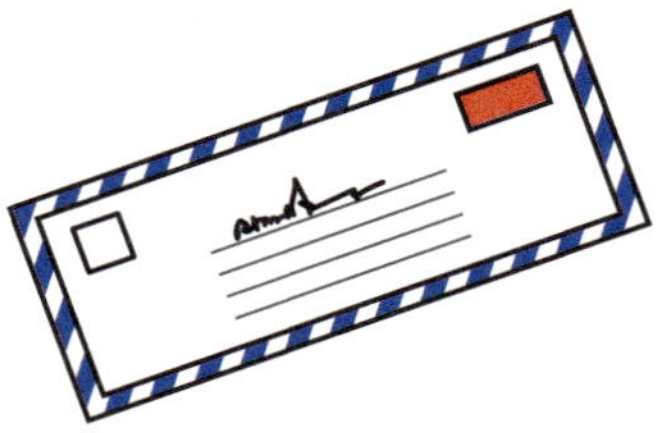

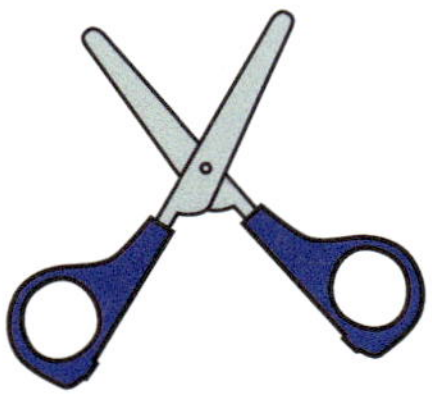

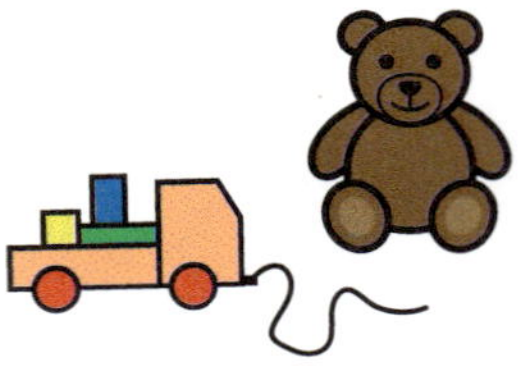

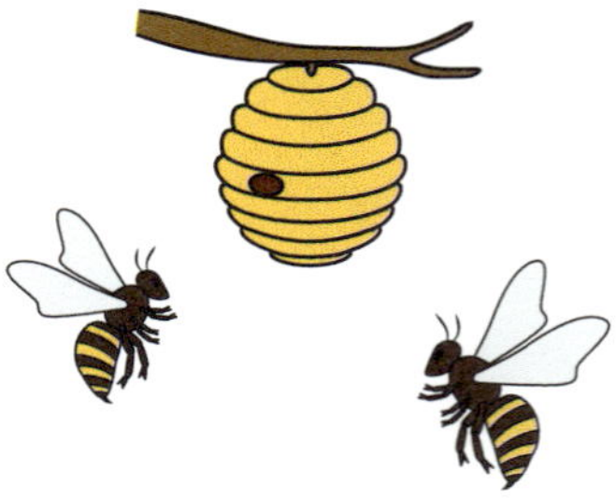

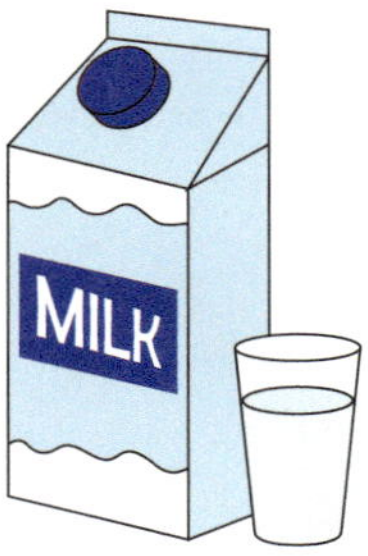

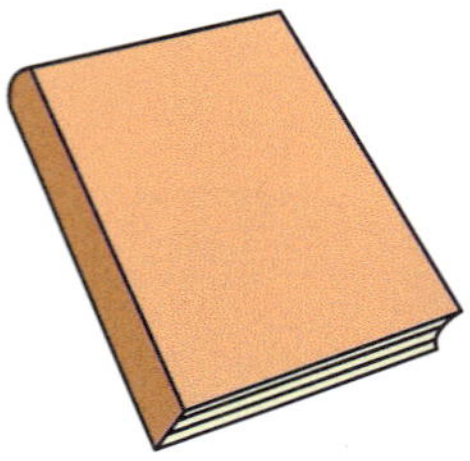

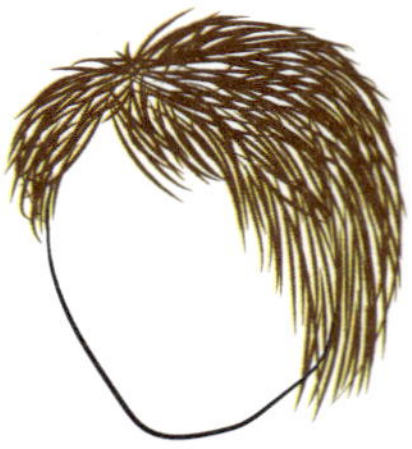

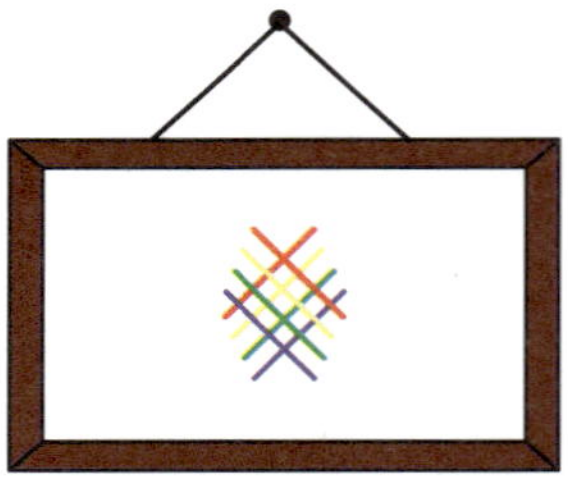

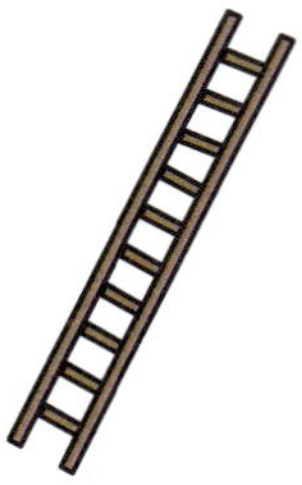

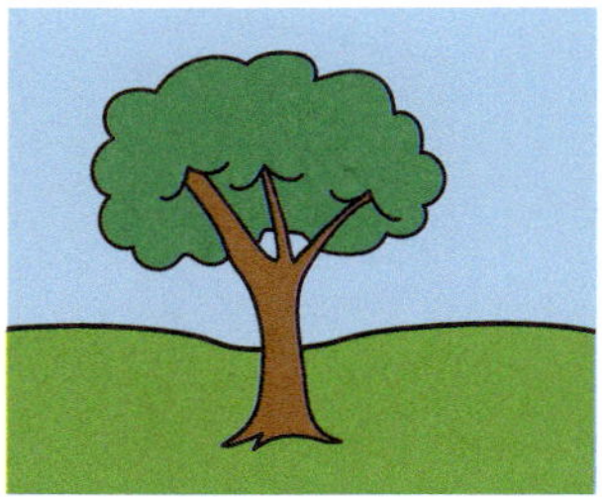

Copyright material from NHS Forth Valley (2020), *Colourful Semantics*, Routledge

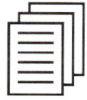

'Where' vocabulary
Home and school

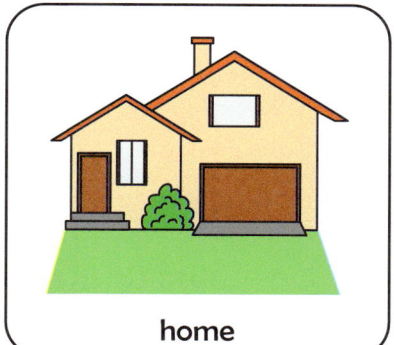

home

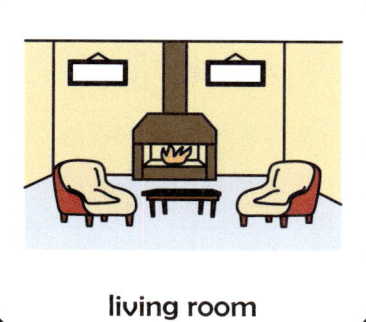

living room

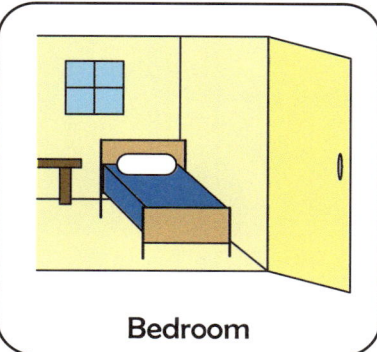

Bedroom

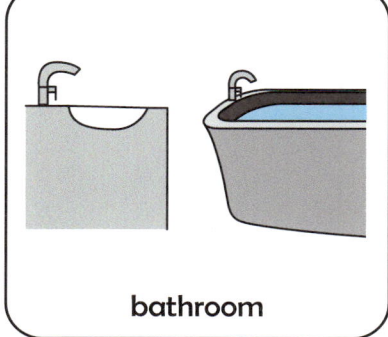

bathroom

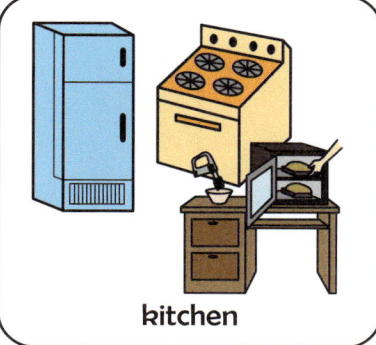

kitchen

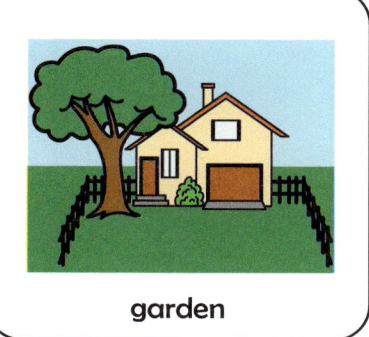

garden

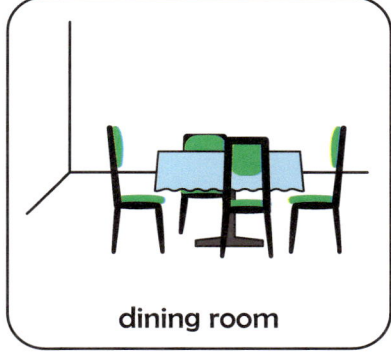

dining room

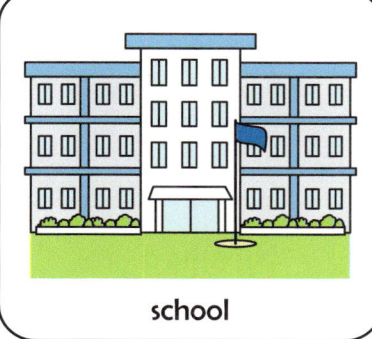

school

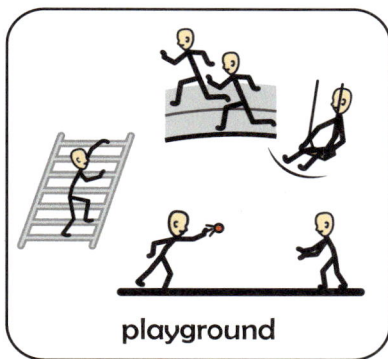

playground

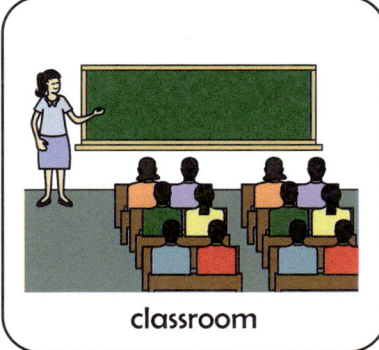

classroom

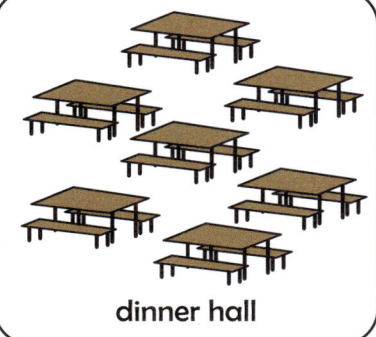

dinner hall

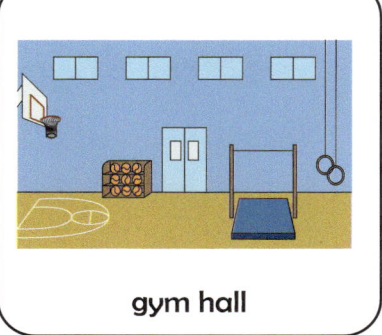

gym hall

Copyright material from NHS Forth Valley (2020), *Colourful Semantics*, Routledge

Day to day and community

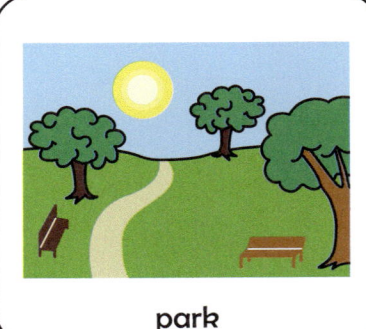

park

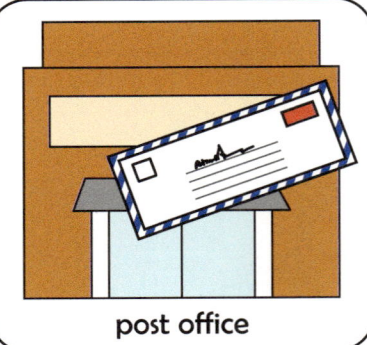

post office

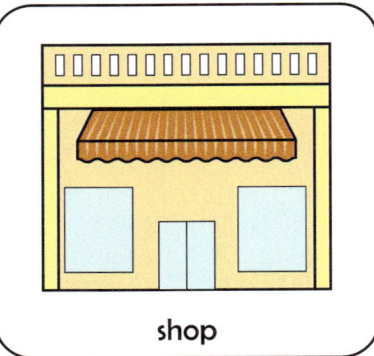

shop

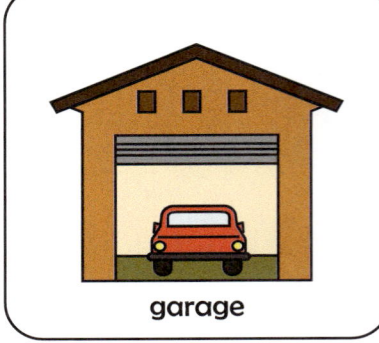

garage

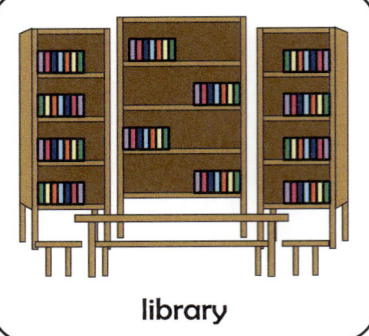

library

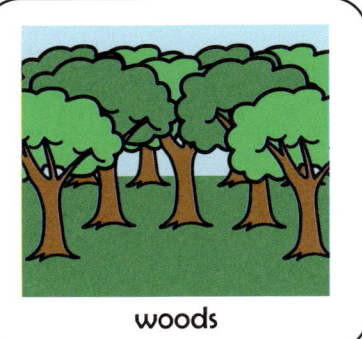

woods

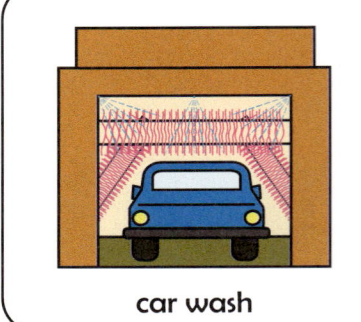

car wash

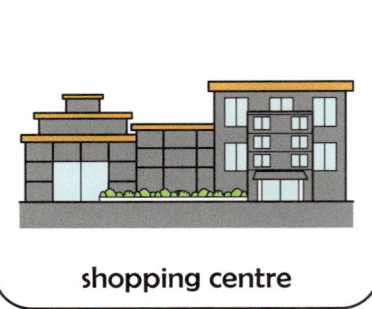

shopping centre

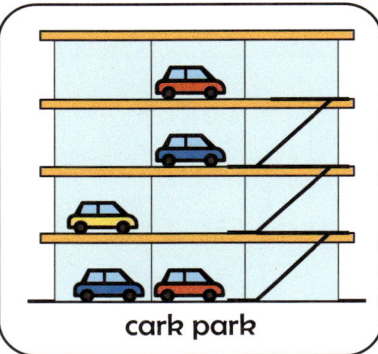

cark park

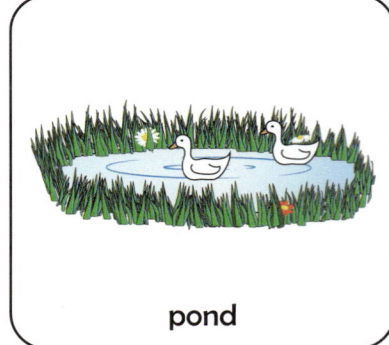

pond

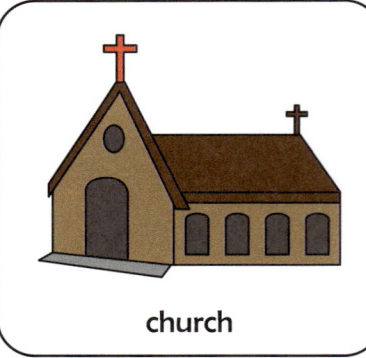

church

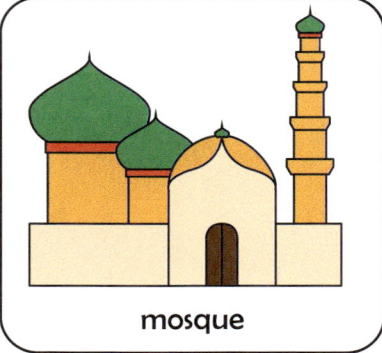

mosque

Copyright material from NHS Forth Valley (2020), *Colourful Semantics*, Routledge

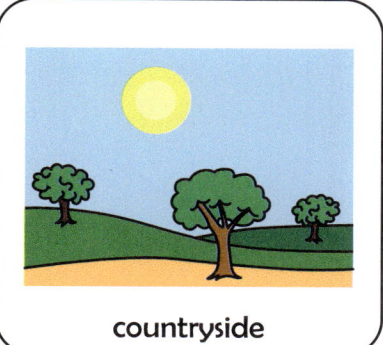

countryside

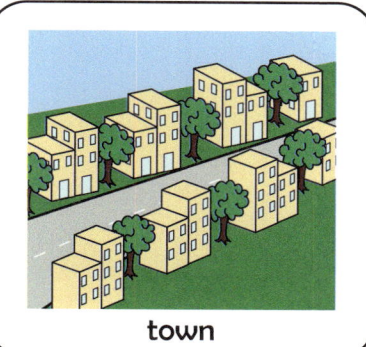

town

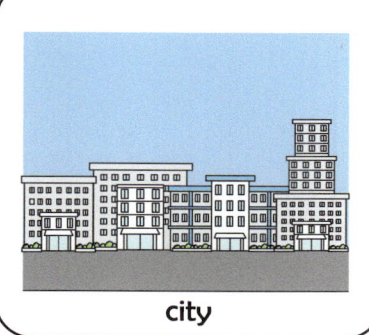

city

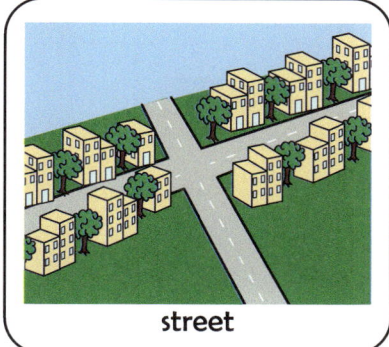

street

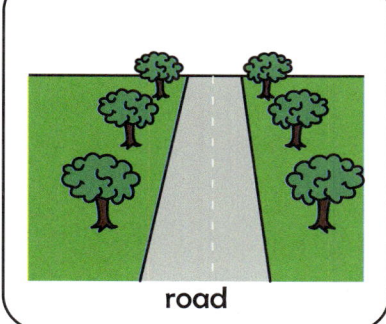

road

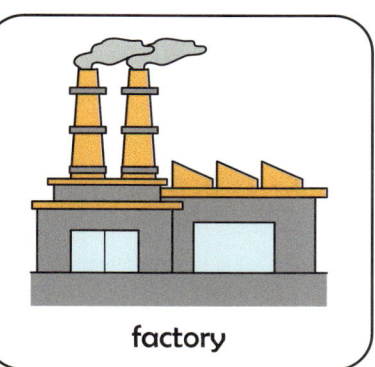

factory

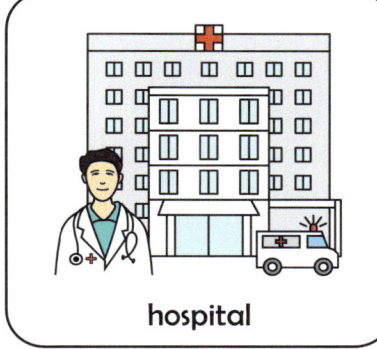

hospital

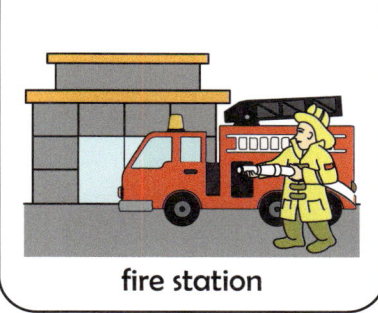

fire station

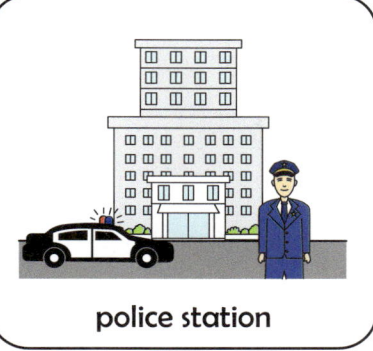

police station

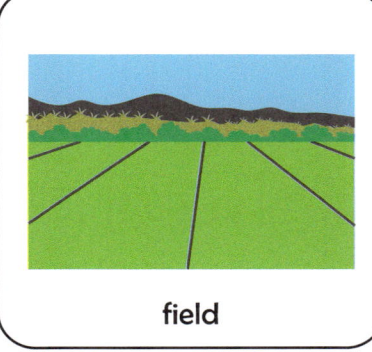

field

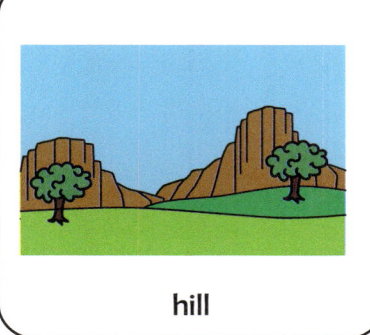

hill

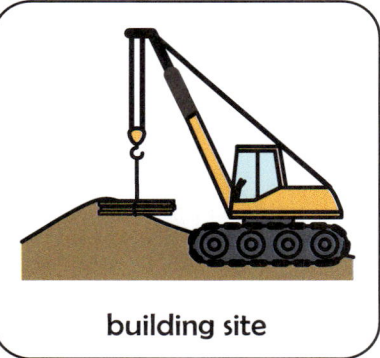

building site

Copyright material from NHS Forth Valley (2020), *Colourful Semantics*, Routledge

Outings, events and holidays

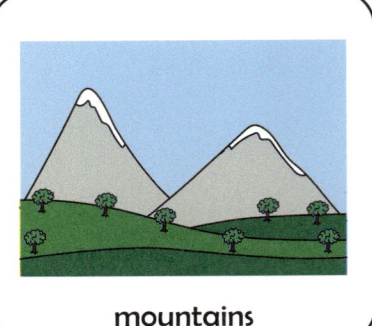

mountains

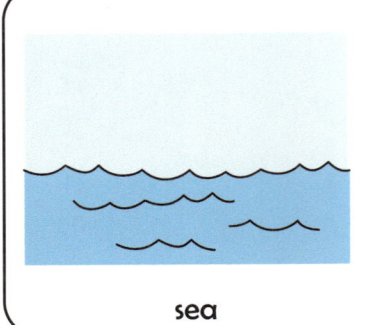

sea

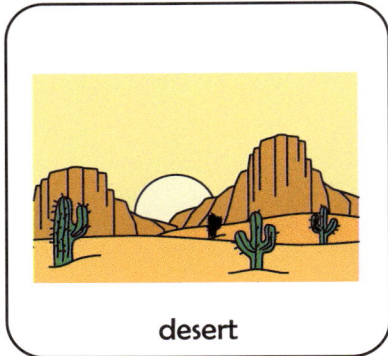

desert

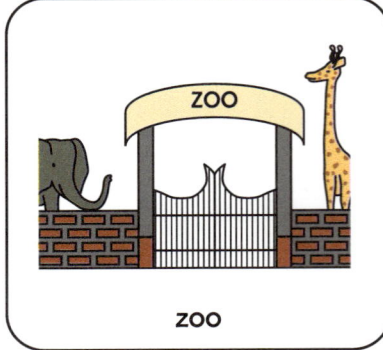

zoo

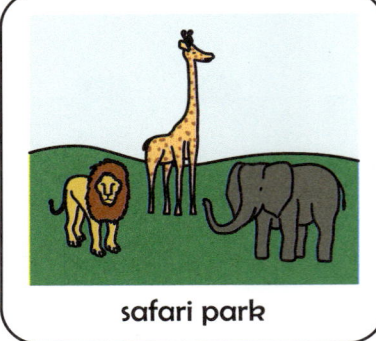

safari park

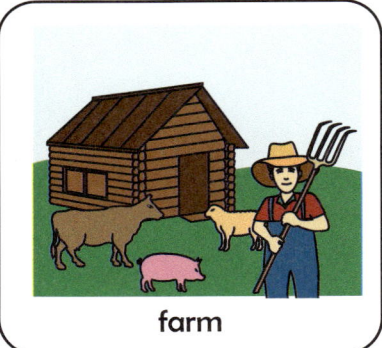

farm

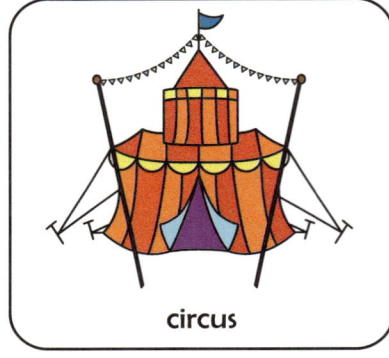

circus

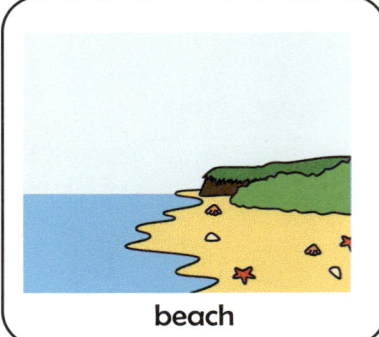

beach

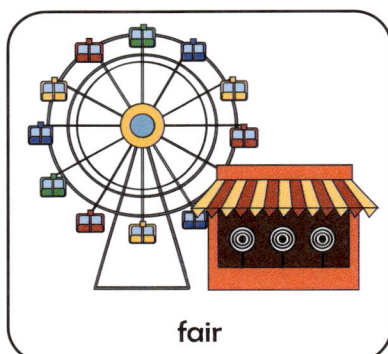

fair

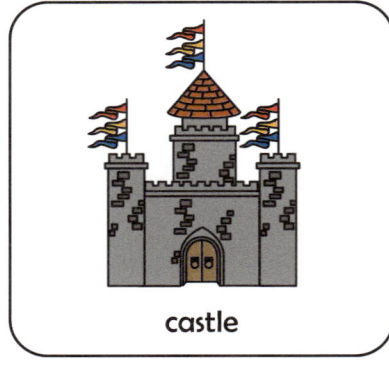

castle

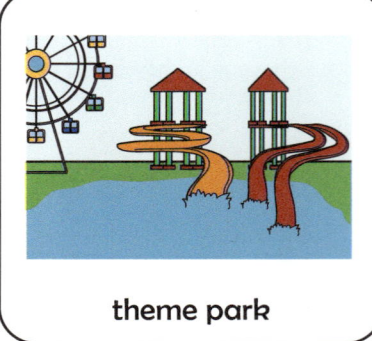

theme park

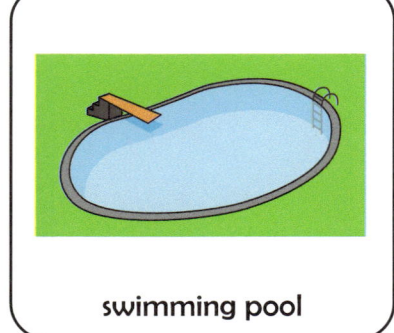

swimming pool

Copyright material from NHS Forth Valley (2020), *Colourful Semantics*, Routledge

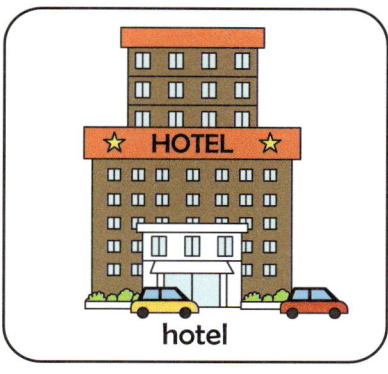

hotel

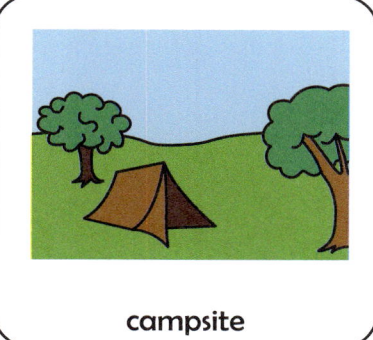

campsite

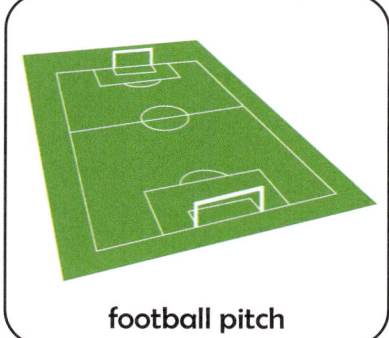

football pitch

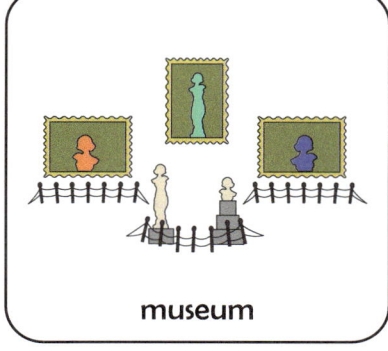

museum

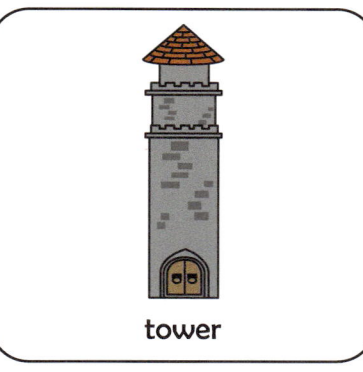

tower

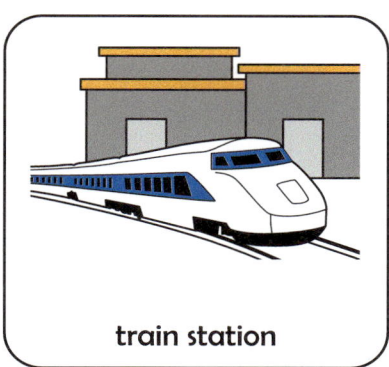

train station

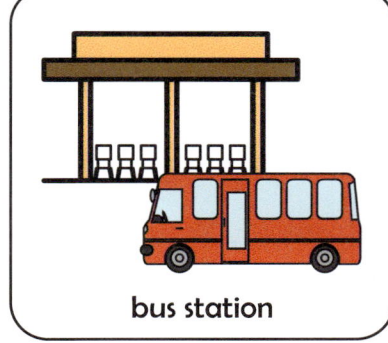

bus station

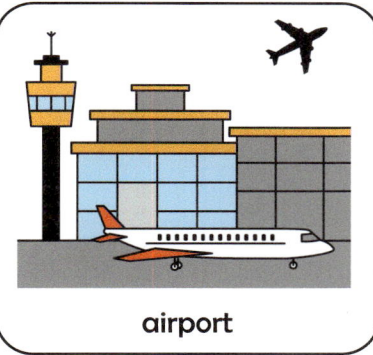

airport

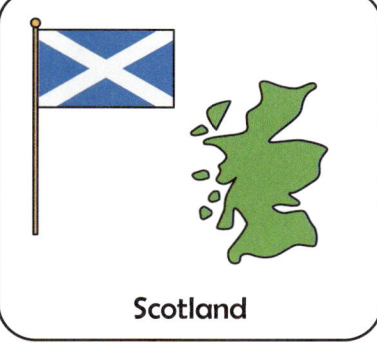

Scotland

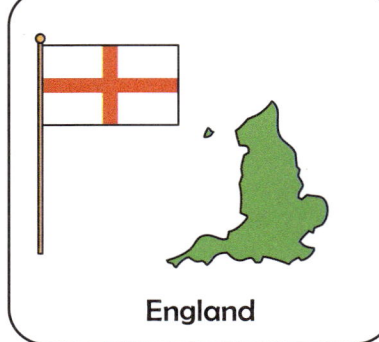

England

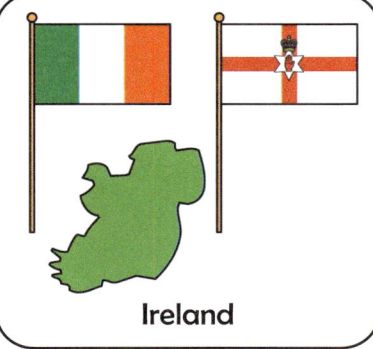

Ireland

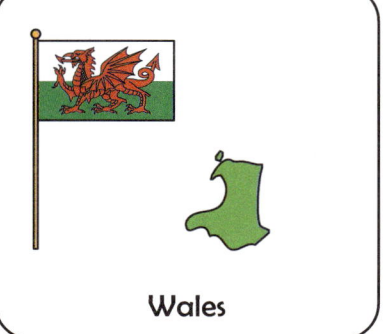

Wales

Copyright material from NHS Forth Valley (2020), *Colourful Semantics*, Routledge

Food/dining and general

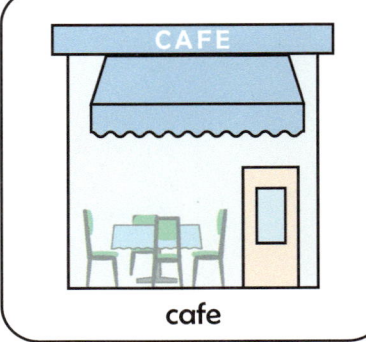
cafe

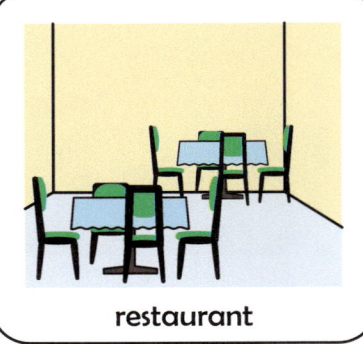
restaurant

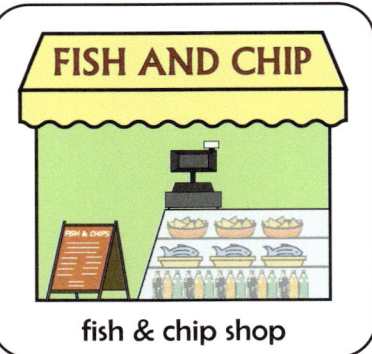
fish & chip shop

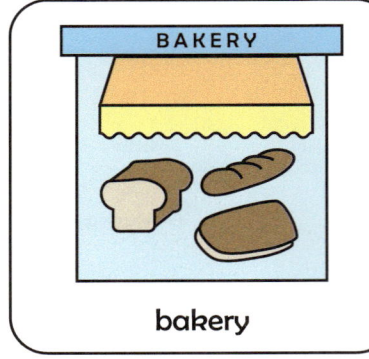
bakery

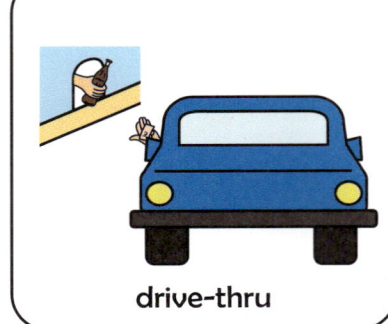
drive-thru

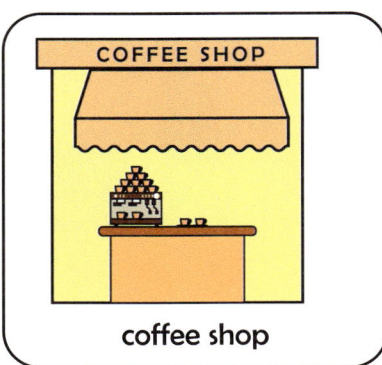
coffee shop

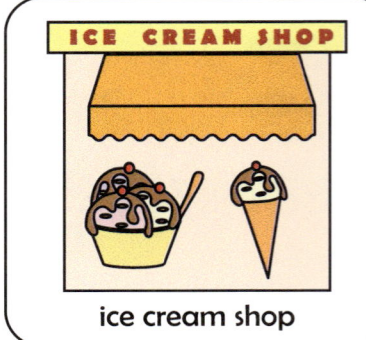
ice cream shop

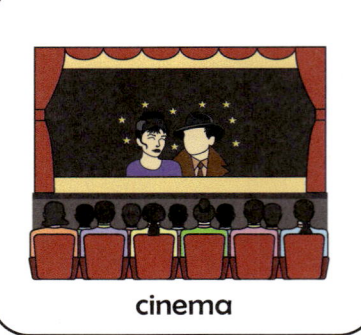
cinema

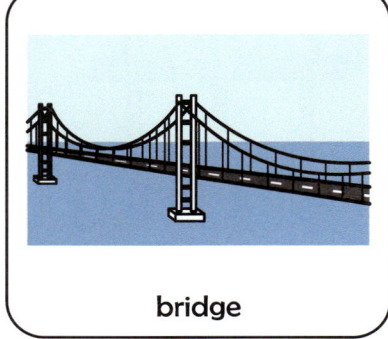
bridge

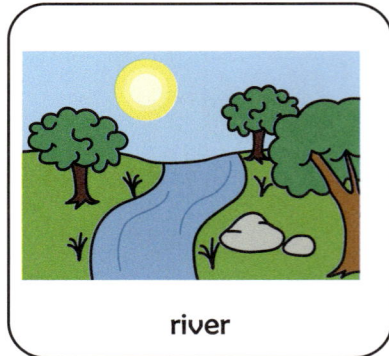
river

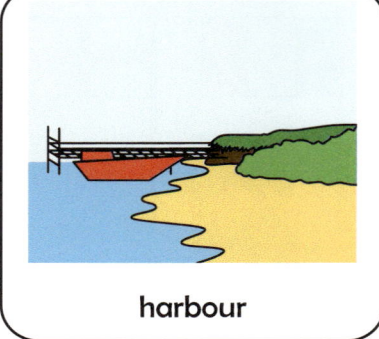
harbour

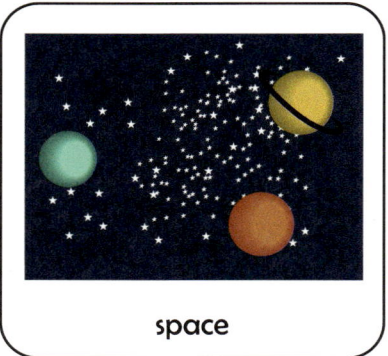
space

Copyright material from NHS Forth Valley (2020), *Colourful Semantics*, Routledge

General places

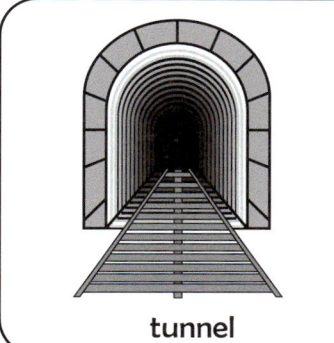

tunnel

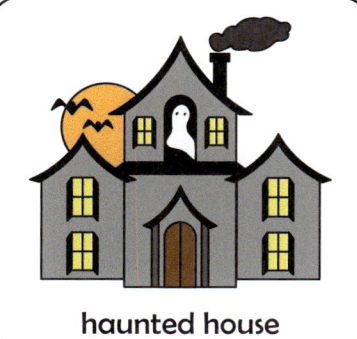

haunted house

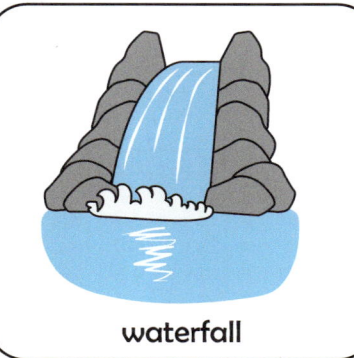

waterfall

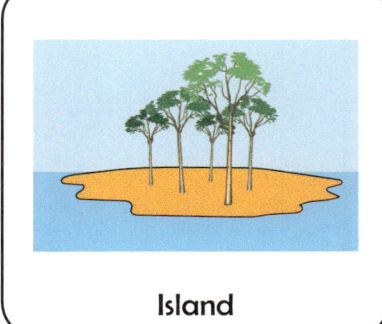

Island

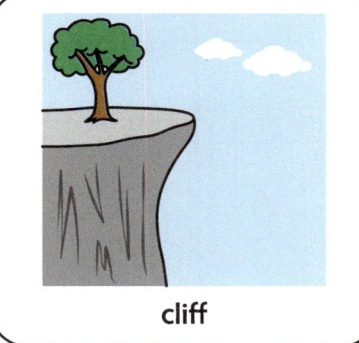

cliff

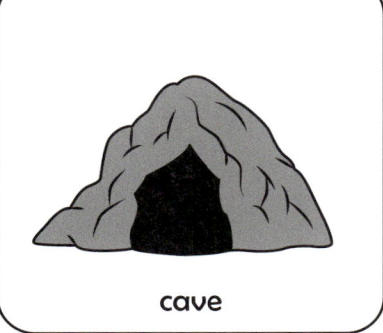

cave

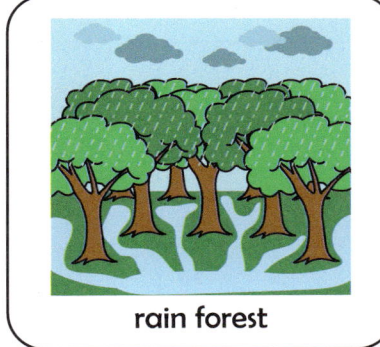

rain forest

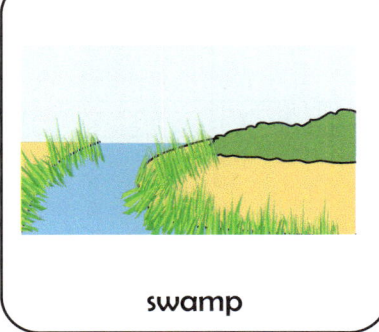

swamp

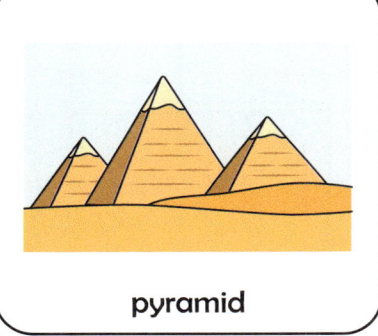

pyramid

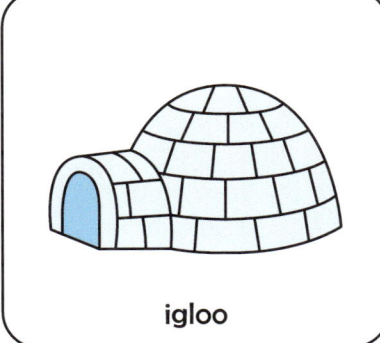

igloo

lighthouse

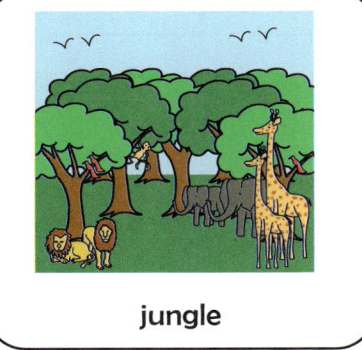

jungle

Copyright material from NHS Forth Valley (2020), *Colourful Semantics*, Routledge

'When' vocabulary
Days

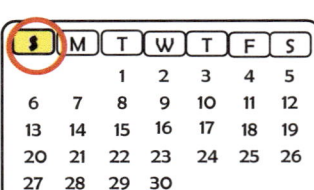

Sunday

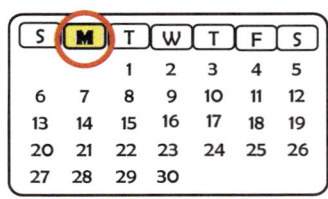

Monday

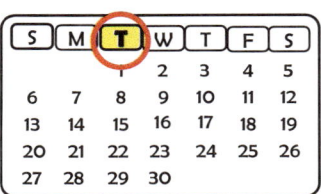

Tuesday

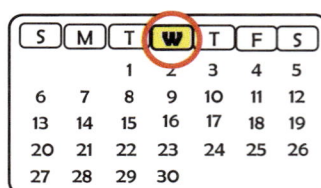

Wednesday

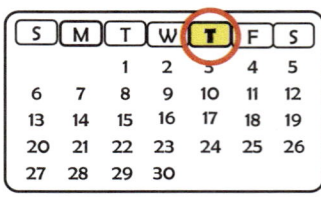

Thursday

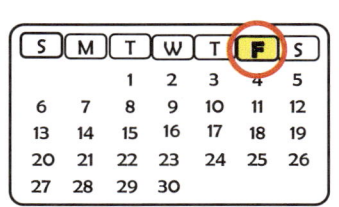

Friday

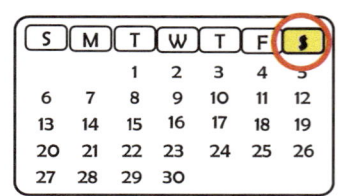

Saturday

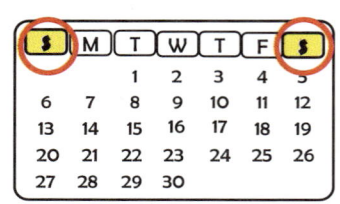

weekend

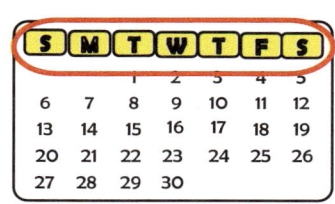

week

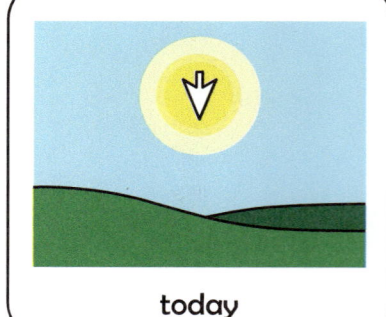

today

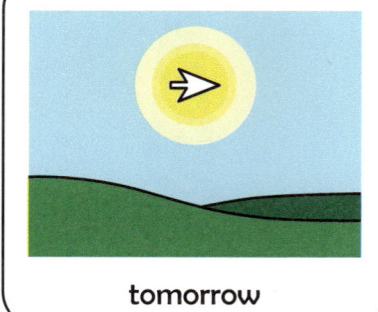

tomorrow

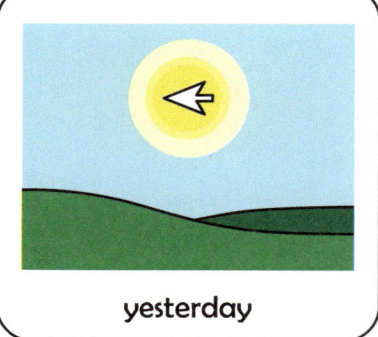

yesterday

Copyright material from NHS Forth Valley (2020), *Colourful Semantics*, Routledge

Months

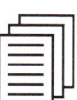

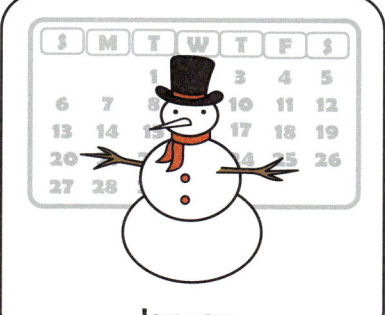

January

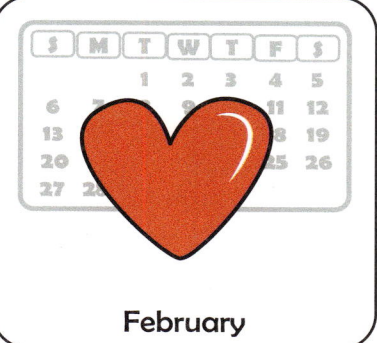

February

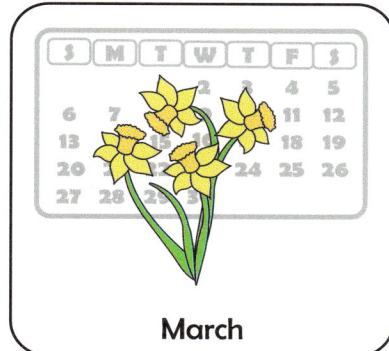

March

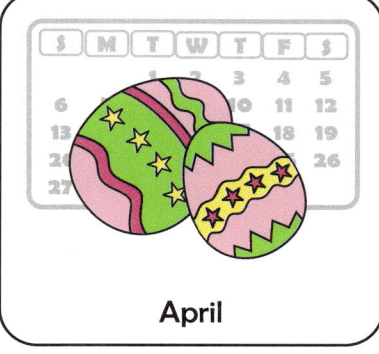

April

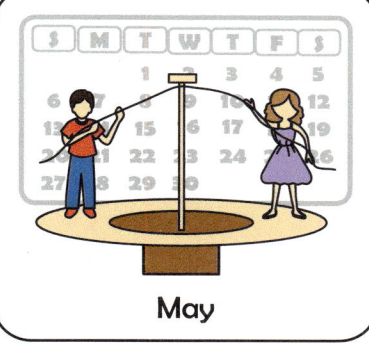

May

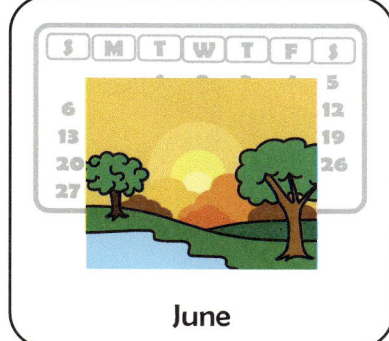

June

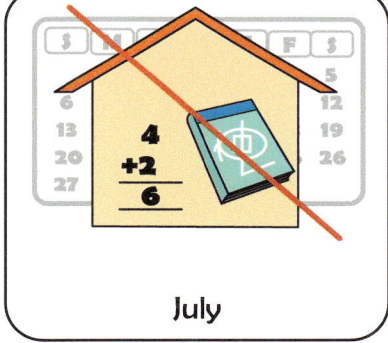

July

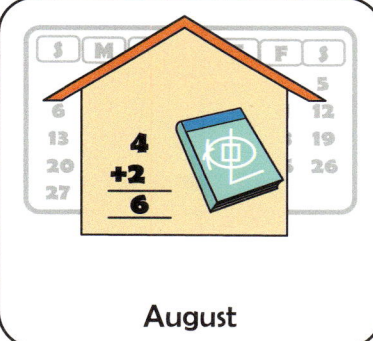

August

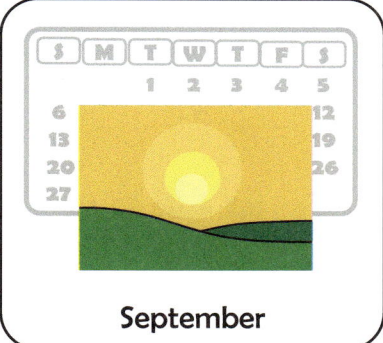

September

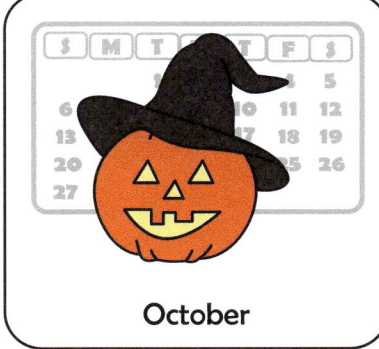

October

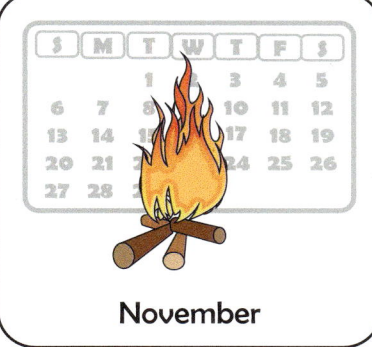

November

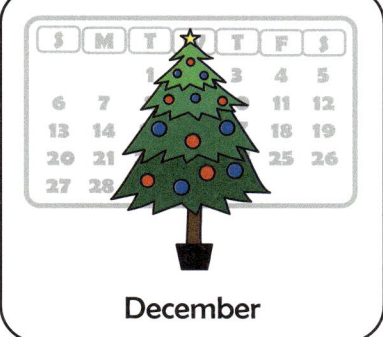

December

Copyright material from NHS Forth Valley (2020), *Colourful Semantics*, Routledge

Annual/special events

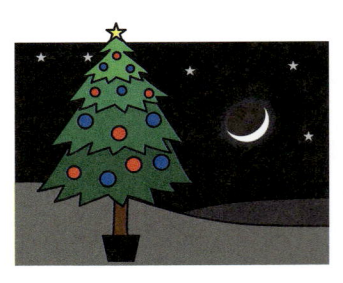

Christmas Eve

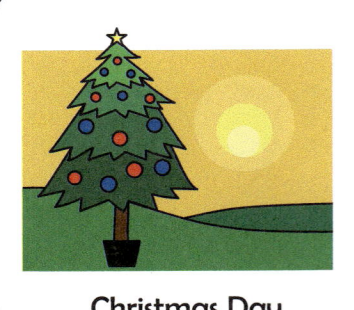

Christmas Day

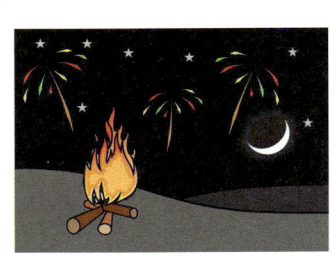

bonfire night

Halloween

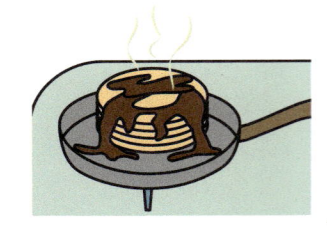

Pancake day

birthday

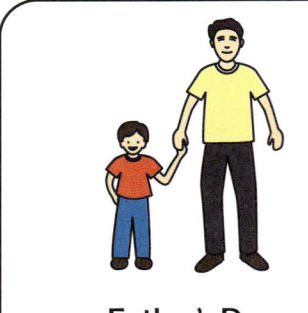

Father's Day

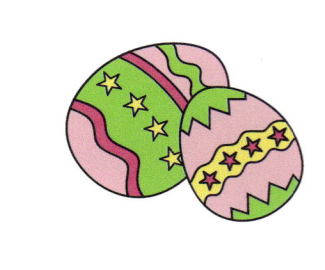

Easter

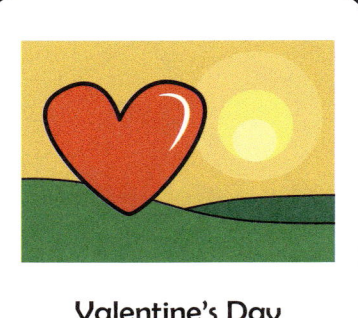

Valentine's Day

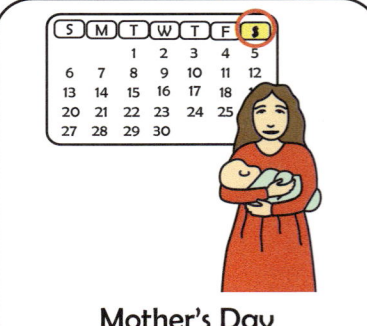

Mother's Day

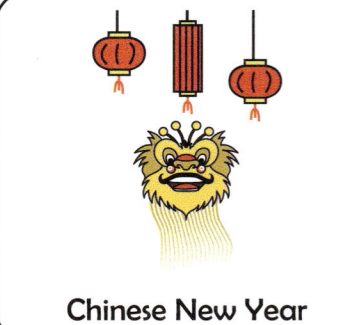

Chinese New Year

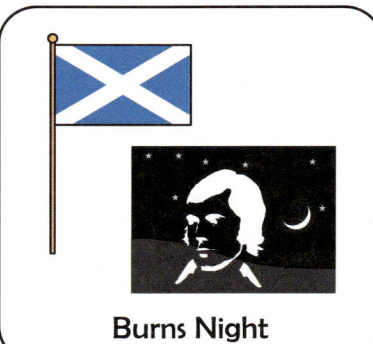

Burns Night

Copyright material from NHS Forth Valley (2020), *Colourful Semantics*, Routledge

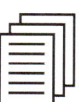

Events/seasons/times of year

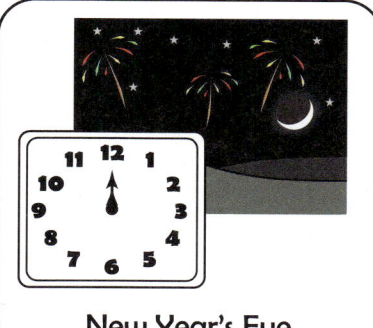

New Year's Eve

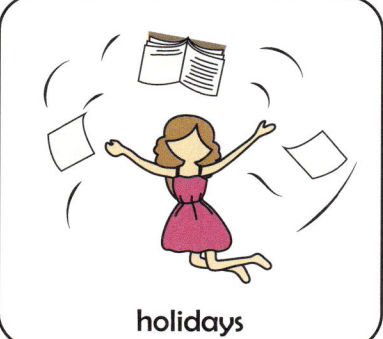

holidays

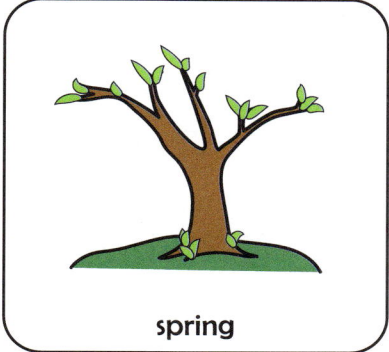

spring

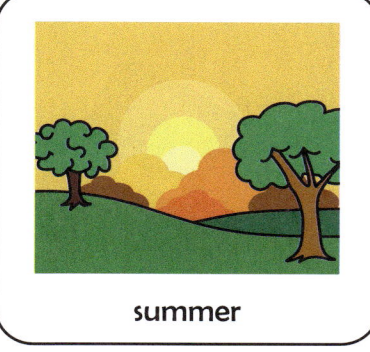

summer

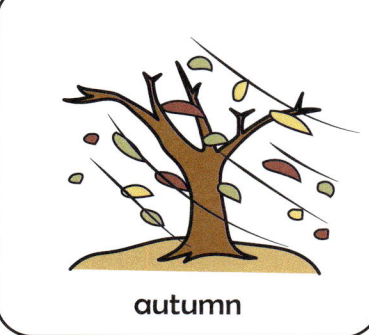

autumn

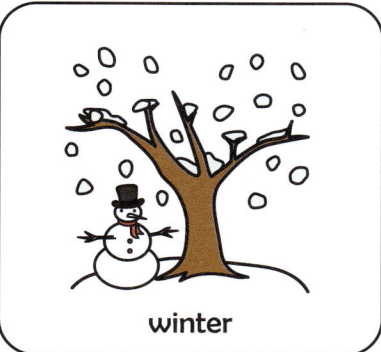

winter

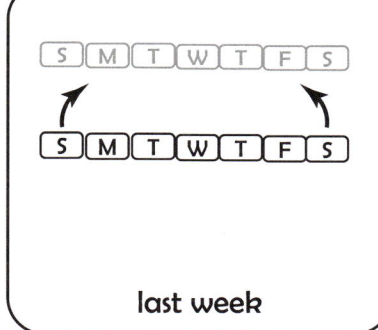

last week

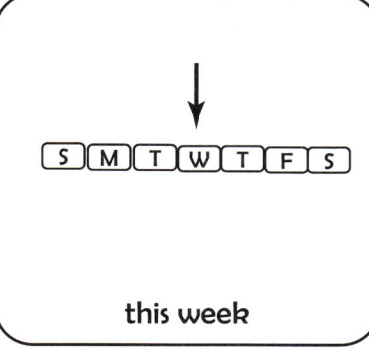

this week

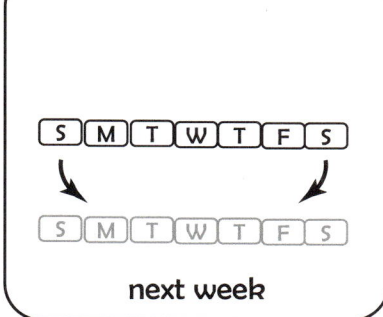

next week

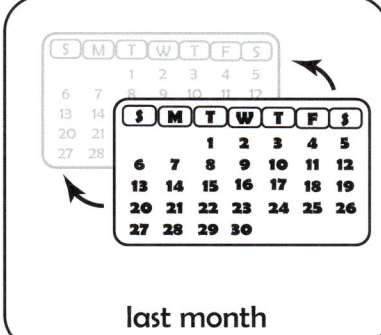

last month

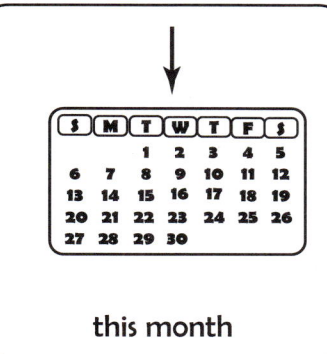

this month

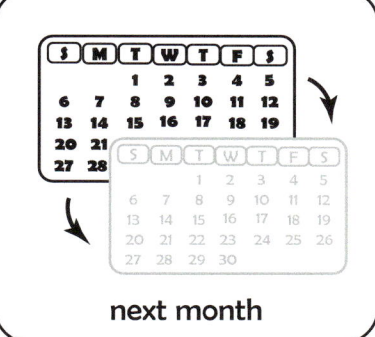

next month

Copyright material from NHS Forth Valley (2020), *Colourful Semantics*, Routledge

Parts of the day/daily routines

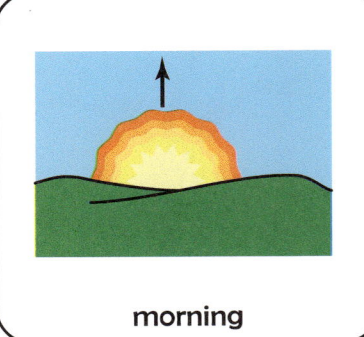

morning

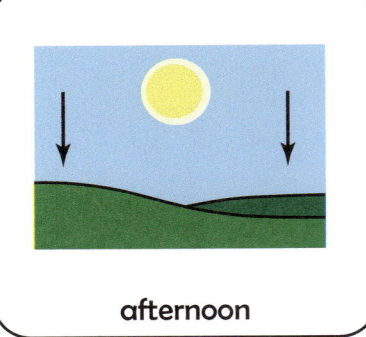

afternoon

evening

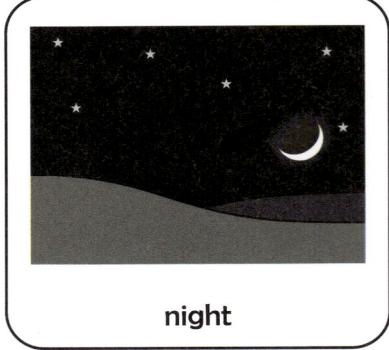

night

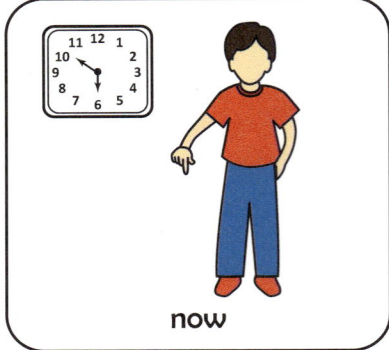

now

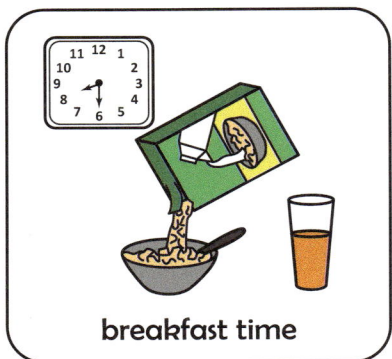

breakfast time

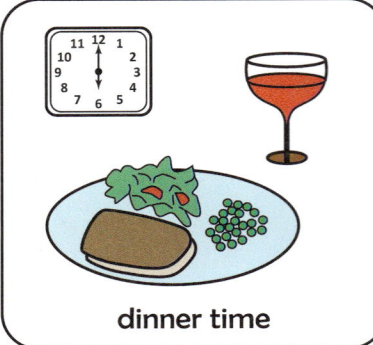

dinner time

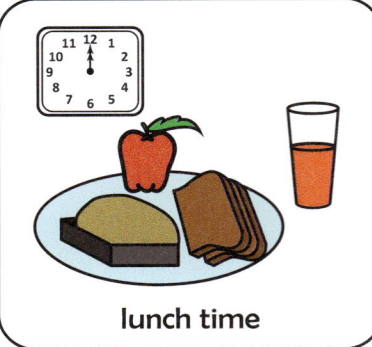

lunch time

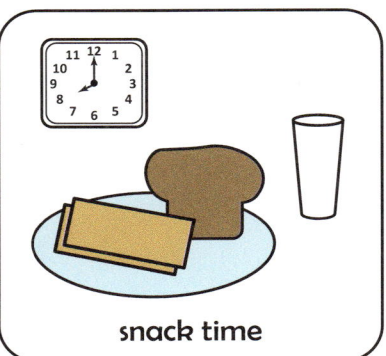

snack time

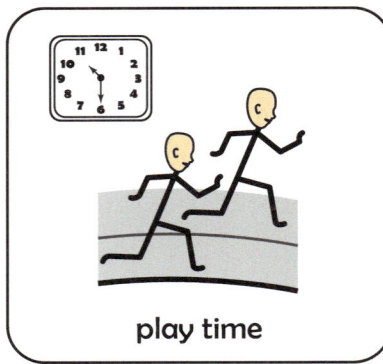

play time

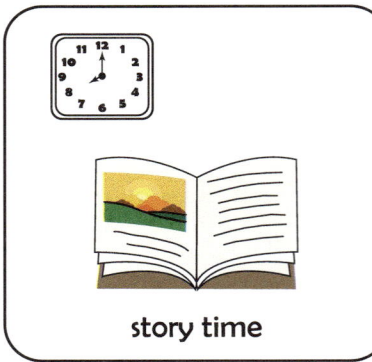

story time

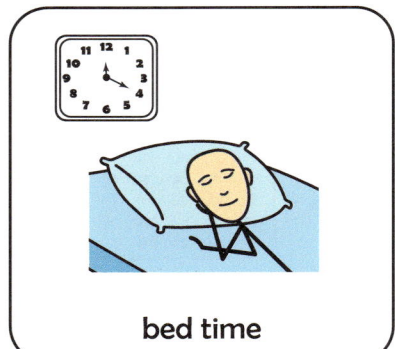

bed time

Copyright material from NHS Forth Valley (2020), *Colourful Semantics*, Routledge

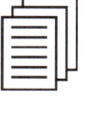

Story ideas

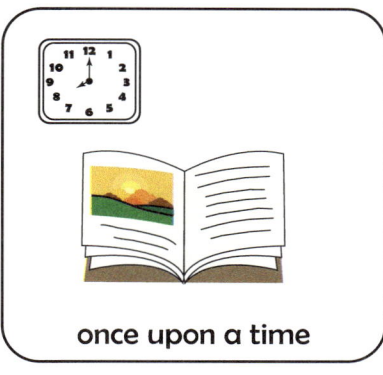

once upon a time

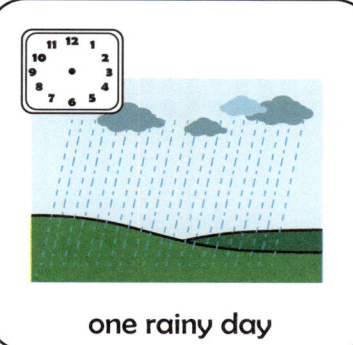

one rainy day

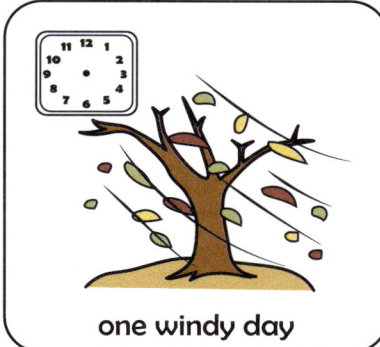

one windy day

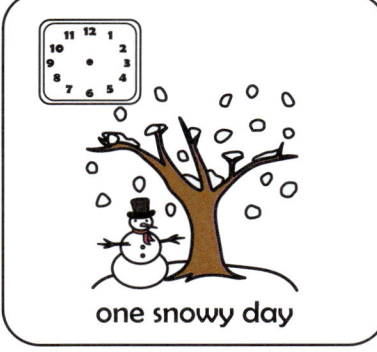

one snowy day

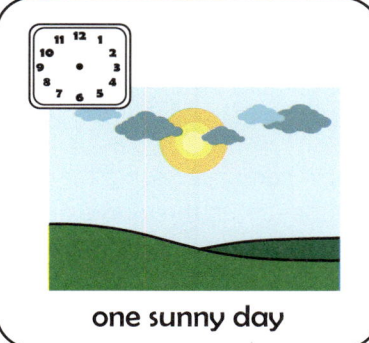

one sunny day

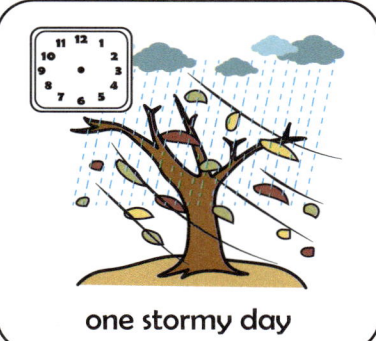

one stormy day

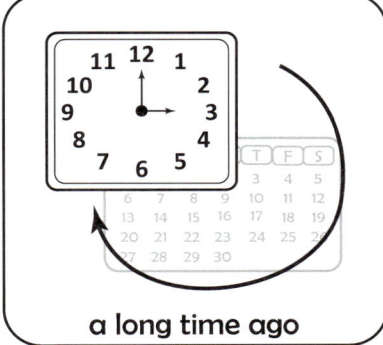

a long time ago

Copyright material from NHS Forth Valley (2020), *Colourful Semantics*, Routledge

Appendix 6
Silly sentences worksheets

Silly sentence worksheets help children at the early stages of writing to begin to transfer spoken language to writing. Two types of worksheets are included in this pack for supporting 'silly sentence' writing: 'Draw a Line' and 'Cut and Stick'.

'Draw a Line' worksheets

These worksheets provide opportunities to practise early writing skills by providing a selection of vocabulary linked to each sentence component, supported with pictures and the written word.

It is helpful to spend time first introducing and discussing the pictured vocabulary with the children and demonstrating completing a worksheet with the whole group or class. Children then complete their own worksheet in the following steps:

- Selecting their favourite word for each sentence component, from the selection given, e.g. their favourite *'who'*, favourite *'doing'* and favourite *'what'*, by either circling it or colouring it in the correct colour.
- Drawing a line between their favourite words and then saying the sentence they made.
- Drawing a picture of the sentence they made in the space underneath or on the back of the worksheet.
- Using the words provided to write their sentence on the lines underneath.
- Colour coding their sentence by underlining the different sentence components in the correct colour.

Below is a completed 'Draw a Line' worksheet, with examples of both use of the current Colourful Semantics colours and the alternative colour coding system.

Copyright material from NHS Forth Valley (2020), *Colourful Semantics*, Routledge

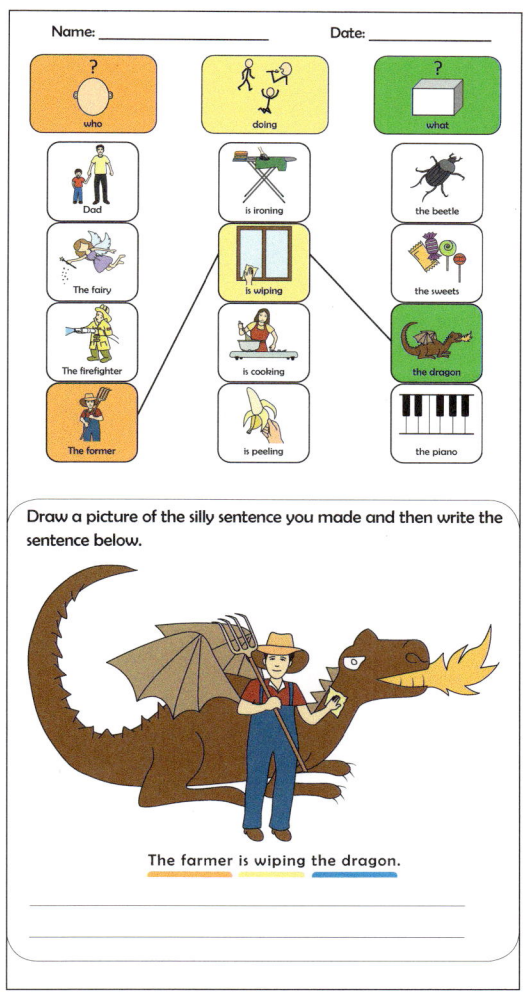

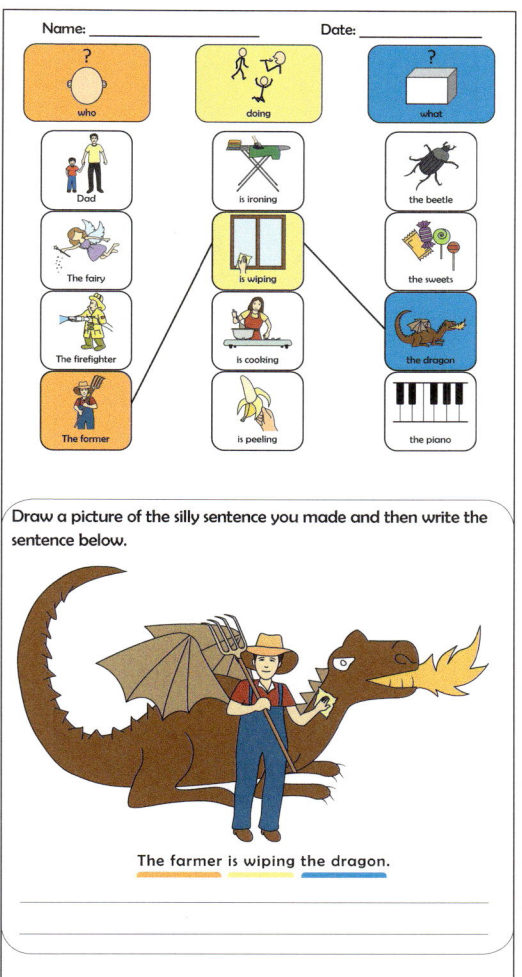

Current Colourful Semantics colours

Adapted Forth Valley colours

Blank 'Draw a Line' worksheets are provided, for use at a range of different ability levels, on pages 192–210.

Copyright material from NHS Forth Valley (2020), *Colourful Semantics*, Routledge

Name: _____ Date: _____

who ?			doing
	The police officer	is eating	
	The witch	is climbing	
	The snowman	is counting	
	Santa	is crying	

Draw a picture of the silly sentence you made and then write the sentence below.

_____

_____

Copyright material from NHS Forth Valley (2020), *Colourful Semantics*, Routledge

'Draw a Line': 'who', 'doing' worksheet 2

Name: _____   Date: _____

who		doing	
?	The farmer	is fighting	
	The elephant	is whispering	
	The monster	is singing	
	The teacher	is drinking	

Draw a picture of the silly sentence you made and then write the sentence below.

_____

_____

Copyright material from NHS Forth Valley (2020), *Colourful Semantics*, Routledge

'Draw a Line': *'who'*, *'doing'* worksheet 3

Name: _____   Date: _____

| who ? | The Queen |
| The astronaut |
| The baby |
| The ghost |

| is swimming | doing |
| is jumping |
| is racing |
| is cleaning |

Draw a picture of the silly sentence you made and then write the sentence below.

_____

_____

Copyright material from NHS Forth Valley (2020), *Colourful Semantics*, Routledge

'Draw a Line': *'who', 'doing'* worksheet 4

Name: _____   Date: _____

who		doing	
?	The hairdresser	is dreaming	
	The boss	is dusting	
	The builder	is mopping	
	The chef	is baking	
	The clown	is talking	

Draw a picture of the silly sentence you made and then write the sentence below.

_____

_____

Copyright material from NHS Forth Valley (2020), *Colourful Semantics*, Routledge

'Draw a Line': *'who', 'doing', 'what'* worksheet 1

Name: _____ Date: _____

who	doing	what
Dad	is ironing	the beetle
The fairy	is wiping	the sweets
The firefighter	is cooking	the dragon
The former	is peeling	the piano

Draw a picture of the silly sentence you made and then write the sentence below.

_____

_____

Copyright material from NHS Forth Valley (2020), *Colourful Semantics*, Routledge

'Draw a Line': *'who', 'doing', 'what'* worksheet 2

Name: _____   Date: _____

who	doing	what
Rudolph	is breaking	the juice
The magician	is phoning	the robot
Granny	is dropping	the ice cream
The postal worker	is fighting	the wallet

Draw a picture of the silly sentence you made and then write the sentence below.

_____

_____

Copyright material from NHS Forth Valley (2020), *Colourful Semantics*, Routledge

'Draw a Line': *'who', 'doing', 'what'* worksheet 3

Name: _____   **Date:** _____

who	doing	what
The superhero	is posting	the cat
The vet	is drawing	the TV
The princess	is following	the pencil
The witch	is hugging	the ballons

Draw a picture of the silly sentence you made and then write the sentence below.

_____

_____

Copyright material from NHS Forth Valley (2020), *Colourful Semantics*, Routledge

'Draw a Line': *'who', 'doing', 'what'* worksheet 4

Name: _____   Date: _____

who	doing	what
The firefighter	is pushing	the beetle
The unicorn	is wiping	the sweets
The bus driver	is cooking	the dragon
The wolf	is peeling	the piano

Draw a picture of the silly sentence you made and then write the sentence below.

_____

_____

Copyright material from NHS Forth Valley (2020), *Colourful Semantics*, Routledge

Name: _____   Date: _____

? who	doing	? what
Santa	is crawling	in the city
The teacher	is sitting	in the garden
Granny	is running	at school
The dog	is crying	at the shop

Draw a picture of the sentence you made and then write the sentence.

_____

_____

Copyright material from NHS Forth Valley (2020), *Colourful Semantics*, Routledge

'Draw a Line': *'who'*, *'doing'*, *'where'* worksheet 2

Name: _____   **Date:** _____

who	doing	what
The angel	is singing	at the beach
The doctor	is climbing	in the living room
The baby	is swimming	in Scotland
The dinosaur	is screaming	at the zoo

Draw a picture of the sentence you made and then write the sentence.

_____

_____

Copyright material from NHS Forth Valley (2020), *Colourful Semantics*, Routledge

Name: _____   **Date:** _____

? who	doing	? what
The man	is crawling	in the park
The nurse	is playing	in the shop
The police officer	is sitting	in the living room
The boy	is crying	in the hospital

Draw a picture of the sentence you made and then write the sentence.

_____

_____

Copyright material from NHS Forth Valley (2020), *Colourful Semantics*, Routledge

'Draw a Line': *'who', 'doing', 'what', 'where'* worksheet 1

Name: _____ **Date:** _____

? who	? doing	? what	? where
The baby	is baking	the penny	in church
The bus driver	is biting	the grapes	at the circus
The singer	is whisking	the envelope	in the cabin
The doctor	is breaking	the desk	at the zoo

Draw a picture of the silly sentence you made and then write the sentence below.

_____

_____

'Draw a Line': *'who', 'doing', 'what', 'where'* worksheet 2

Name: _____   **Date:** _____

who	doing	what	where
The former	is cleaning	the train	in scotland
The vampire	is chewing	the fish and chips	in the dinner hall
The prince	is flushing	the glitter	at the North Pole
The ghost	is building	the watermelon	in outer space

Draw a picture of the silly sentence you made and then write the sentence below.

_____

_____

Copyright material from NHS Forth Valley (2020), *Colourful Semantics*, Routledge

'Draw a Line': *'who', 'doing', 'what', 'where'* worksheet 3

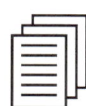

Name: _____   **Date:** _____

? who	? doing	? what	? where
The vet	is climbing	the giraffe	in the library
The soldier	is cutting	the book	in the car wash
The boy	is cooking	the boat	in the gym hall
The lady	is painting	the window	in the castle

Draw a picture of the silly sentence you made and then write the sentence below.

_____

_____

Copyright material from NHS Forth Valley (2020), *Colourful Semantics*, Routledge

'Draw a Line': *'who', 'doing', 'what', 'where'* worksheet 4

Name: _____   Date: _____

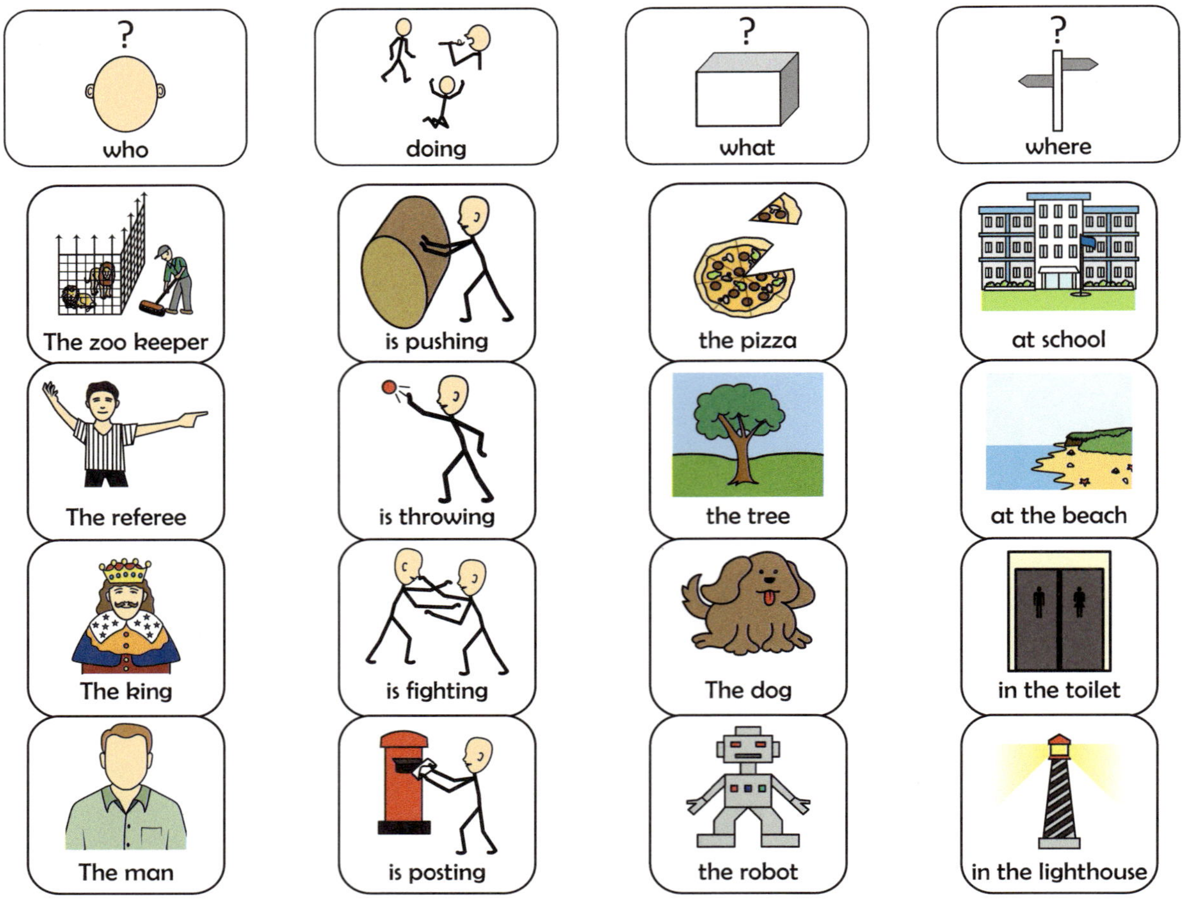

who	doing	what	where
The zoo keeper	is pushing	the pizza	at school
The referee	is throwing	the tree	at the beach
The king	is fighting	The dog	in the toilet
The man	is posting	the robot	in the lighthouse

Draw a picture of the silly sentence you made and then write the sentence below.

_____

_____

Copyright material from NHS Forth Valley (2020), *Colourful Semantics*, Routledge

'Draw a Line': *'who'*, *'doing'*, *'what'*, *'where'*, *'when'* worksheet 1

Name: _____

Date: _____

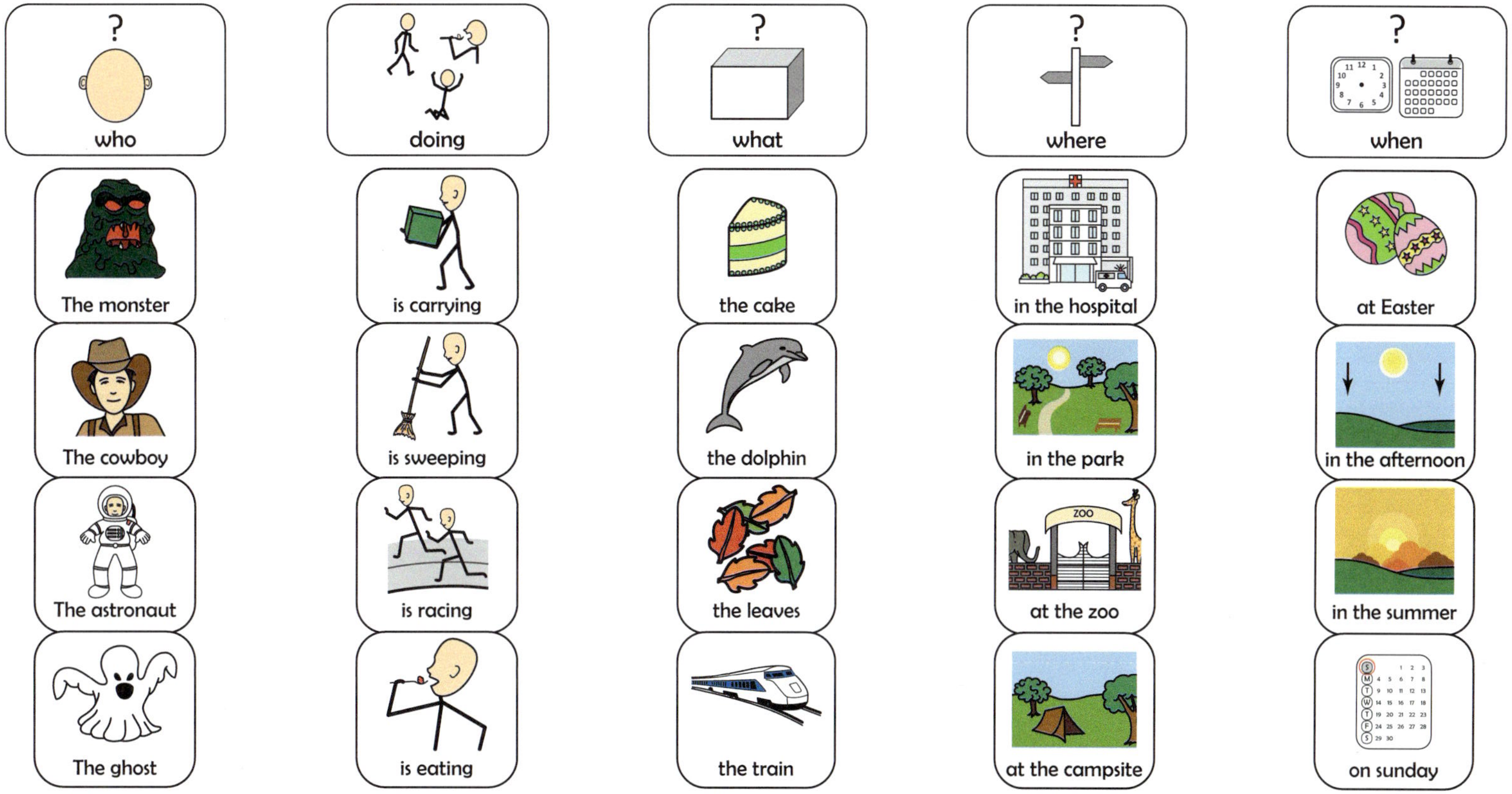

who

?:

The monster

The cowboy

The astronaut

The ghost

doing

?:

is carrying

is sweeping

is racing

is eating

what

?:

the cake

the dolphin

the leaves

the train

where

?:

in the hospital

in the park

at the zoo

at the campsite

when

?:

at Easter

in the afternoon

in the summer

on sunday

Write the sentence you made below and then draw a picture of the sentence on the back of this page.

_____

_____

Copyright material from NHS Forth Valley (2020), *Colourful Semantics*, Routledge

'Draw a Line': *'who', 'doing', 'what', 'where', 'when'* worksheet 2

Name: _____

Date: _____

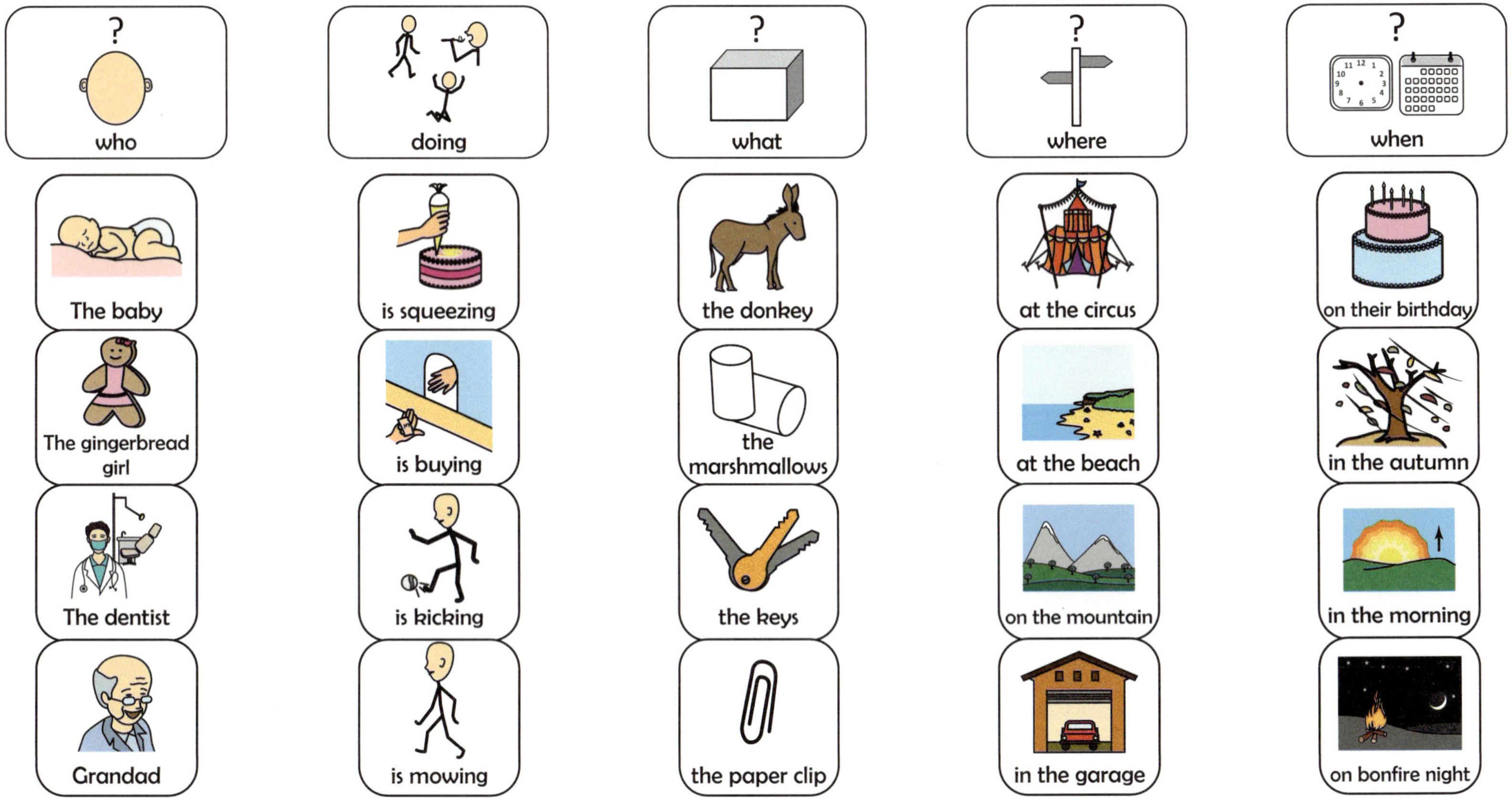

who ?
- The baby
- The gingerbread girl
- The dentist
- Grandad

doing ?
- is squeezing
- is buying
- is kicking
- is mowing

what ?
- the donkey
- the marshmallows
- the keys
- the paper clip

where ?
- at the circus
- at the beach
- on the mountain
- in the garage

when ?
- on their birthday
- in the autumn
- in the morning
- on bonfire night

Write the sentence you made below and then draw a picture of the sentence on the back of this page.

_____
_____
_____

Copyright material from 'NHS Forth Valley (2020), *Colourful Semantics*, Routledge

'Draw a Line': *'who'*, *'doing'*, *'what'*, *'where'*, *'when'* worksheet 3

Name: _____

Date: _____

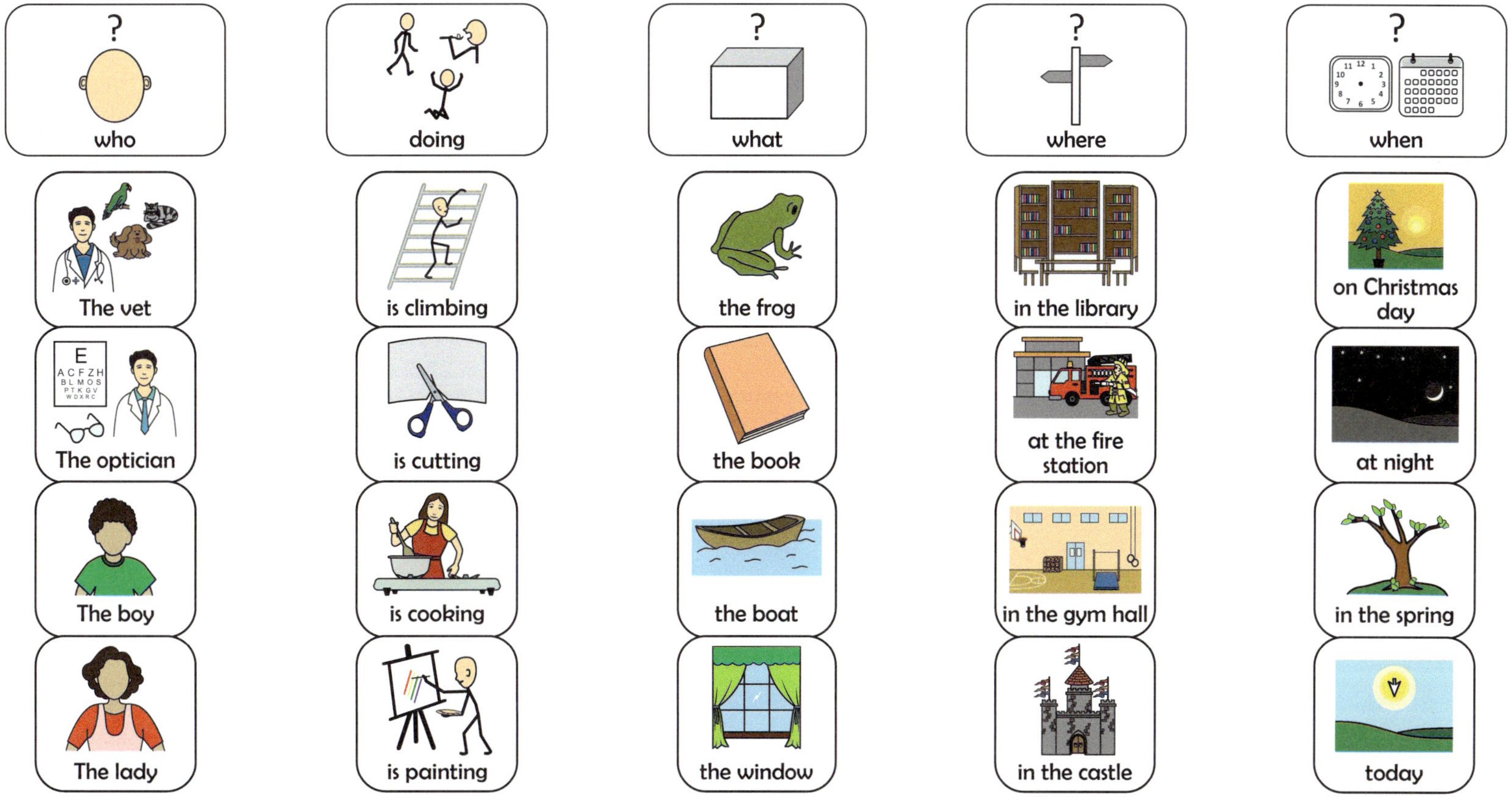

who

? | The vet | The optician | The boy | The lady

doing

? | is climbing | is cutting | is cooking | is painting

what

? | the frog | the book | the boat | the window

where

? | in the library | at the fire station | in the gym hall | in the castle

when

? | on Christmas day | at night | in the spring | today

Write the sentence you made below and then draw a picture of the sentence on the back of this page.

_____

_____

Copyright material from NHS Forth Valley (2020), *Colourful Semantics*, Routledge

'Draw a Line': *'who', 'doing', 'what', 'where', 'when'* worksheet 4

Name: _____

Date: _____

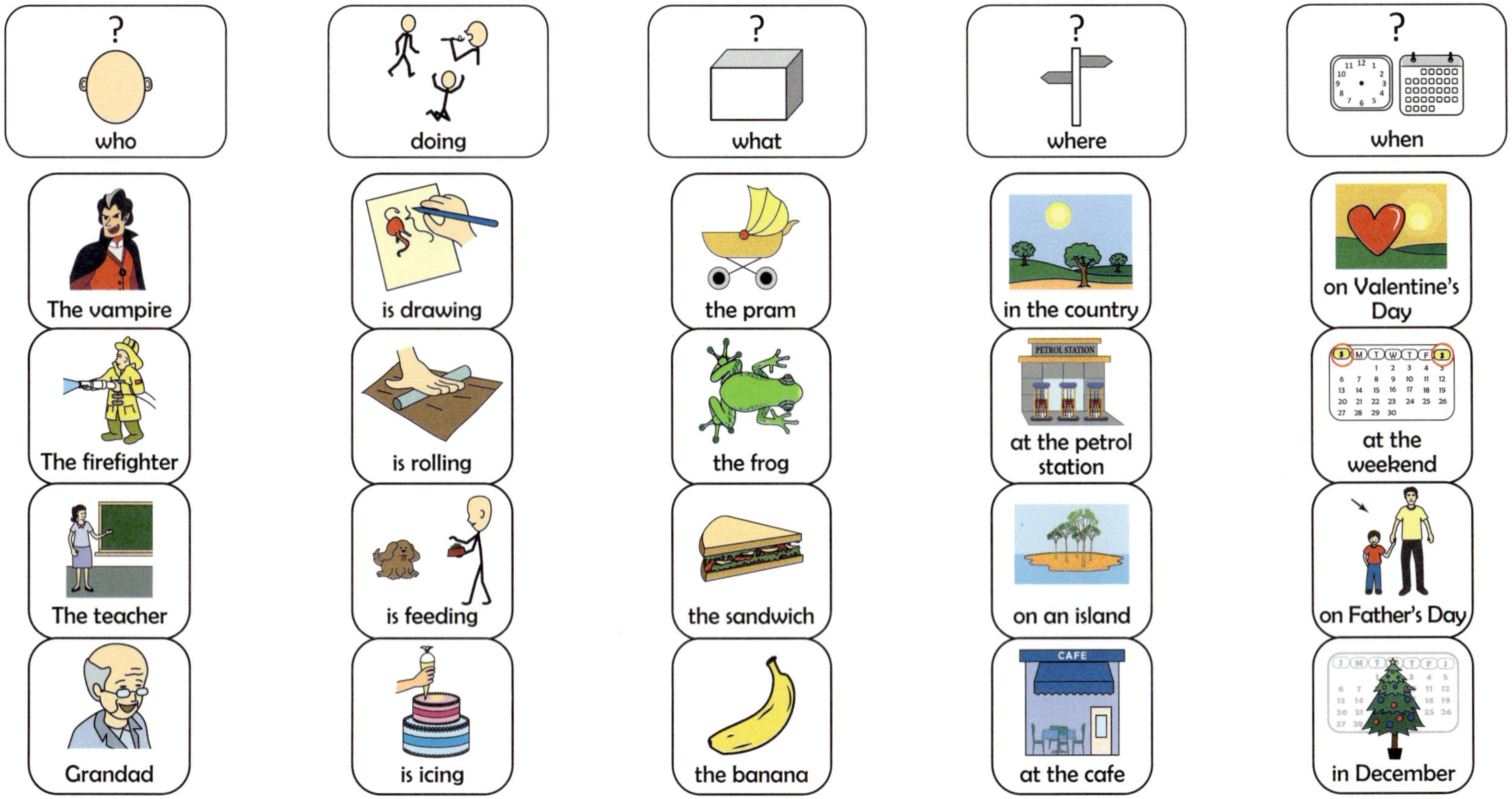

who

The vampire

The firefighter

The teacher

Grandad

doing

is drawing

is rolling

is feeding

is icing

what

the pram

the frog

the sandwich

the banana

where

in the country

at the petrol station

on an island

at the cafe

when

on Valentine's Day

at the weekend

on Father's Day

in December

Write the sentence you made below and then draw a picture of the sentence on the back of this page.

_____

_____

Copyright material from NHS Forth Valley (2020), *Colourful Semantics*, Routledge

'Cut and Stick' worksheets

'Cut and Stick' worksheets are an alternative way to practise early writing and creation of 'silly sentences'. These are more challenging than 'Draw a Line', as children need to work out which pictures go with each component of the sentence, so they can put it in the right place in the sentence, e.g. knowing that 'the nurse' is a 'who', or that 'is jumping' is a 'doing'. As with 'Draw a Line' worksheets, it is important to spend time first introducing and discussing the pictured vocabulary with the children and demonstrating how to complete a worksheet with the whole group or class. Children then complete their own worksheet in the following steps:

- Cut along the marked line and cut out all the vocabulary pictures from the top of the worksheet.

- Decide which sentence component each word is, e.g. which words are 'who', which are 'doing' etc. and mark each picture with the correct colour for that sentence component, e.g. orange for 'who' pictures.

- Practise making different sentences by placing the vocabulary pictures on the correct box on the box template underneath, then point to the pictures left to right while saying the sentence.

- Select their favourite word for each sentence component, e.g. their favourite 'who', favourite 'doing' and favourite 'where', and stick each one onto the correct place on the box template.

- Say the sentence they made.

- Write the sentence.

- Colour code the written sentence by underlining the sentence components in their correct colour.

- Drawing a picture of the sentence they created on the back of the worksheet.

Below is an example of how to complete a 'Cut and Stick' worksheet for 'who' and 'doing'.

Copyright material from NHS Forth Valley (2020), *Colourful Semantics*, Routledge

Cut out the pictures. Make some silly sentences. Glue your favourite 'who' and 'doing' words onto the boxes below to make a sentence. Then write the sentence underneath.

The king

is jumping

The girl

is sleeping

is drawing

The nurse

Name: _____   Date: _____

?
who

doing

_____
_____

Now draw a picture of the silly sentence you made on the back!

Name: _____   Date: _____

The king

is sleeping

The king is sleeping.

_____

Now draw a picture of the silly sentence you made on the back!

Blank 'Cut and Stick' worksheets are provided, for use at a range of different ability levels, on pages 213–231.

Copyright material from NHS Forth Valley (2020), *Colourful Semantics*, Routledge

'Cut and Stick': 'who', 'doing' worksheet 1

Cut out the pictures. Make some silly sentences. Glue your favourite 'who' and 'doing' words onto the boxes below to make a sentence. Then write the sentence underneath.

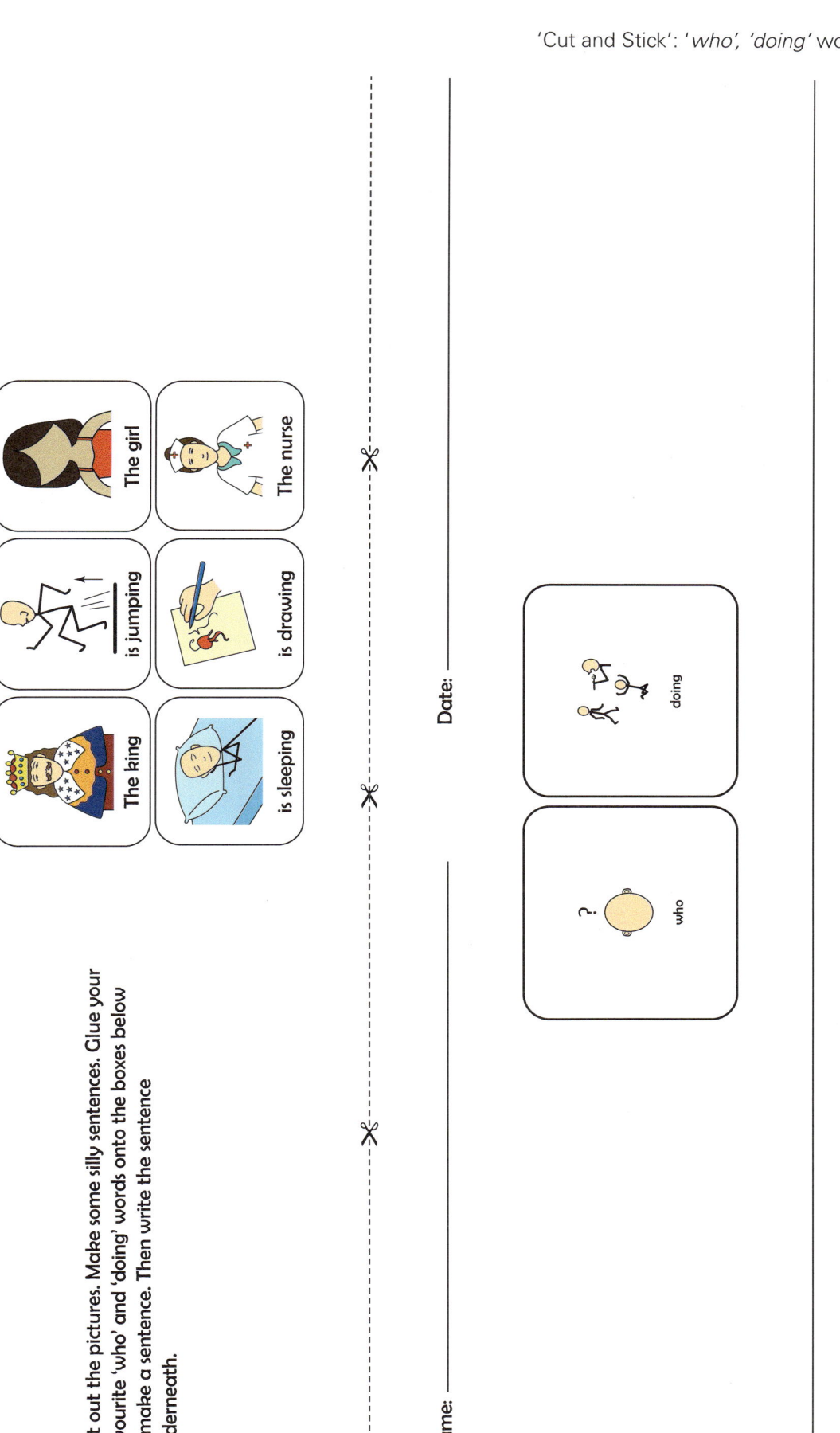

The girl

is jumping

The king

The nurse

is drawing

is sleeping

Name:

Date:

who

doing

Now draw a picture of the silly sentence you made on the back!

Copyright material from NHS Forth Valley (2020), *Colourful Semantics*, Routledge

'Cut and Stick': 'who', 'doing' worksheet 2

Cut out the pictures. Make some silly sentences. Glue your favourite 'who' and 'doing' words onto the boxes below to make a sentence. Then write the sentence underneath.

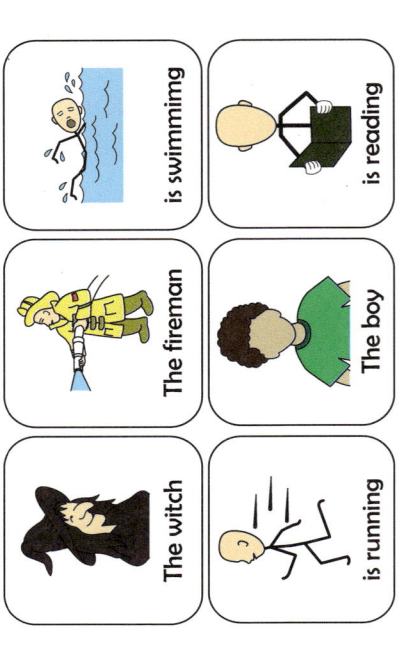

Name:

Date:

who

doing

Now draw a picture of the silly sentence you made on the back!

Copyright material from NHS Forth Valley (2020), *Colourful Semantics*, Routledge

'Cut and Stick': '*who*', '*doing*' worksheet 3

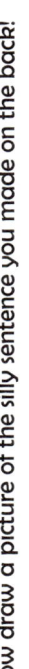

Cut out the pictures. Make some silly sentences. Glue your favourite 'who' and 'doing' words onto the boxes below to make a sentence. Then write the sentence underneath.

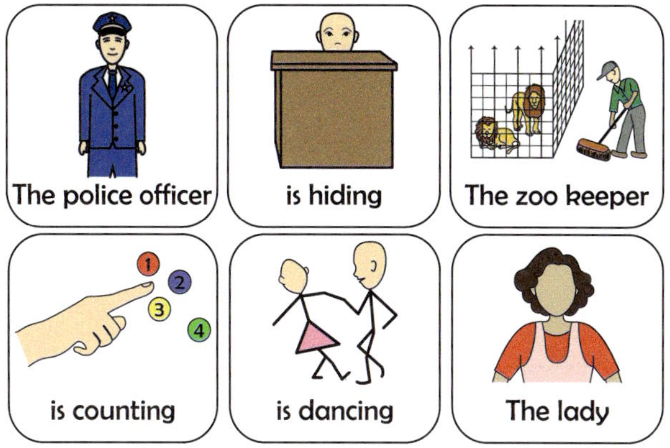

The zoo keeper

The lady

is hiding

is dancing

The police officer

is counting

Name:

Date:

who

doing

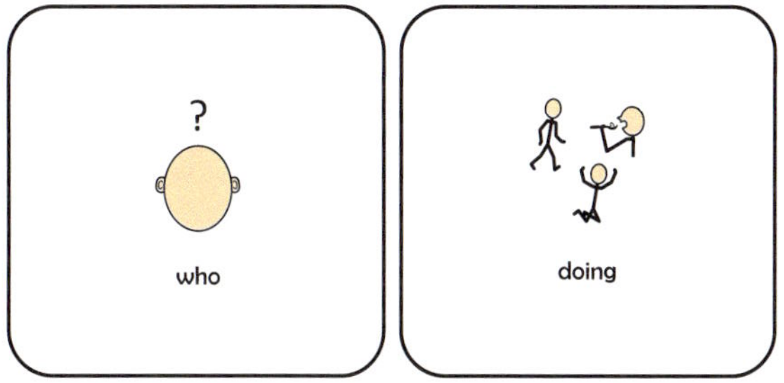

Now draw a picture of the silly sentence you made on the back!

Copyright material from NHS Forth Valley (2020), *Colourful Semantics*, Routledge

'Cut and Stick': *'who'*, *'doing'*, *'what'* worksheet 1

Cut out the pictures. Make some silly sentences.
Glue your favourite 'who', 'doing' and 'what'
words onto the boxes below to make a sentence.
Then write the sentence underneath.

The firefighter

is painting

the flower

the TV

is licking

The wizard

is watching

The cup

The boy

Date:

who

doing

what

Name:

Now draw a picture of the silly sentence you made on the back!

Copyright material from NHS Forth Valley (2020), *Colourful Semantics*, Routledge

'Cut and Stick': 'who', 'doing', 'what' worksheet 2

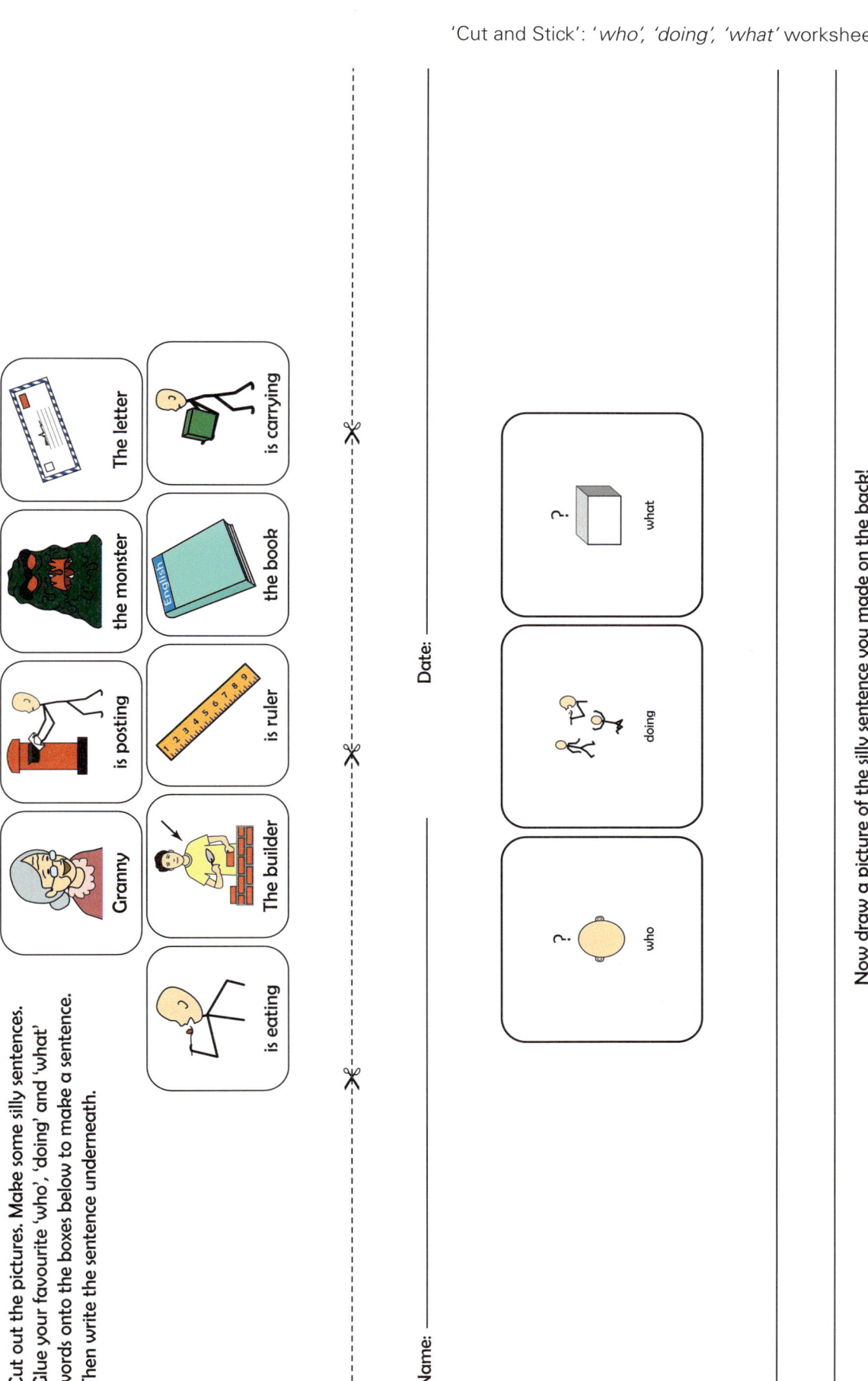

Cut out the pictures. Make some silly sentences.
Glue your favourite 'who', 'doing' and 'what'
words onto the boxes below to make a sentence.
Then write the sentence underneath.

The letter

is carrying

the monster

the book

is posting

is ruler

Granny

The builder

is eating

Name:

Date:

who

doing

what

Now draw a picture of the silly sentence you made on the back!

Copyright material from NHS Forth Valley (2020), *Colourful Semantics*, Routledge

'Cut and Stick': *'who'*, *'doing'*, *'what'* worksheet 3

Cut out the pictures. Make some silly sentences.
Glue your favourite 'who', 'doing' and 'what'
words onto the boxes below to make a sentence.
Then write the sentence underneath.

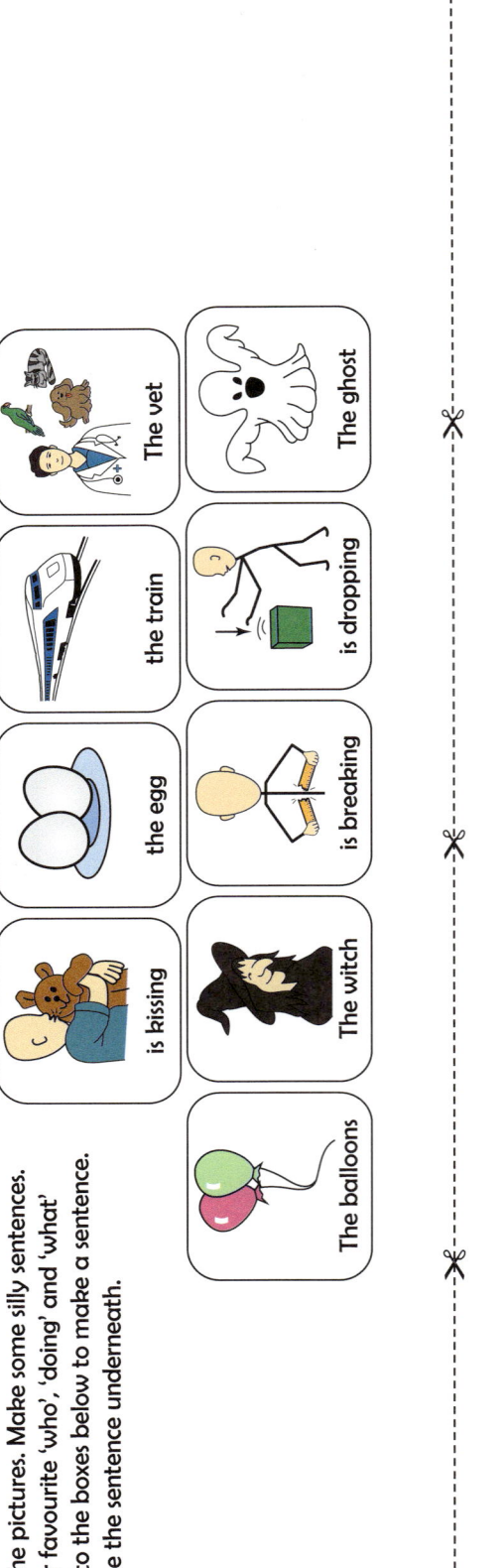

The vet

The ghost

the train

is dropping

the egg

is breaking

is kissing

The witch

The balloons

Name: _____

Date: _____

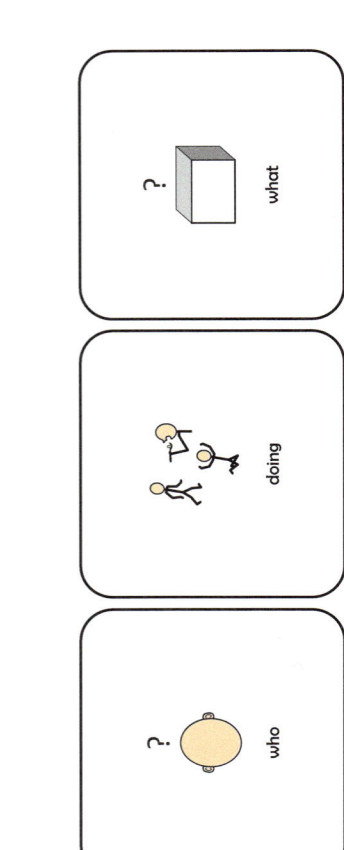

who

doing

what

Now draw a picture of the silly sentence you made on the back!

Copyright material from NHS Forth Valley (2020), *Colourful Semantics*, Routledge

'Cut and Stick': *'who'*, *'doing'*, *'where'* worksheet 1

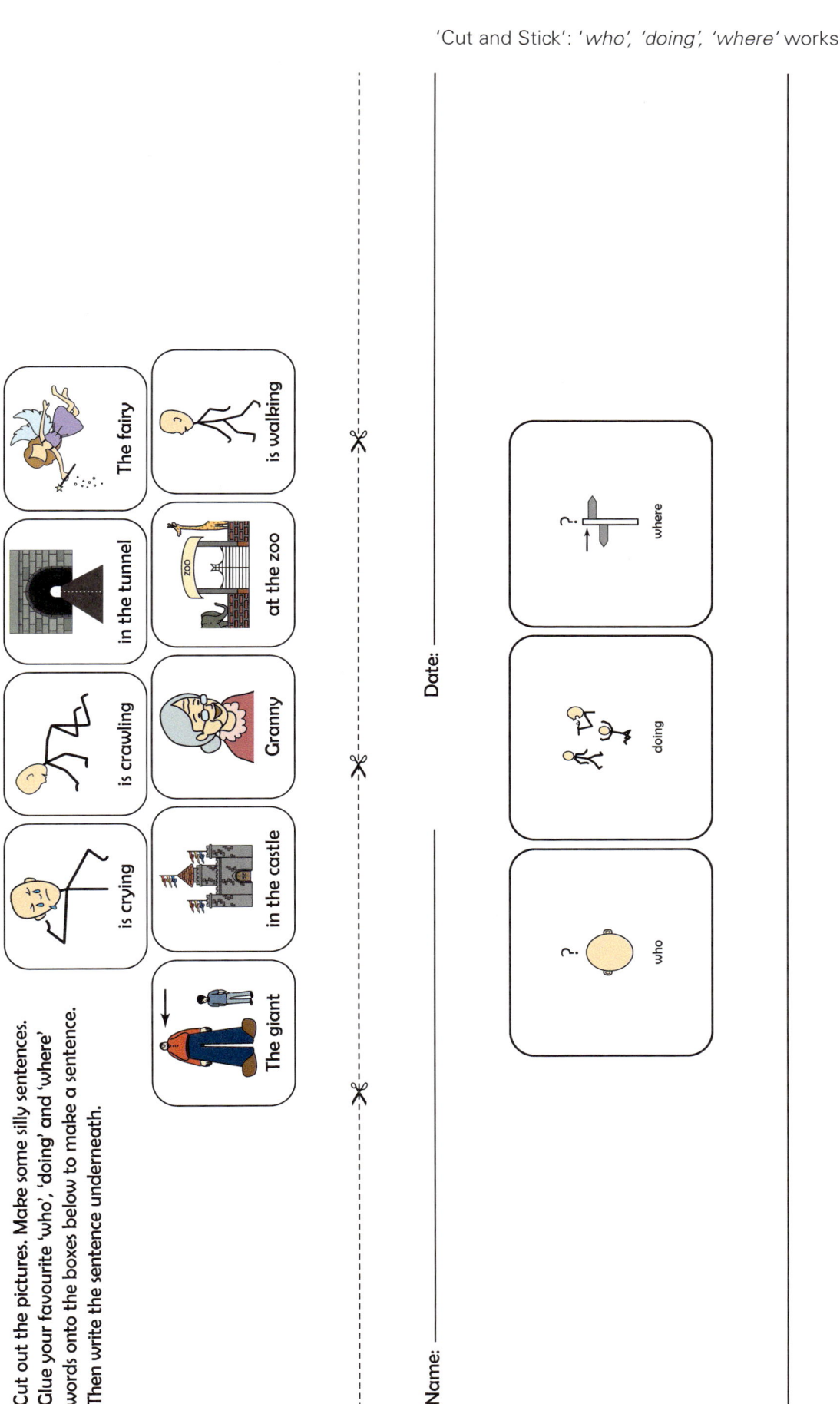

Cut out the pictures. Make some silly sentences. Glue your favourite 'who', 'doing' and 'where' words onto the boxes below to make a sentence. Then write the sentence underneath.

The fairy

is walking

in the tunnel

at the zoo

is crawling

Granny

is crying

in the castle

The giant

Name: _____

Date: _____

who

doing

where

Now draw a picture of the silly sentence you made on the back!

Copyright material from NHS Forth Valley (2020), *Colourful Semantics*, Routledge

'Cut and Stick': *'who'*, *'doing'*, *'where'* worksheet 2

Cut out the pictures. Make some silly sentences.
Glue your favourite 'who', 'doing' and 'where'
words onto the boxes below to make a sentence.
Then write the sentence underneath.

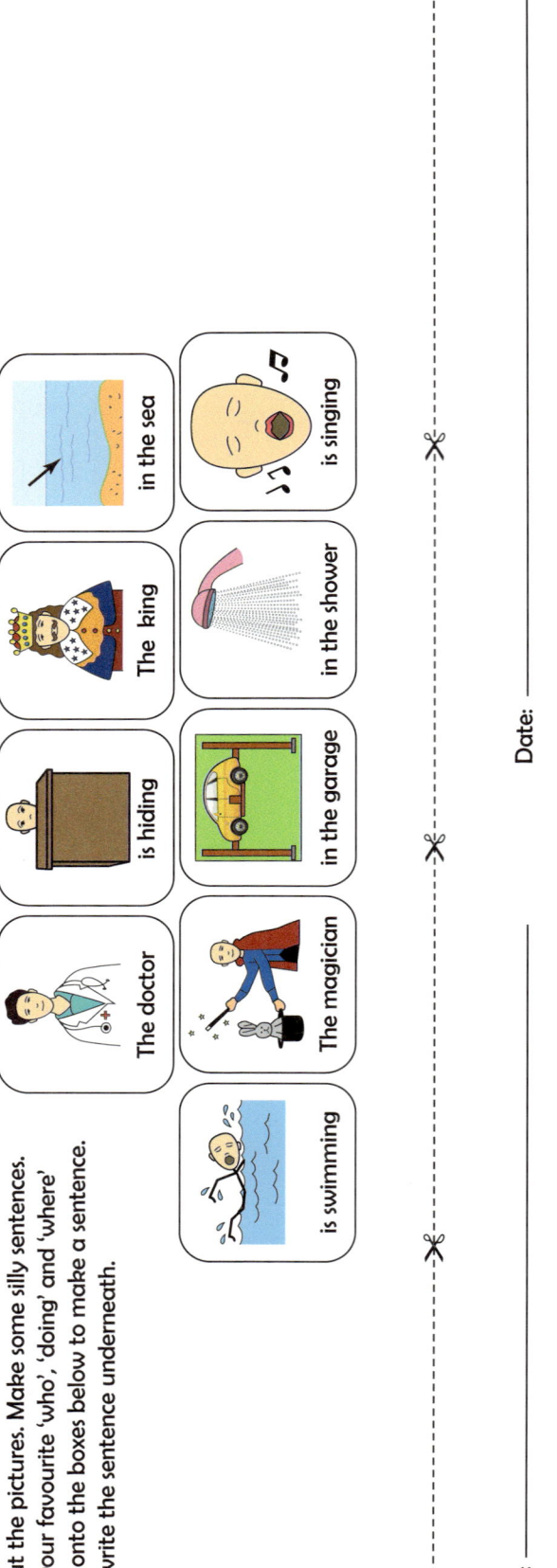

in the sea

is singing

The king

in the shower

is hiding

in the garage

The doctor

The magician

is swimming

Name: _____

Date: _____

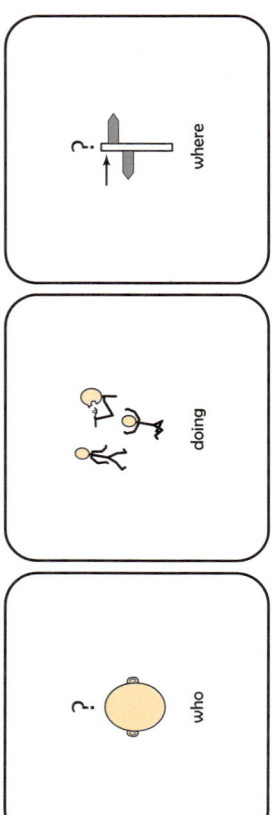

who

doing

where

Now draw a picture of the silly sentence you made on the back!

Copyright material from NHS Forth Valley (2020), *Colourful Semantics*, Routledge

'Cut and Stick': *'who'*, *'doing'*, *'where'* worksheet 3

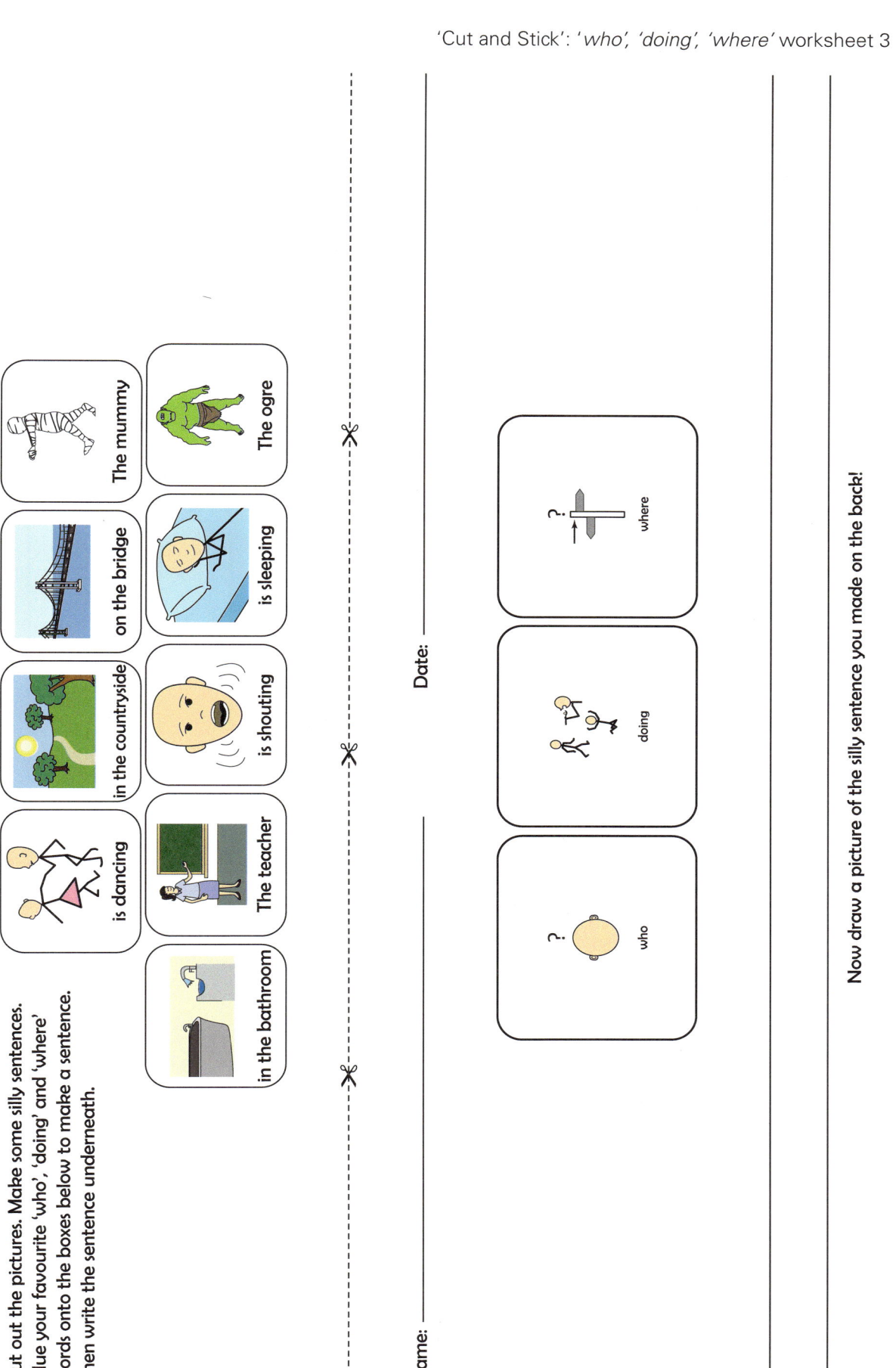

Cut out the pictures. Make some silly sentences.
Glue your favourite 'who', 'doing' and 'where'
words onto the boxes below to make a sentence.
Then write the sentence underneath.

The mummy

The ogre

on the bridge

is sleeping

in the countryside

is shouting

is dancing

The teacher

in the bathroom

Name:

Date:

who

doing

where

Now draw a picture of the silly sentence you made on the back!

Copyright material from NHS Forth Valley (2020), *Colourful Semantics*, Routledge

'Cut and Stick': *'who'*, *'doing'*, *'what'*, *'where'* worksheet 1

Cut out the pictures. Make some silly sentences. Glue your favourite 'who', 'doing', 'what' and 'where' words onto the boxes below to make a sentence. Then write the sentence underneath.

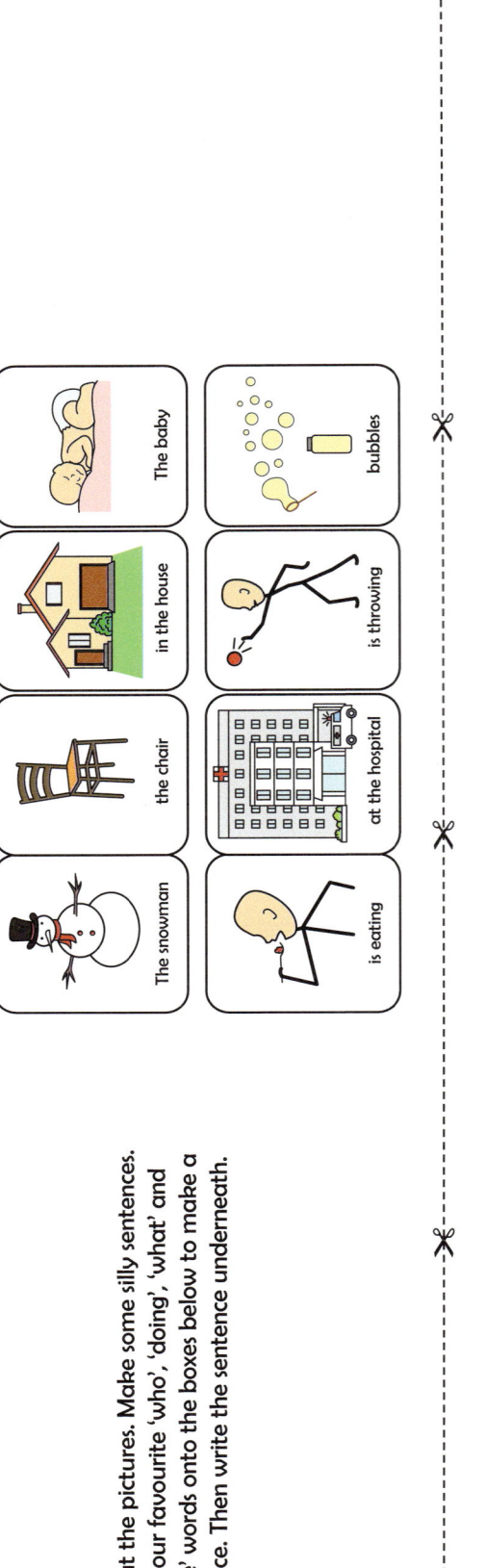

Name: _____

Date: _____

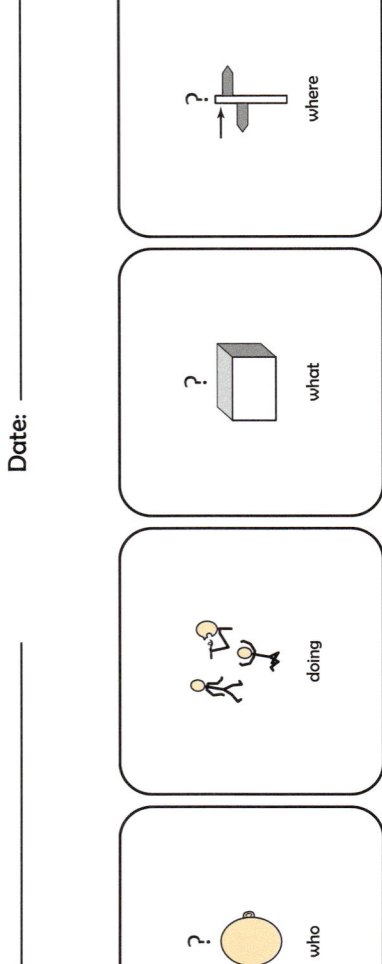

Now draw a picture of the silly sentence you made on the back!

Copyright material from NHS Forth Valley (2020), *Colourful Semantics*, Routledge

'Cut and Stick': 'who', 'doing', 'what', 'where' worksheet 2

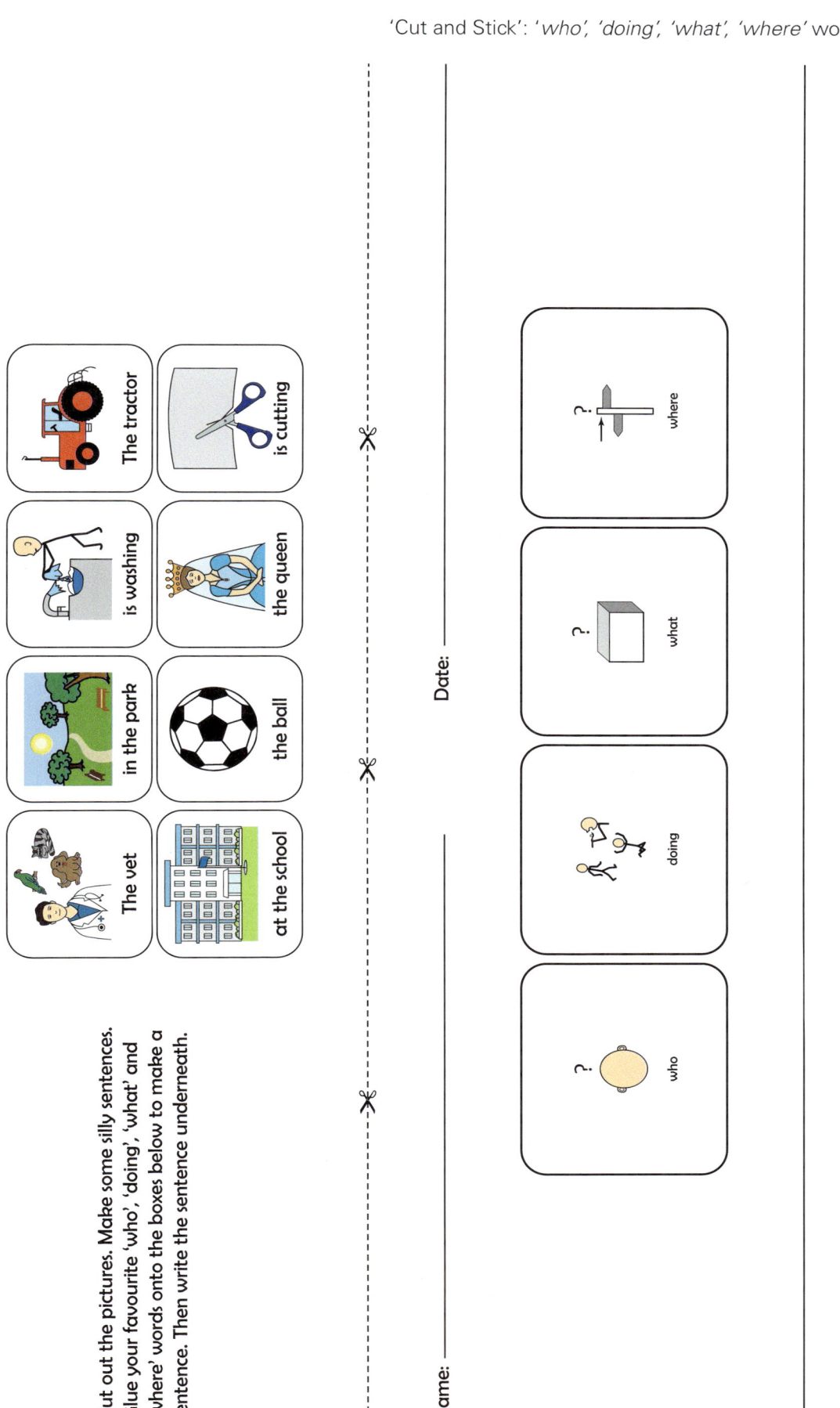

Cut out the pictures. Make some silly sentences. Glue your favourite 'who', 'doing', 'what' and 'where' words onto the boxes below to make a sentence. Then write the sentence underneath.

The tractor

is cutting

is washing

the queen

in the park

the ball

The vet

at the school

Name: _____

Date: _____

who

doing

what

where

Now draw a picture of the silly sentence you made on the back!

Copyright material from NHS Forth Valley (2020), *Colourful Semantics*, Routledge

'Cut and Stick': 'who', 'doing', 'what', 'where' worksheet 3

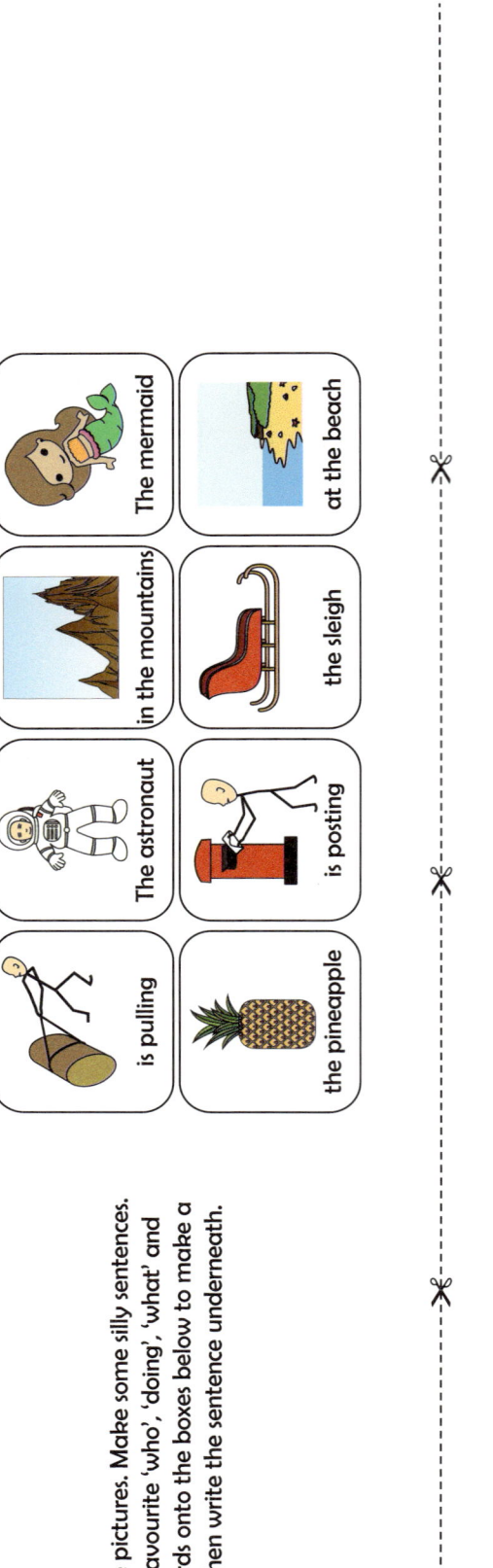

Cut out the pictures. Make some silly sentences. Glue your favourite 'who', 'doing', 'what' and 'where' words onto the boxes below to make a sentence. Then write the sentence underneath.

Name:

Date:

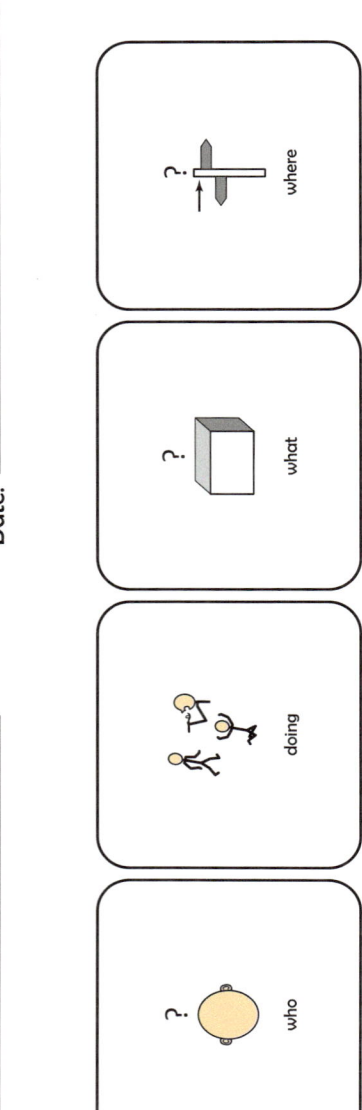

Now draw a picture of the silly sentence you made on the back!

Copyright material from NHS Forth Valley (2020), *Colourful Semantics*, Routledge

'Cut and Stick': *'who'*, *'doing'*, *'what'*, *'where'*, *'when'* worksheet 1

Cut out the pictures. Make some silly sentences.
Glue your favourite 'who', 'doing', 'what', 'where'
and 'when' words onto the boxes below to make
a sentence. Then write the sentence underneath.

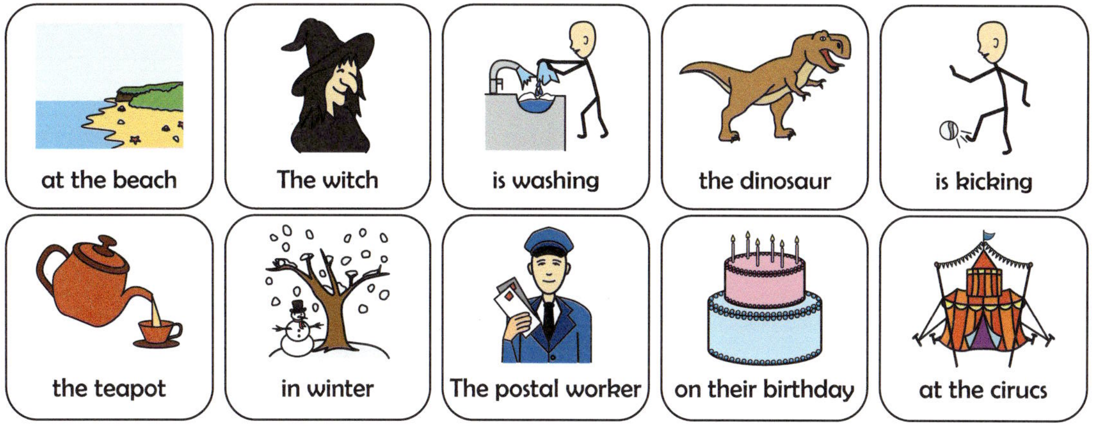

is kicking

at the cirucs

the dinosaur

on their birthday

is washing

The postal worker

The witch

in winter

at the beach

the teapot

Name: _____

Date: _____

who

doing

what

where

when

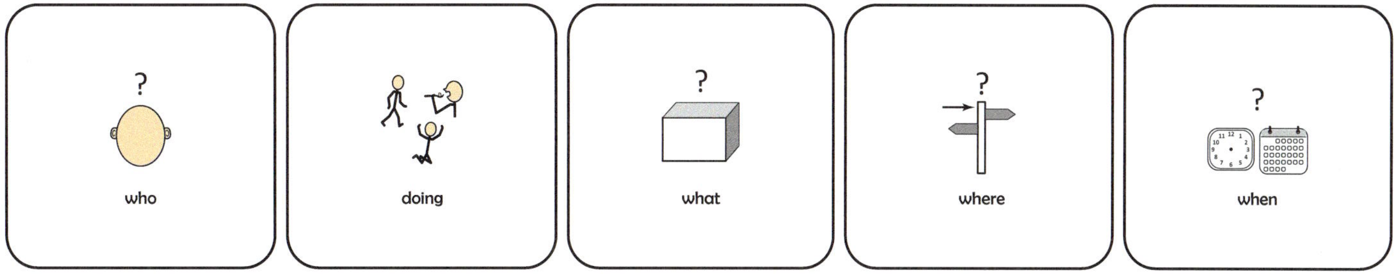

Now draw a picture of the silly sentence you made on the back!

Copyright material from NHS Forth Valley (2020), *Colourful Semantics*, Routledge

'Cut and Stick': *'who', 'doing', 'what', 'where'* and *'when'* worksheet 2

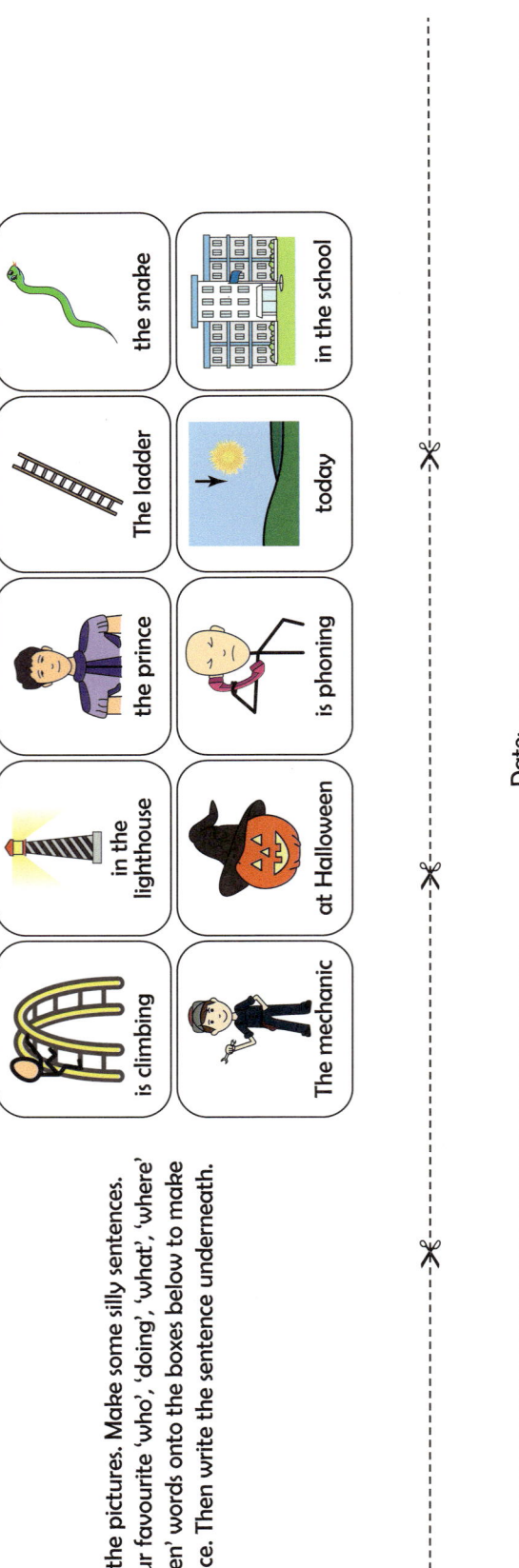

Cut out the pictures. Make some silly sentences.
Glue your favourite 'who', 'doing', 'what', 'where' and 'when' words onto the boxes below to make a sentence. Then write the sentence underneath.

the snake

in the school

The ladder

today

the prince

is phoning

in the lighthouse

at Halloween

is climbing

The mechanic

Name: _____

Date: _____

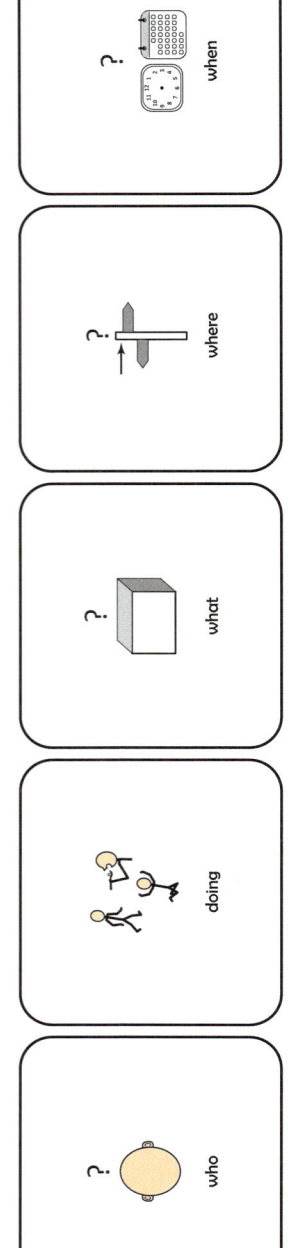

who

doing

what

where

when

Now draw a picture of the silly sentence you made on the back!

Copyright material from NHS Forth Valley (2020), *Colourful Semantics*, Routledge

'Cut and Stick': *'who', 'doing', 'what', 'where', 'when'* worksheet 3

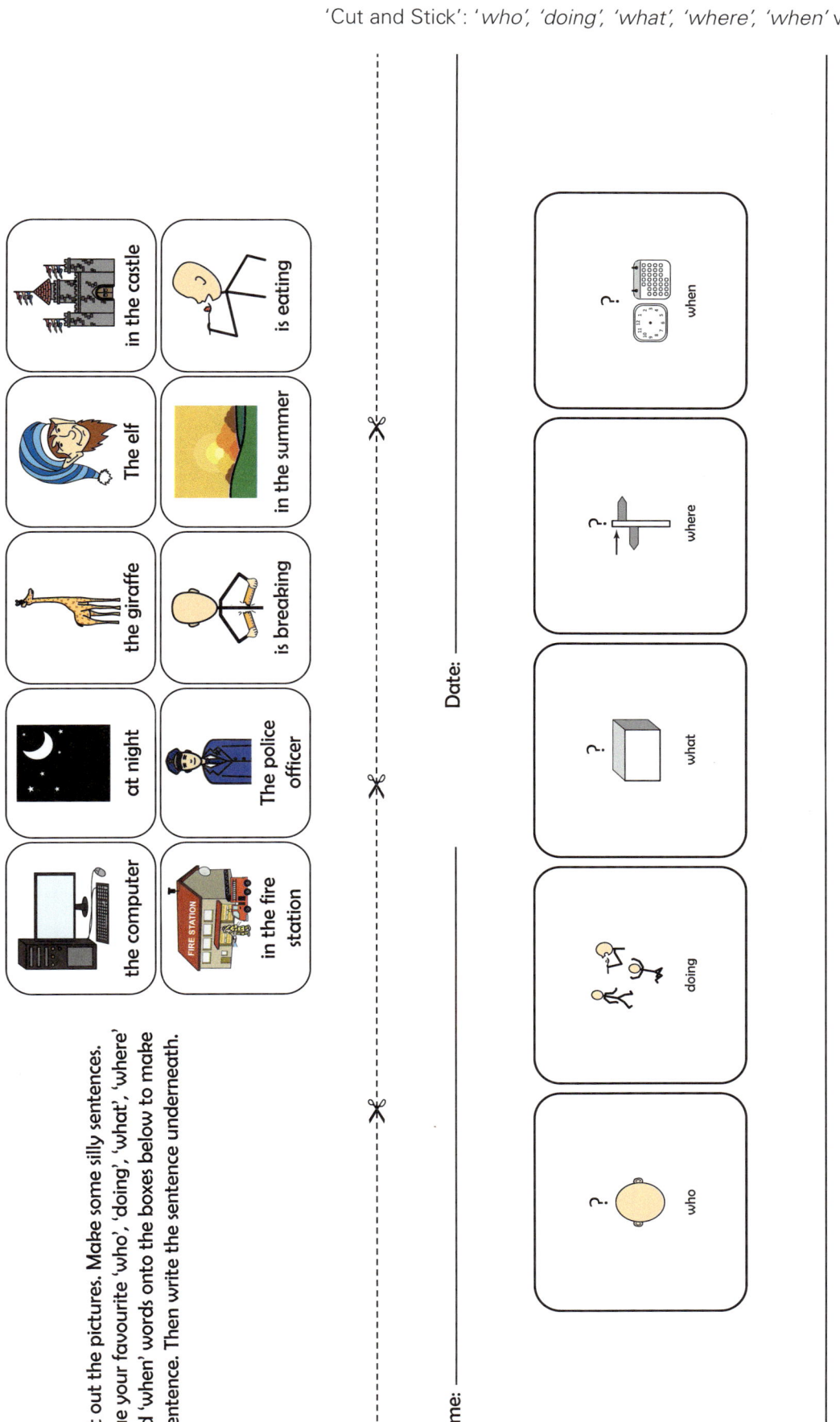

Cut out the pictures. Make some silly sentences.
Glue your favourite 'who', 'doing', 'what', 'where' and 'when' words onto the boxes below to make a sentence. Then write the sentence underneath.

in the castle

is eating

The elf

in the summer

the giraffe

is breaking

at night

The police officer

the computer

in the fire station

Name:

Date:

who

doing

what

where

when

Now draw a picture of the silly sentence you made on the back!

Copyright material from NHS Forth Valley (2020), *Colourful Semantics*, Routledge

'Cut and Stick': *'who', 'doing', 'what', 'to who'* worksheet 1

Cut out the pictures. Make some silly sentences.
Glue your favourite 'who', 'doing', 'what' and 'to who' words onto the boxes below to make a sentence. Then write the sentence underneath.

to the dragon

to the wolf

the homework

is showing

The witch

a rocket

The scuba diver

is giving

Name:

Date:

who

doing

what

to who

Now draw a picture of your favourite silly sentence on the back!

Copyright material from NHS Forth Valley (2020), *Colourful Semantics*, Routledge

'Cut and Stick': *'who'*, *'doing'*, *'what'*, *'to who'* worksheet 2

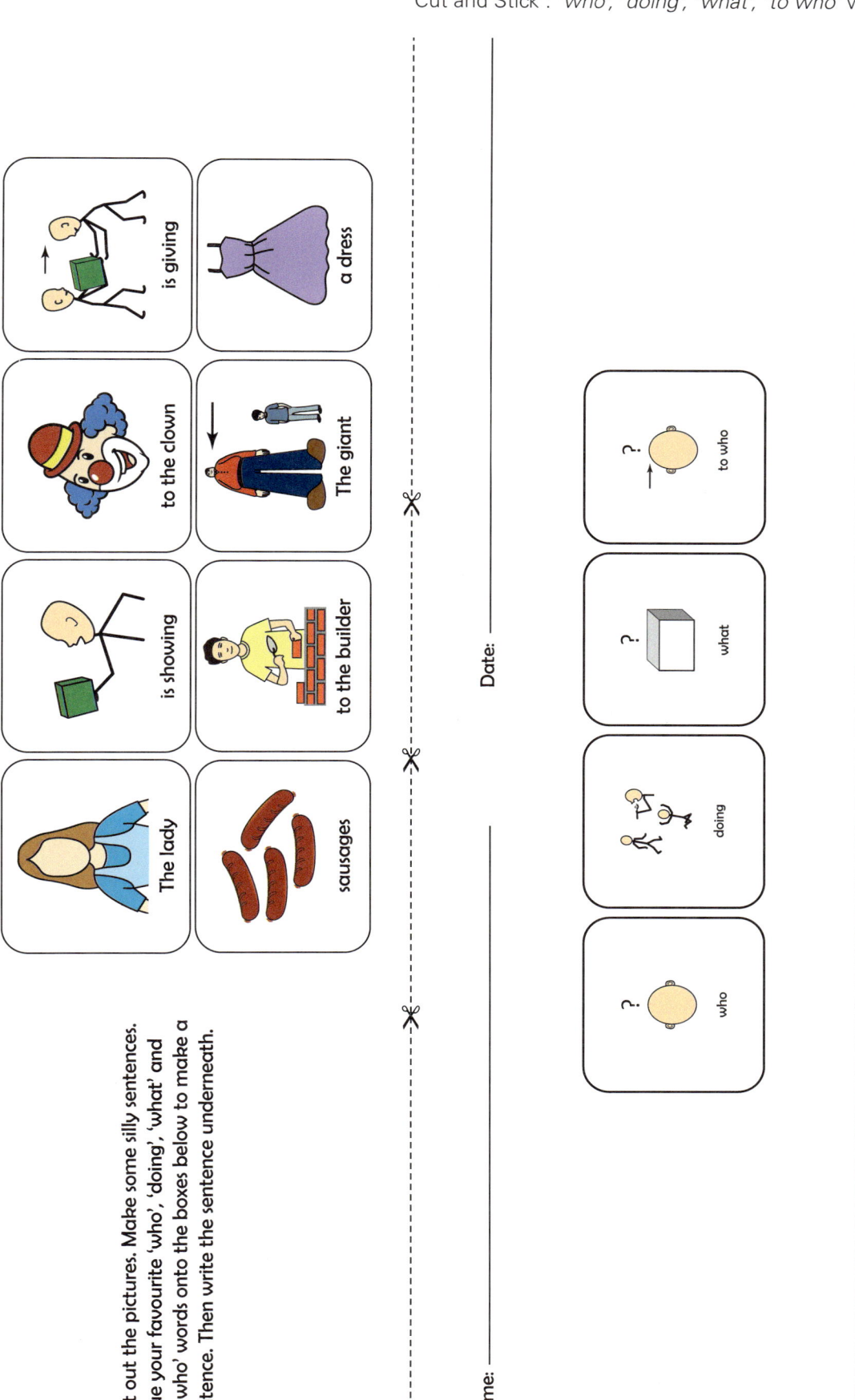

Cut out the pictures. Make some silly sentences. Glue your favourite 'who', 'doing', 'what' and 'to who' words onto the boxes below to make a sentence. Then write the sentence underneath.

is giving

a dress

to the clown

The giant

is showing

to the builder

The lady

sausages

Name: _____

Date: _____

who

doing

what

to who

Now draw a picture of your favourite silly sentence on the back!

Copyright material from NHS Forth Valley (2020), *Colourful Semantics*, Routledge

'Cut and Stick': *'who'*, *'doing'*, *'what'*, *'to who'*, *'where'* worksheet 1

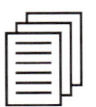

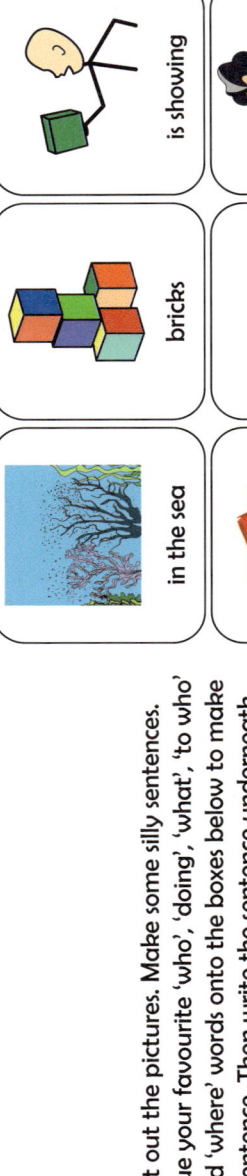

Cut out the pictures. Make some silly sentences.
Glue your favourite 'who', 'doing', 'what', 'to who'
and 'where' words onto the boxes below to make
a sentence. Then write the sentence underneath.

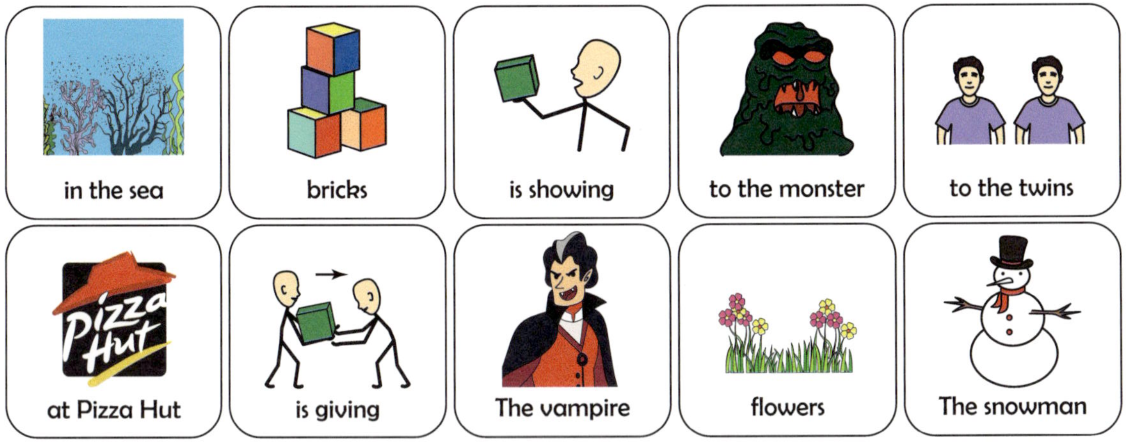

Name:

Date:

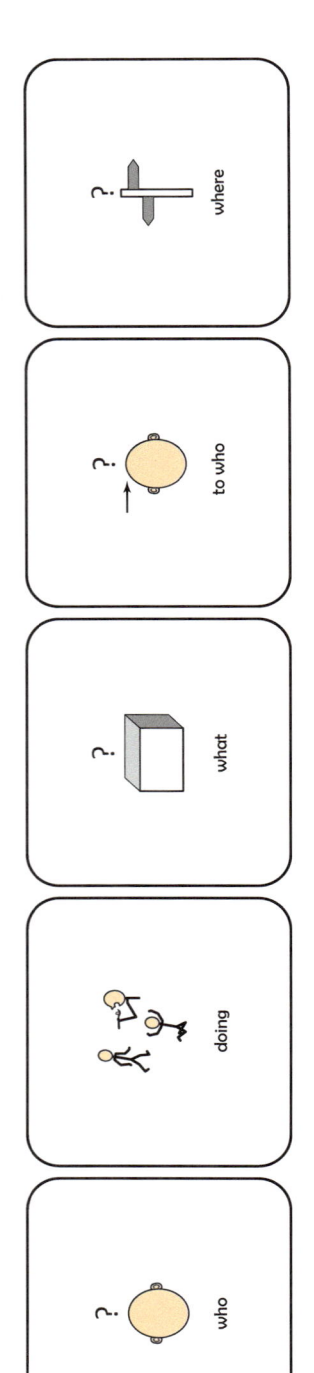

Now draw a picture of your favourite silly sentence on the back!

Copyright material from NHS Forth Valley (2020), *Colourful Semantics*, Routledge

'Cut and Stick': *'who', 'doing', 'what', 'to who', 'where'* worksheet 2

a ladybird

at the zoo

in outer space

The pilot

a cake

is showing

Superman

is giving

to the ballerina

to the teacher

Cut out the pictures. Make some silly sentences.
Glue your favourite 'who', 'doing', 'what', 'to who'
and 'where' words onto the boxes below to make
a sentence. Then write the sentence underneath.

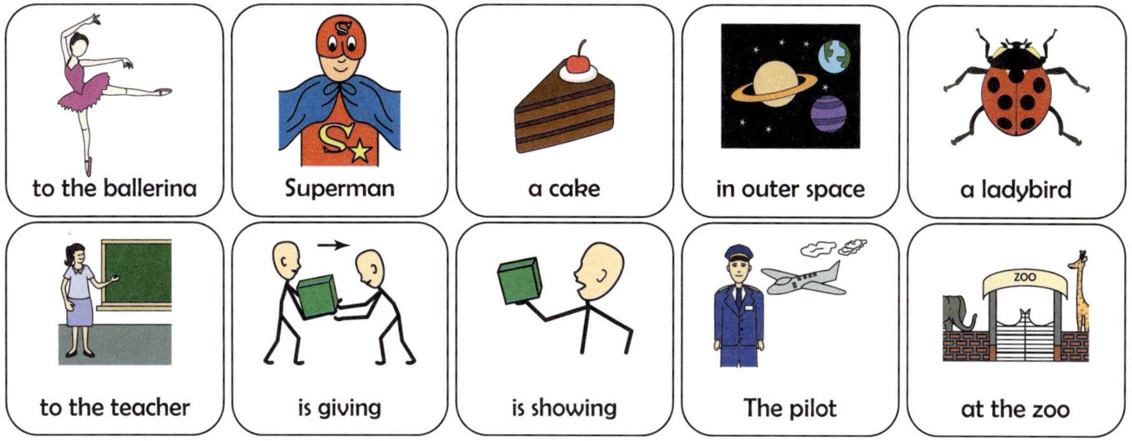

Date: _____

Name: _____

where

to who

what

doing

who

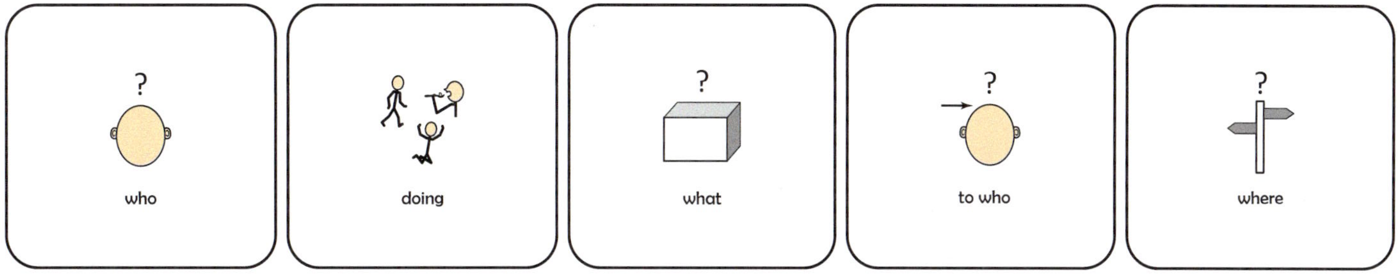

Now draw a picture of your favourite silly sentence on the back!

Copyright material from NHS Forth Valley (2020), *Colourful Semantics*, Routledge

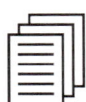

Appendix 7

Picture description and sequencing worksheets

This section provides sample worksheets for writing about one picture or a picture sequence and demonstrates how worksheets could be differentiated for the ability levels of different children. Three suggested levels of difficulty are provided for each worksheet to show how this might be done.

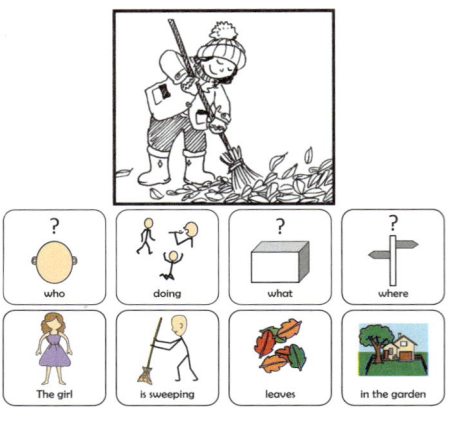

Level 1: Cue card sentence template provided; vocabulary pictures provided in the correct order to make the sentence, from left to right

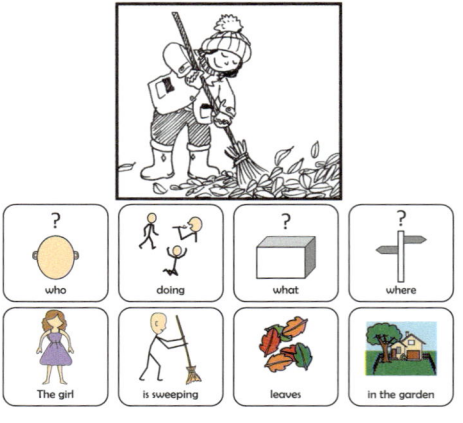

Level 2: Cue card sentence template provided; vocabulary pictures provided in a mixed up order left to right, requiring learners to reorder the vocabulary to make the sentence

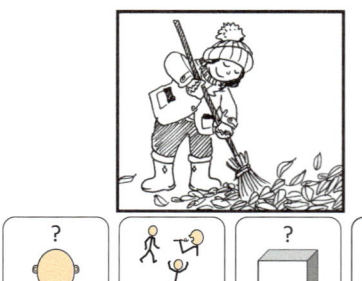

Level 3: Only the cue card sentence template is provided, to challenge children to generate their own vocabulary for their sentence

Copyright material from NHS Forth Valley (2020), *Colourful Semantics*, Routledge

Worksheet: Autumn Leaves

Name: _____ Date: _____

Write a sentence about the autumn leaves picture. Colour the question words and small pictures in the correct colours first to help you. After writing the sentence, underline the 'who', 'doing', 'what' and 'where' words in the correct colour.

?		?	?
who	doing	what	where
The girl	is sweeping	leaves	in the garden

_____

_____

_____

Copyright material from NHS Forth Valley (2020), *Colourful Semantics*, Routledge

Worksheet: Autumn Leaves

Name: _____   Date: _____

Write a sentence about the autumn leaves picture. Colour the question words and small pictures in the correct colours first to help you. Then work out which order the words in the sentence should come in. After writing your sentence, underline the 'who', 'doing', 'what' and 'where' words in the correct colour.

who	doing	what	where
leaves	is sweeping	in the garden	The girl

_____

_____

_____

_____

Copyright material from NHS Forth Valley (2020), *Colourful Semantics*, Routledge

Worksheet: Autumn Leaves

Name: _____   Date: _____

Write a sentence about the autumn leaves picture, using the question words below for ideas. Colour the question words the correct colours first to help you. After writing your sentence, underline the 'who', 'doing', 'what' and 'where' words in the correct colour.

? who	? doing	? what	? where

_____

_____

_____

_____

_____

_____

Copyright material from NHS Forth Valley (2020), *Colourful Semantics*, Routledge

Worksheet: Easter Eggs

Name: _____   Date: _____

Write a sentence about the Easter eggs picture. Colour the question words and small pictures in the correct colours first to help you. After writing the sentence, underline the 'who', 'doing', 'what' and 'where' words in the correct colour.

?		?	?
who	doing	what	where
The girl	is buying	Easter eggs	at the sweet shop

_____

_____

_____

_____

Copyright material from NHS Forth Valley (2020), *Colourful Semantics*, Routledge

Worksheet: Easter Eggs

Name: _____ Date: _____

Write a sentence about the Easter eggs picture. Colour the question words and small pictures in the correct colours first to help you. Then work out the correct order for the words in the sentence. After writing your sentence, underline the 'who', 'doing', 'what' and 'where' words in the correct colour.

? who	? doing	? what	? where
at the sweet shop	is buying	The girl	Easter eggs

_____

_____

_____

_____

Copyright material from NHS Forth Valley (2020), *Colourful Semantics*, Routledge

Worksheet: Easter Eggs

Name: _____   Date: _____

Write a sentence about the Easter eggs picture, using the question words below for ideas. Colour the question words the correct colours first to help you. After writing your sentence, underline the 'who', 'doing', 'what' and 'where' words in the correct colour.

? who	? doing	? what	? where

_____

_____

_____

_____

_____

_____

Copyright material from NHS Forth Valley (2020), *Colourful Semantics*, Routledge

'Who', 'doing', 'what', 'where' worksheet template

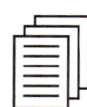

Name: _____   **Date:** _____

who	doing	what	where
?		?	?

_____

_____

_____

_____

_____

Copyright material from NHS Forth Valley (2020), *Colourful Semantics*, Routledge

Worksheet: The Airport

Name: _____   Date: _____

Write a sentence about the airport picture. Colour the question words and small pictures in the correct colours first to help you. After writing the sentence, underline the 'who', 'doing', 'what', 'where' and 'when' words in the correct colour.

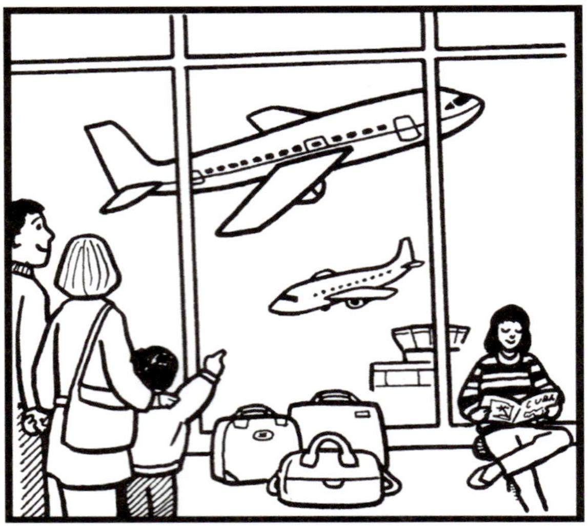

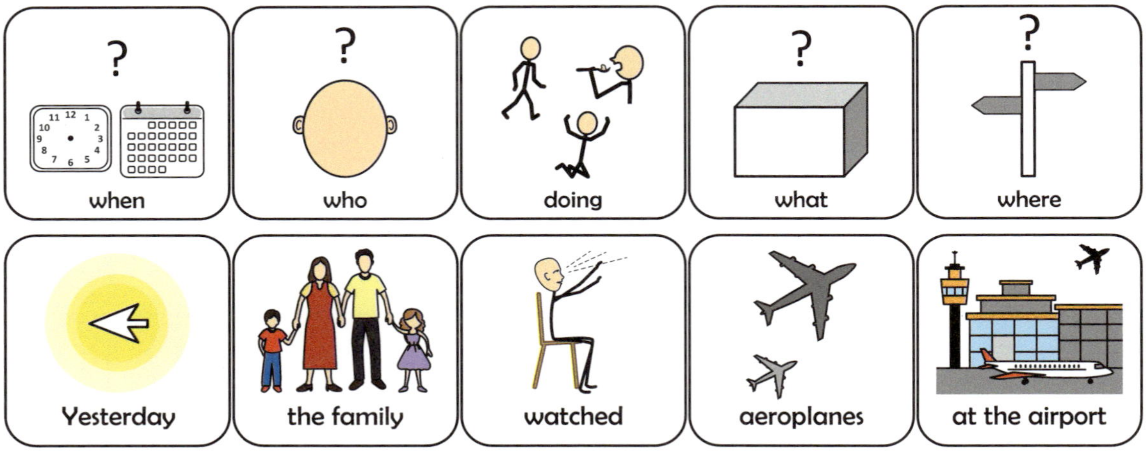

? when	? who	doing	? what	? where

Yesterday	the family	watched	aeroplanes	at the airport

_____

_____

_____

_____

Copyright material from NHS Forth Valley (2020), *Colourful Semantics*, Routledge

Worksheet: The Airport

Name: _____   Date: _____

Write a sentence about the airport picture. Colour the question words and small pictures in the correct colours first to help you. Then work out which order the words in the sentence should come in. After writing your sentence, underline the 'who', 'doing', 'what', 'where' and 'when' words in the correct colour.

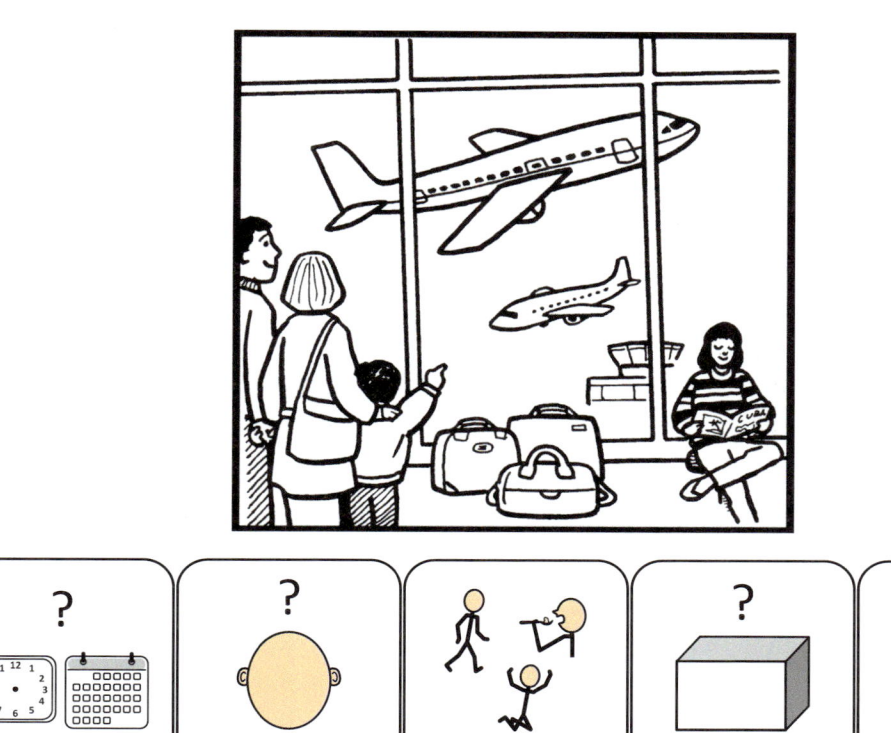

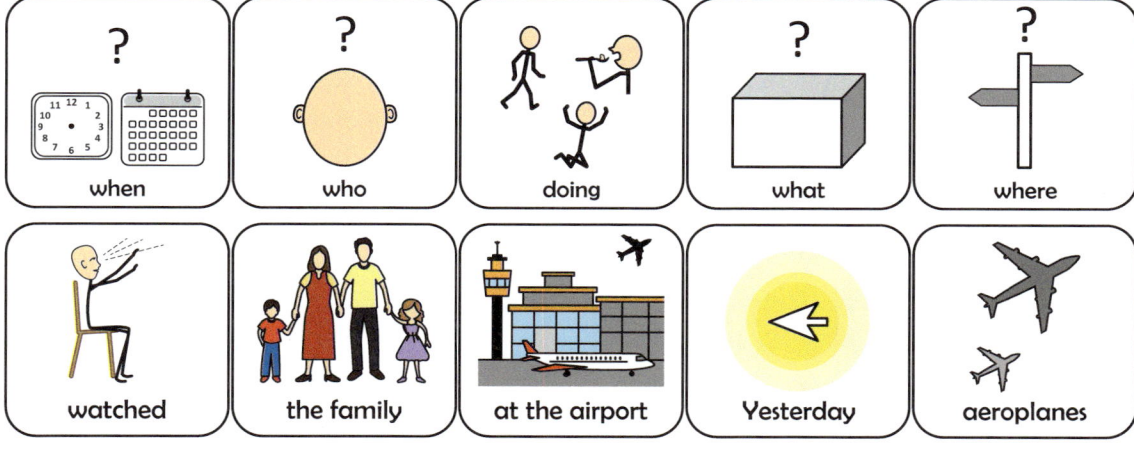

| when | who | doing | what | where |
| watched | the family | at the airport | Yesterday | aeroplanes |

_____

_____

_____

_____

Copyright material from NHS Forth Valley (2020), *Colourful Semantics*, Routledge

Worksheet: The Airport

Name: _____   Date: _____

Write a sentence about the airport picture, using the question words below for ideas. Colour the question words the correct colours first to help you. After writing your sentence, underline the 'who', 'doing', 'what', 'where' and 'when' words in the correct colour.

?	?	?	?	?
when	who	doing	what	where

_____

_____

_____

_____

_____

Copyright material from NHS Forth Valley (2020), *Colourful Semantics*, Routledge

Worksheet: Playing in the Snow

Name: _____   Date: _____

Write a sentence about the playing in the snow picture. Colour the question words and small pictures in the correct colours first to help you. After writing the sentence, underline the 'who', 'doing', 'what', 'where' and 'when' words in the correct colour.

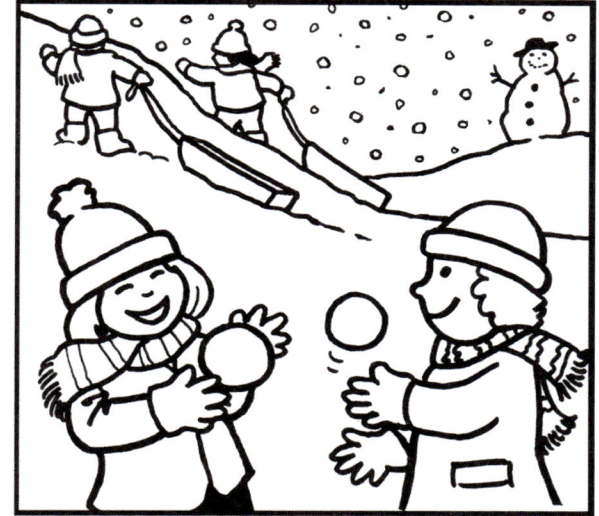

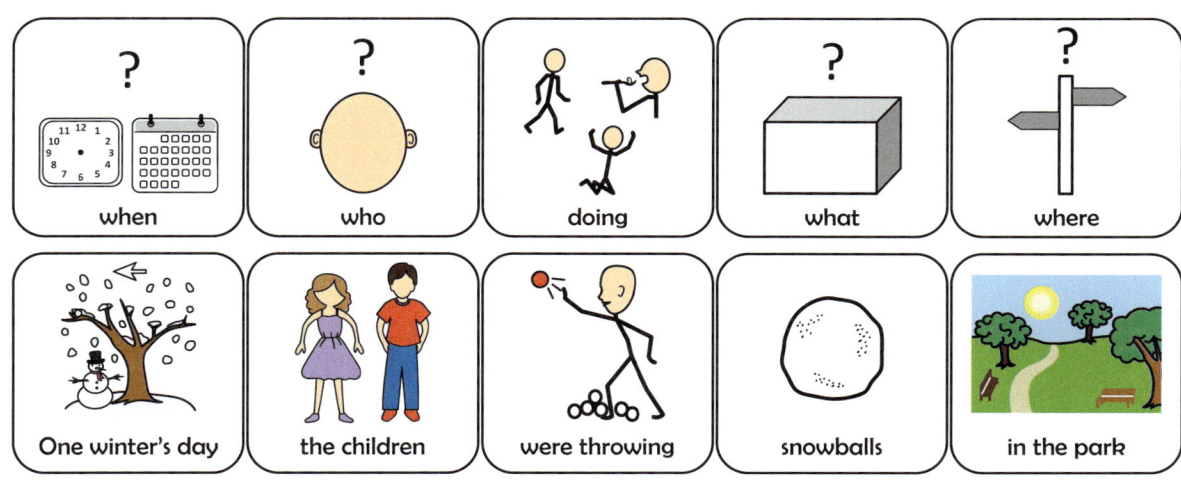

_____

_____

_____

_____

Worksheet: Playing in the Snow

Name: _____   Date: _____

Write a sentence about the playing in the snow picture. Colour the question words and small pictures in the correct colours first to help you. Then work out which order the words in the sentence should come in. After writing your sentence, underline the 'who', 'doing', 'what', 'where' and 'when' words in the correct colour.

? when	? who	doing	? what	? where
snowballs	in the park	One winter's day	were throwing	the children

_____

_____

_____

_____

Copyright material from NHS Forth Valley (2020), *Colourful Semantics*, Routledge

Worksheet: Playing in the Snow

Name: _____   Date: _____

Write a sentence about the playing in the snow picture, using the question words below
for ideas. Colour the question words the correct colours first to help you. After writing your
sentence, underline the 'who', 'doing', 'what', 'where' and 'when' words in the correct colour.

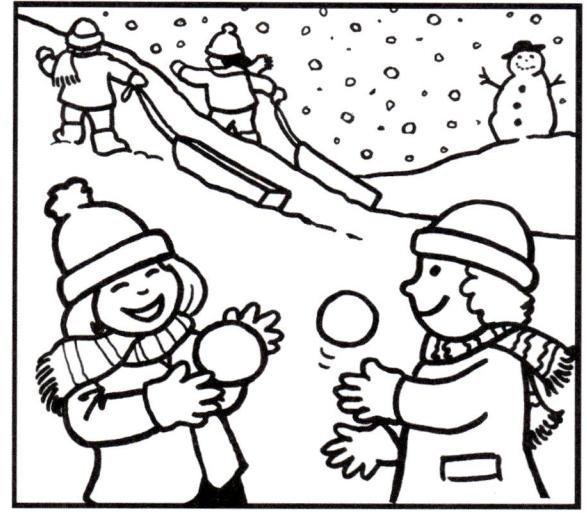

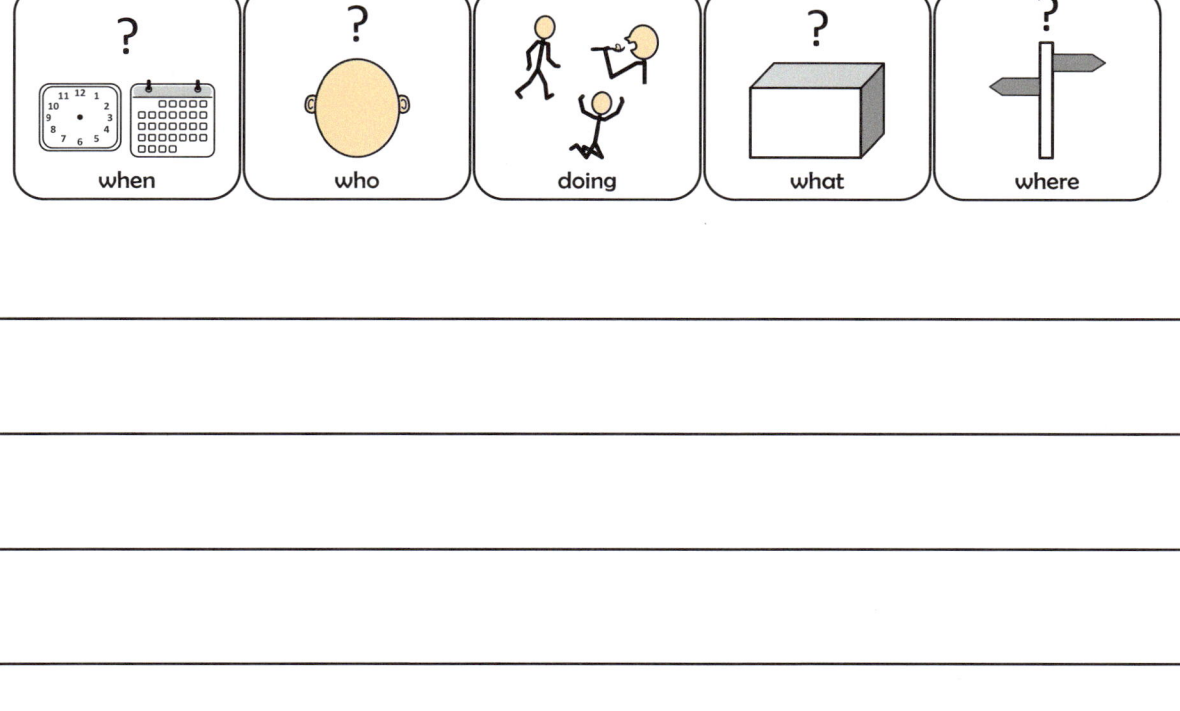

_____

_____

_____

_____

_____

_____

Copyright material from NHS Forth Valley (2020), *Colourful Semantics*, Routledge

'when', 'who', 'doing', 'what', 'where' worksheet template

Name: _____ **Date:** _____

? when	? who	doing	? what	? where

_____

_____

_____

_____

_____

Copyright material from NHS Forth Valley (2020), *Colourful Semantics*, Routledge

Worksheet: Firefighters

Name: _____   Date: _____

Write a sentence about the firefighters picture. Colour the question words and small pictures in the correct colours first to help you. After writing the sentence, underline the 'when', 'who', 'doing', 'what', 'where' and 'why' words in the correct colour.

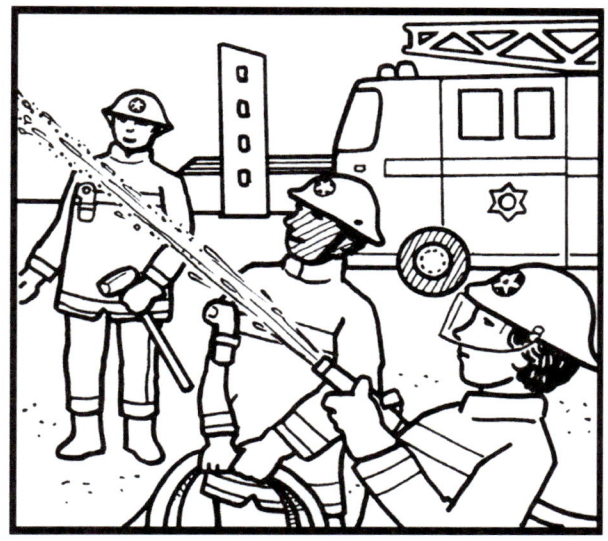

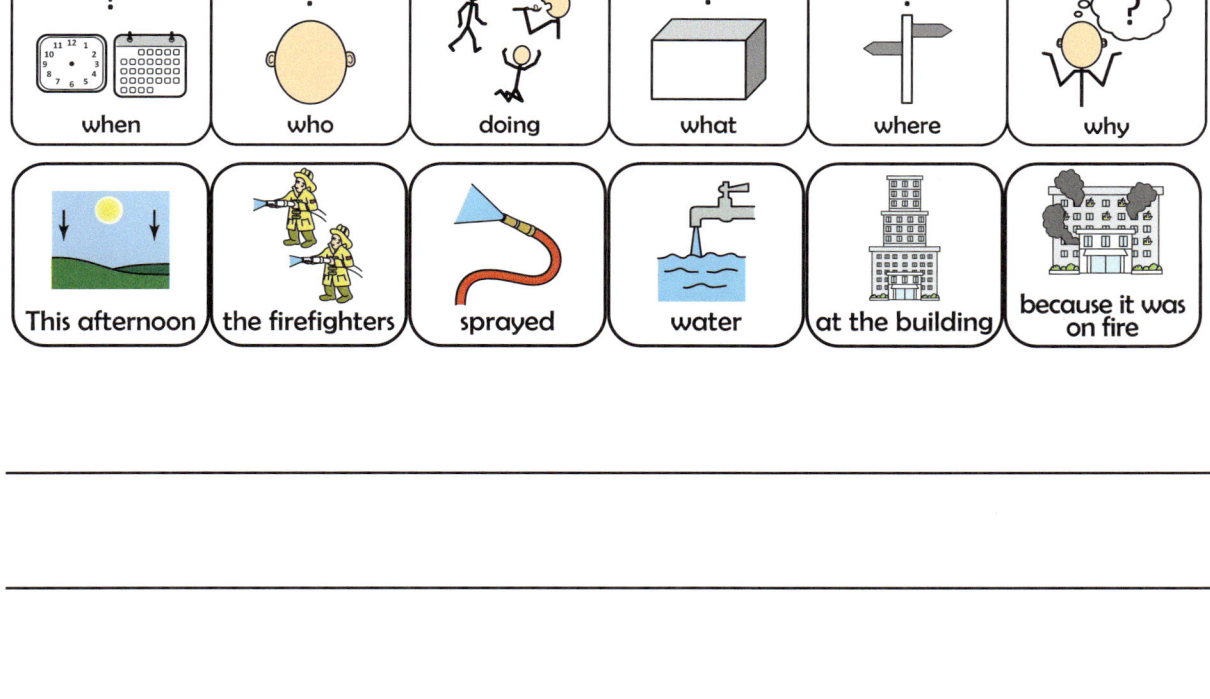

? when	? who	? doing	? what	? where	? why
This afternoon	the firefighters	sprayed	water	at the building	because it was on fire

_____

_____

_____

_____

Copyright material from NHS Forth Valley (2020), *Colourful Semantics*, Routledge

Worksheet: Firefighters

Name: _____   Date: _____

Write a sentence about the firefighters picture. Colour the question words and small pictures in the correct colours first to help you. Then work out which order the words in the sentence should come in. After writing your sentence, underline the 'when', 'who', 'doing', 'what', 'where' and 'why' words in the correct colour.

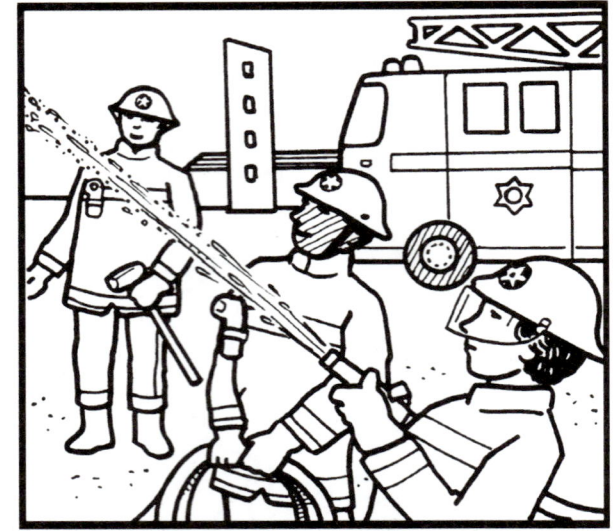

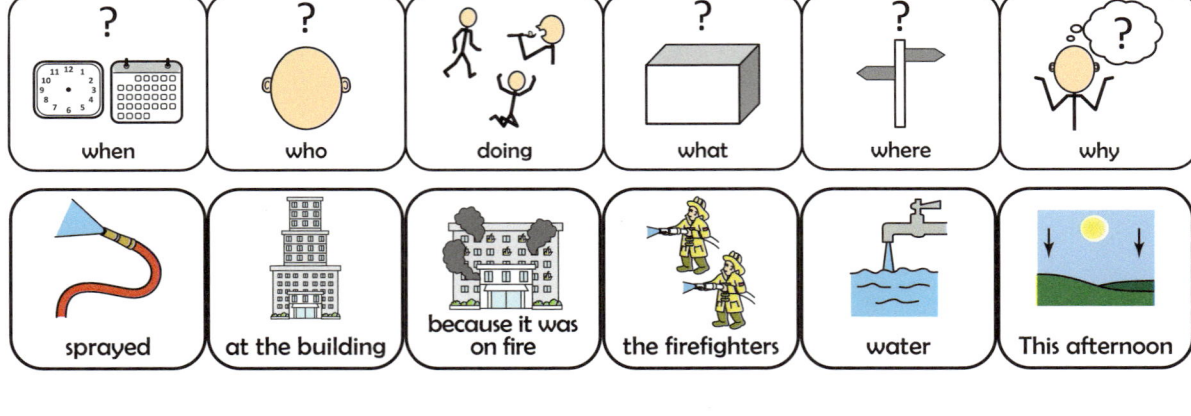

| when | who | doing | what | where | why |

| sprayed | at the building | because it was on fire | the firefighters | water | This afternoon |

_____

_____

_____

_____

Copyright material from NHS Forth Valley (2020), *Colourful Semantics*, Routledge

Worksheet: Firefighters

Name: _____   Date: _____

Write a sentence about the firefighters picture, using the question words below for ideas. Colour the question words the correct colours first to help you. After writing your sentence, underline the 'when', 'who', 'doing', 'what', 'where' and 'why' words in the correct colour.

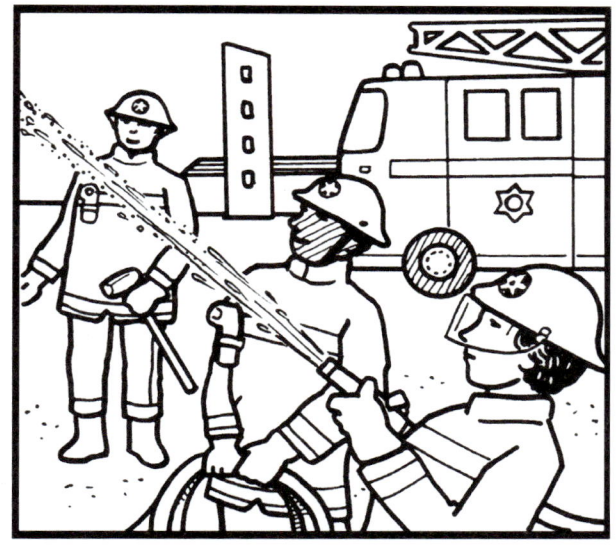

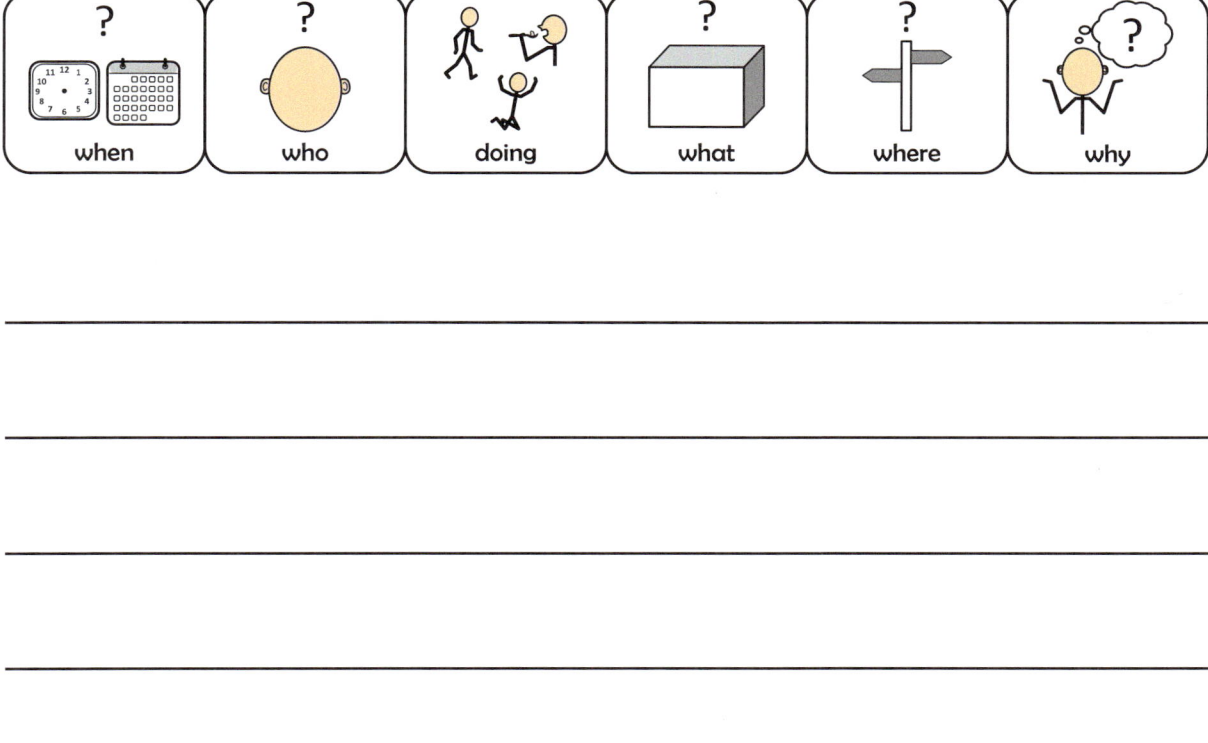

| when | who | doing | what | where | why |

_____

_____

_____

_____

_____

Sequencing Worksheet: Bedtime

Name: _____   Date: _____

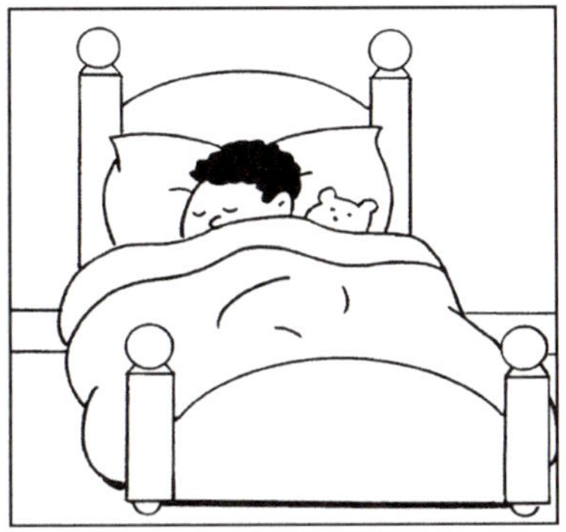

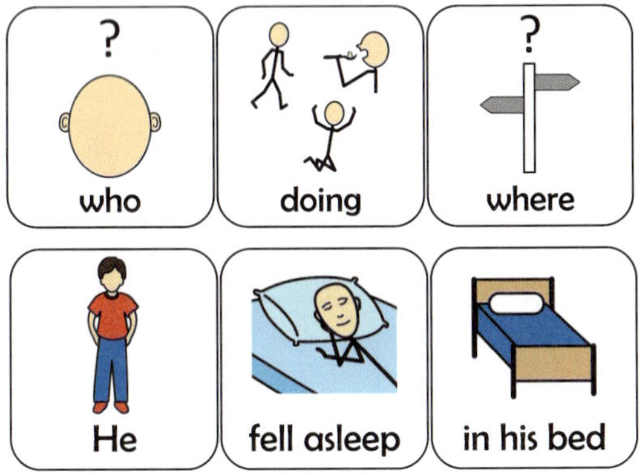

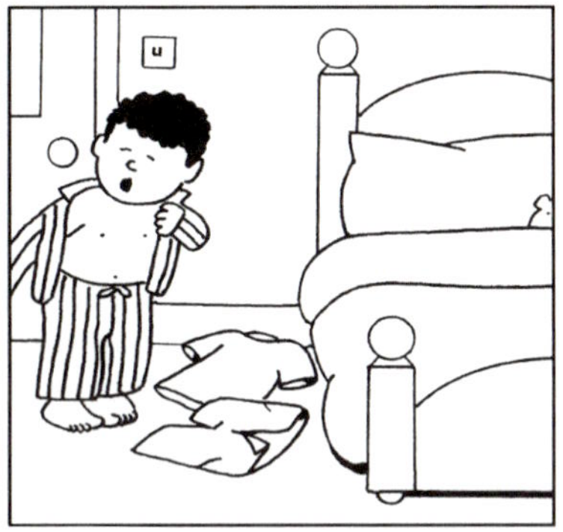

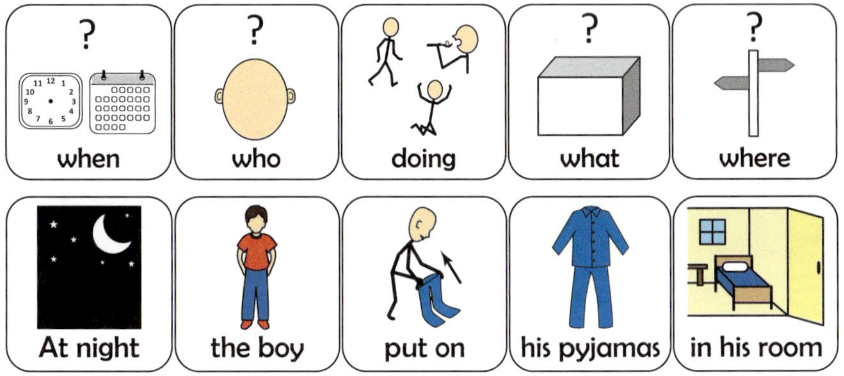

Copyright material from NHS Forth Valley (2020), *Colourful Semantics*, Routledge

Sequencing Worksheet: Bedtime

Name: _____ Date: _____

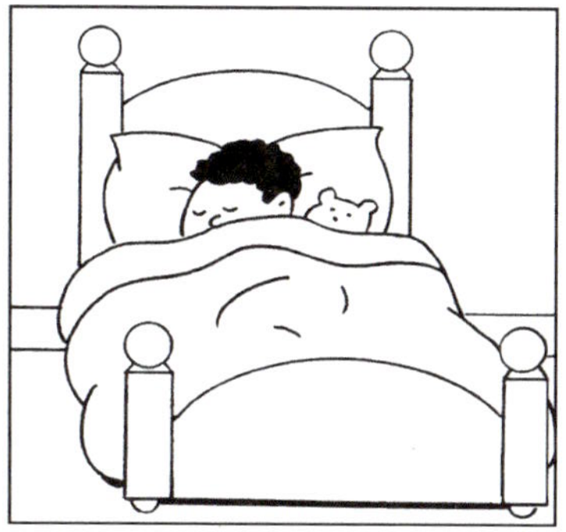

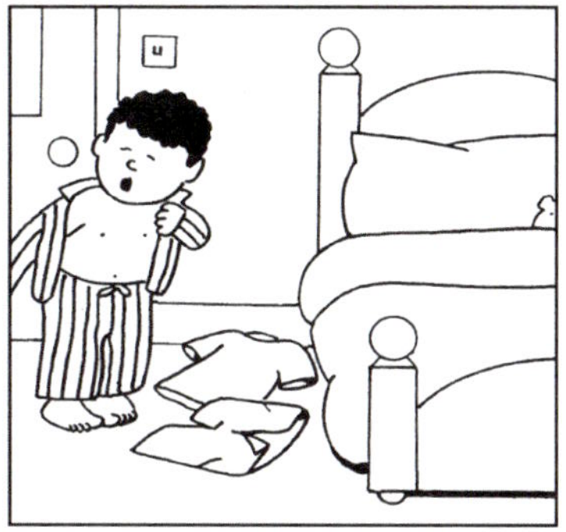

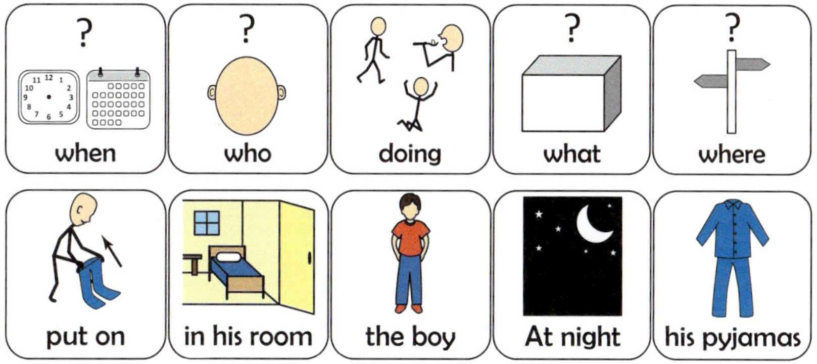

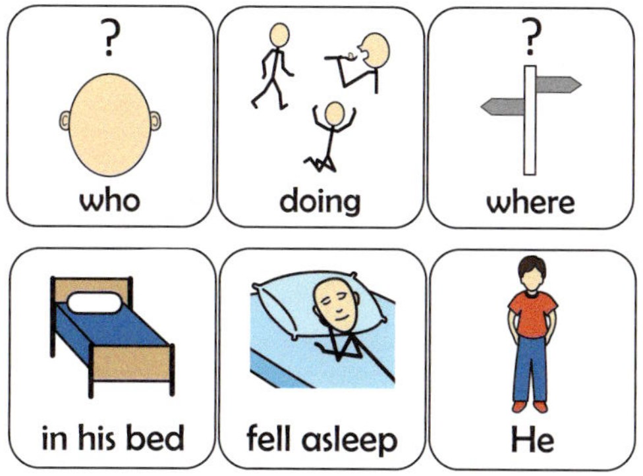

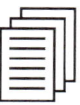

First picture symbols:

where | doing | who
what | |
when | |

his pyjamas | At night | the boy
in his room | put on

Second picture symbols:

where | doing | who
He | fell asleep | in his bed

Copyright material from NHS Forth Valley (2020), *Colourful Semantics*, Routledge

Sequencing Worksheet: Bedtime

Name: _____

Date: _____

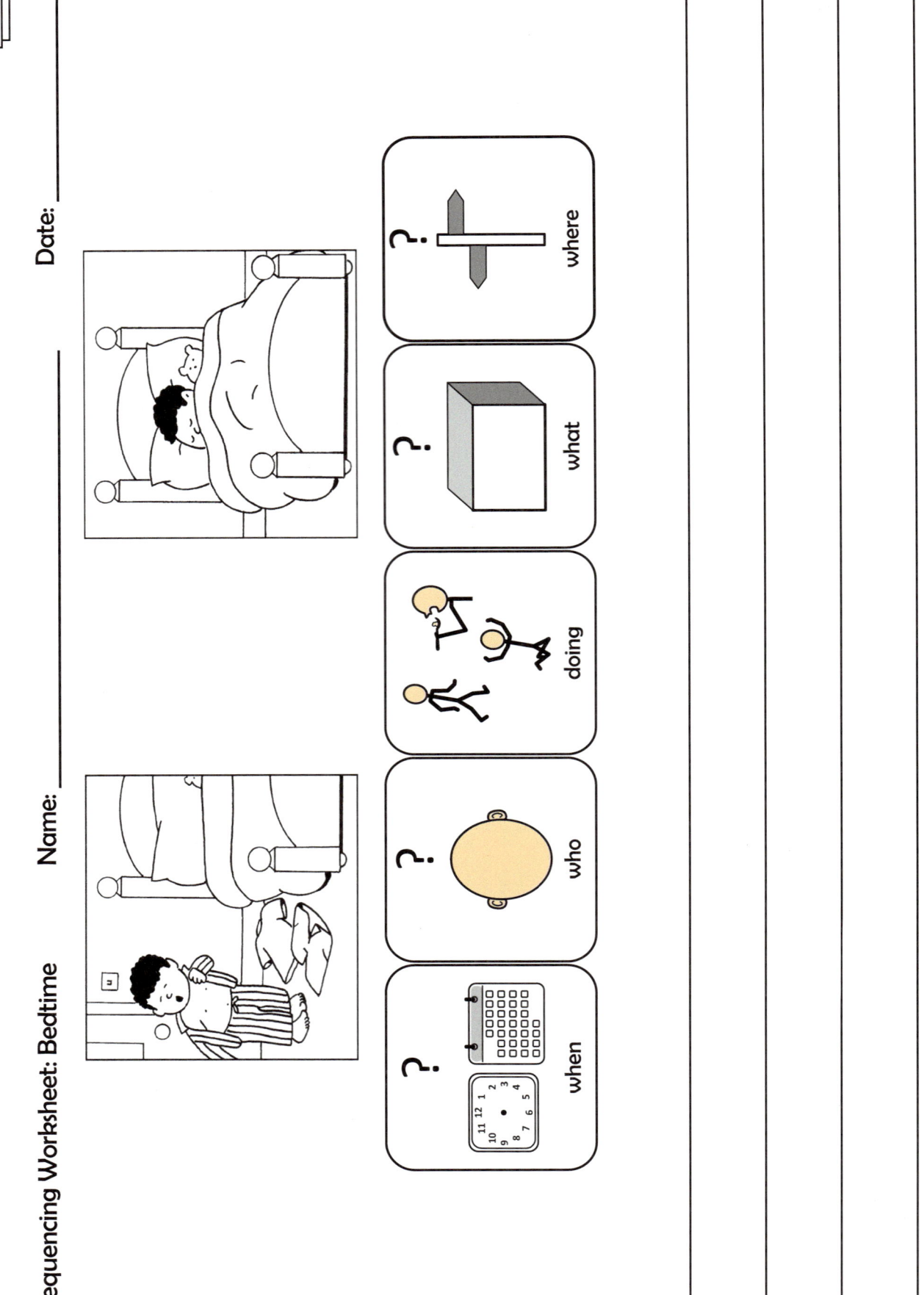

Copyright material from NHS Forth Valley (2020), *Colourful Semantics*, Routledge

Sequencing Worksheet: The Picnic

Name: _____   Date: _____

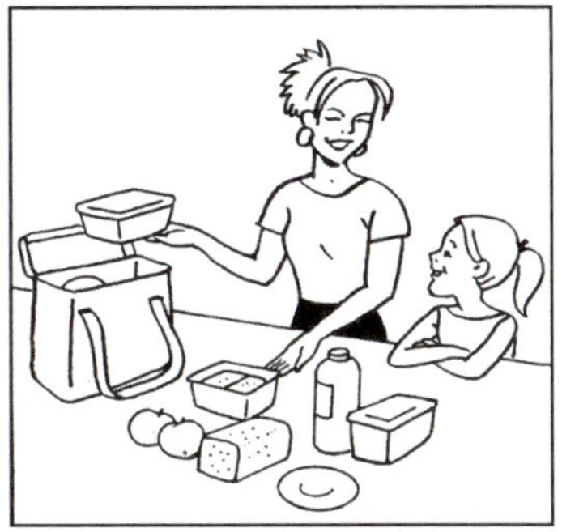

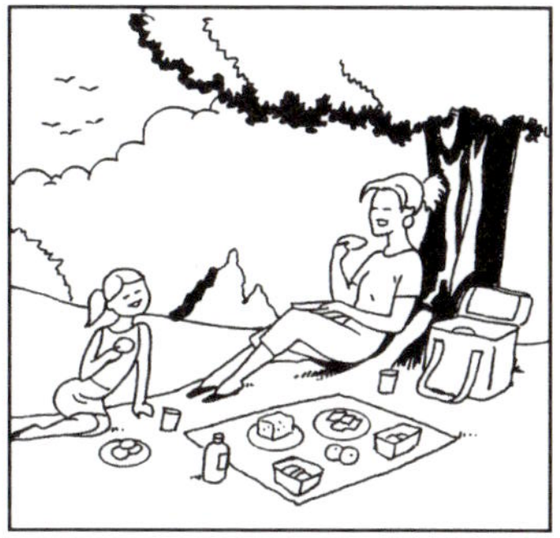

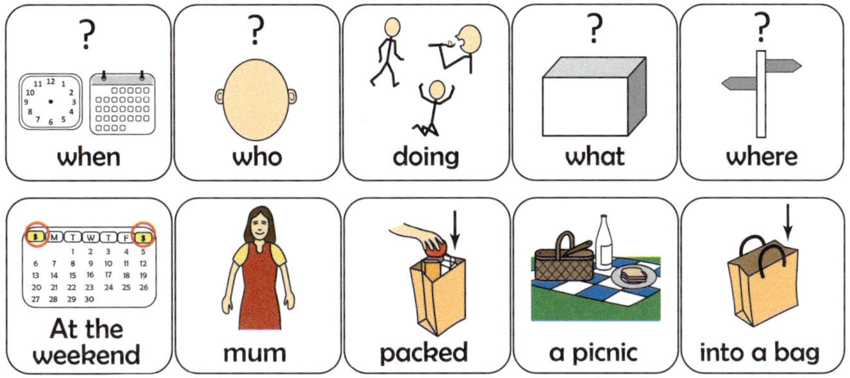

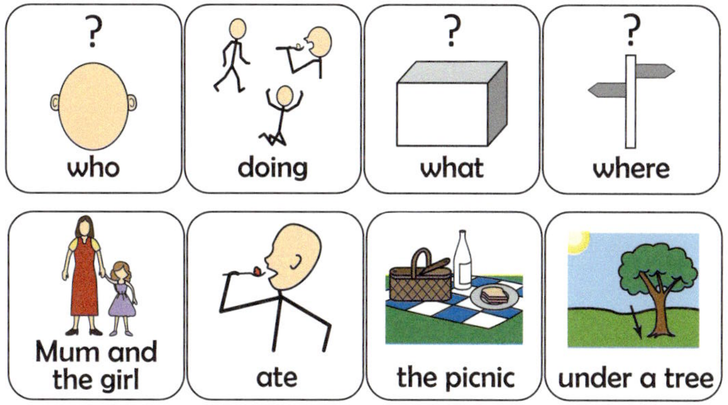

where ? | what ? | doing | who ?

under a tree | the picnic | ate | Mum and the girl

where ? | what ? | doing | who ? | when ?

into a bag | a picnic | packed | mum | At the weekend

Copyright material from NHS Forth Valley (2020), *Colourful Semantics*, Routledge

Sequencing Worksheet: The Picnic   Name: _____   Date: _____

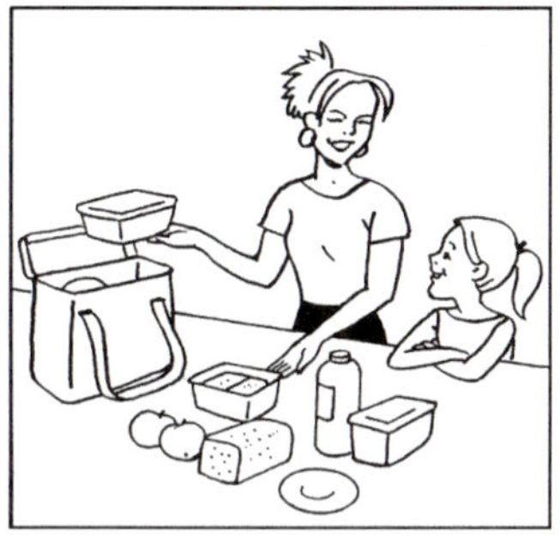

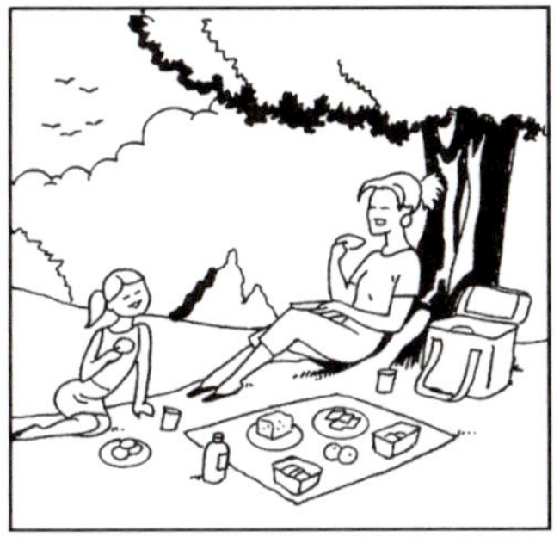

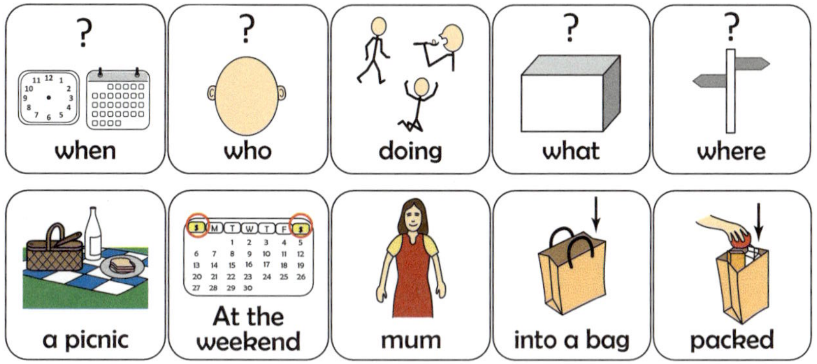

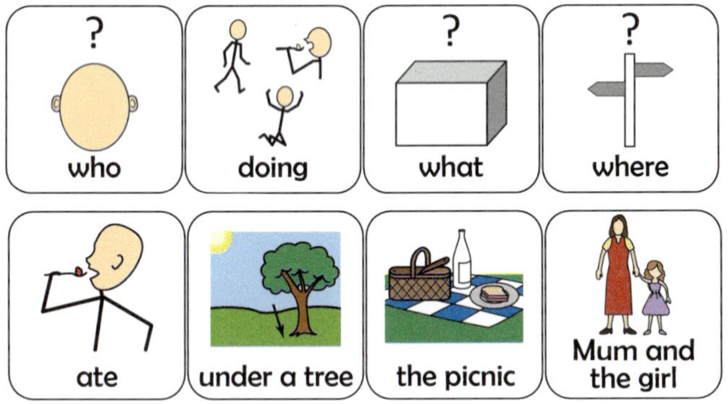

where · ?   what · ?   doing   who · ?

Mum and the girl   the picnic   under a tree   ate

where · ?   what · ?   doing   who · ?   when · ?

packed   into a bag   mum   At the weekend   a picnic

Copyright material from NHS Forth Valley (2020), *Colourful Semantics*, Routledge

Sequencing Worksheet: The Picnic   Name: Date:

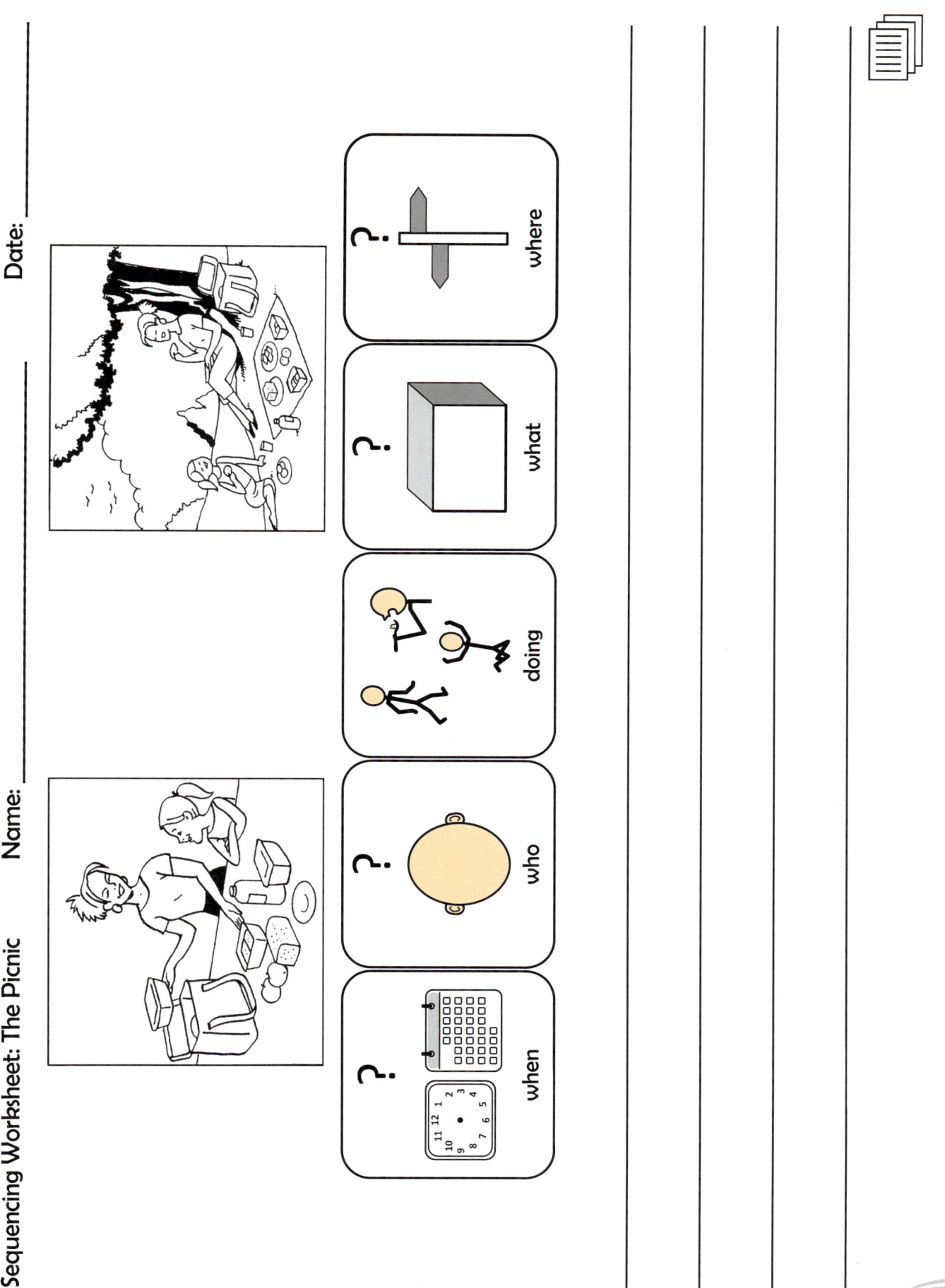

where   what   doing   who   when

Copyright material from NHS Forth Valley (2020), *Colourful Semantics*, Routledge

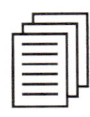

Date:

Sequencing Worksheet: Ice Cream   Name:

who	doing	what	where
why	where		
to eat it	to the park	ran	He

when	who	doing	what	where
In summer	the boy	bought	an ice cream	at the ice cream van

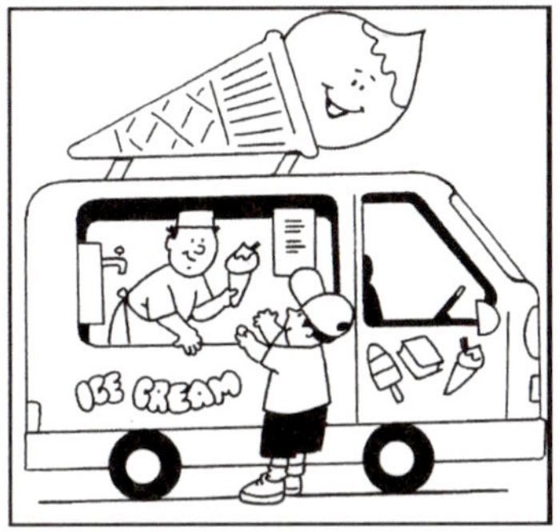

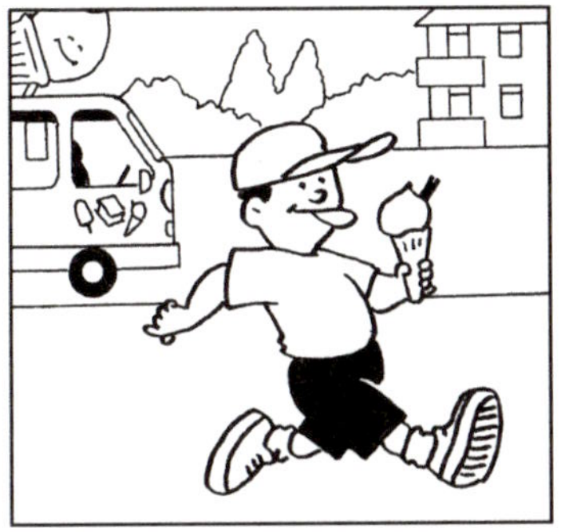

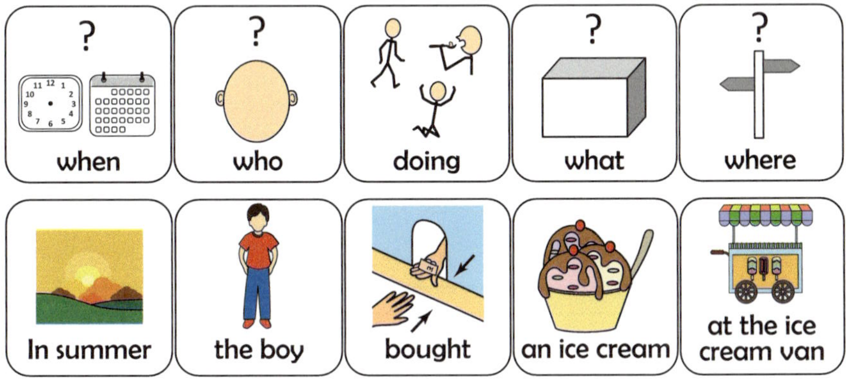

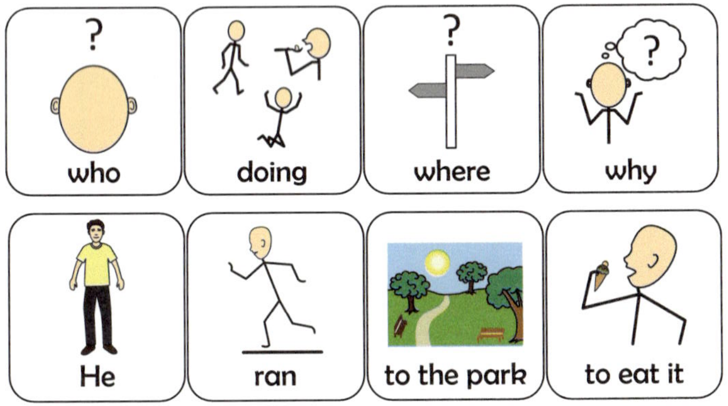

Copyright material from NHS Forth Valley (2020), *Colourful Semantics*, Routledge

Sequencing Worksheet: Ice Cream   Name: _____   Date: _____

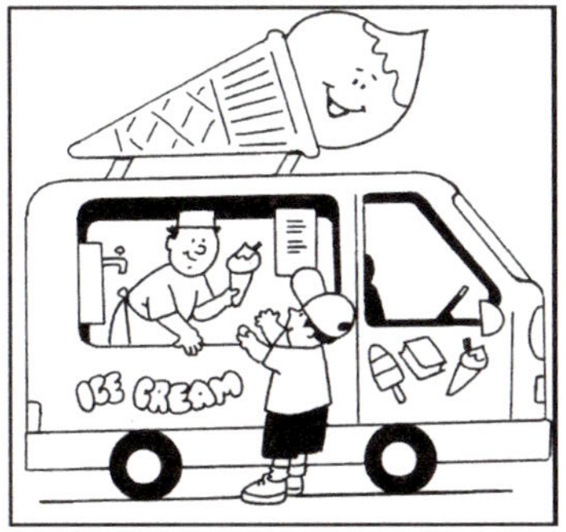

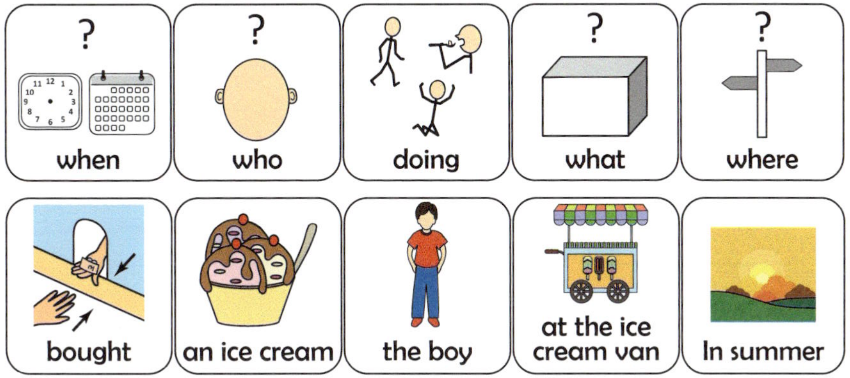

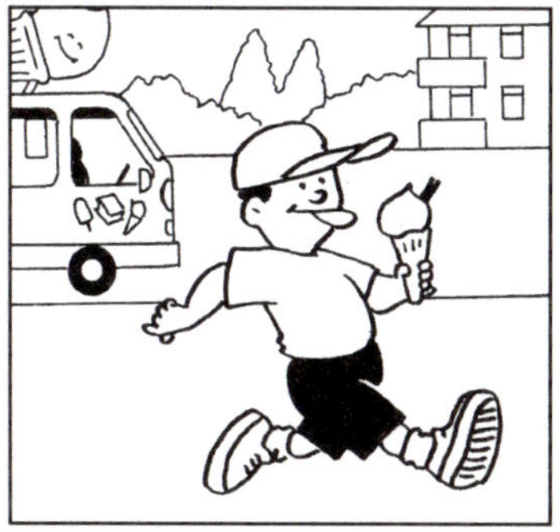

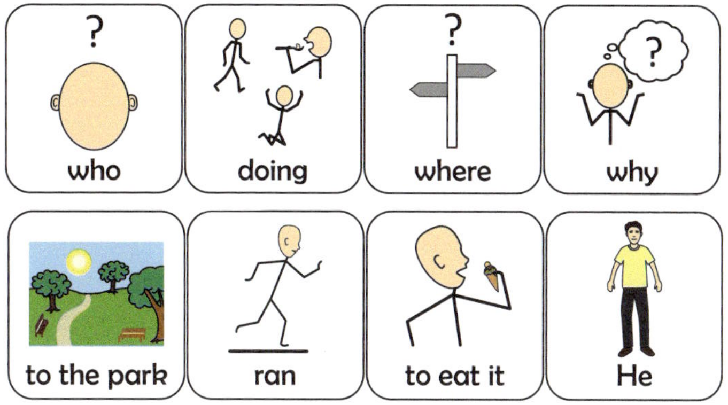

why	where	doing	who
He	to eat it	ran	to the park

where	what	doing	who	when
In summer	at the ice cream van	the boy	an ice cream	bought

Sequencing Worksheet: Ice Cream

Name: _____

Date: _____

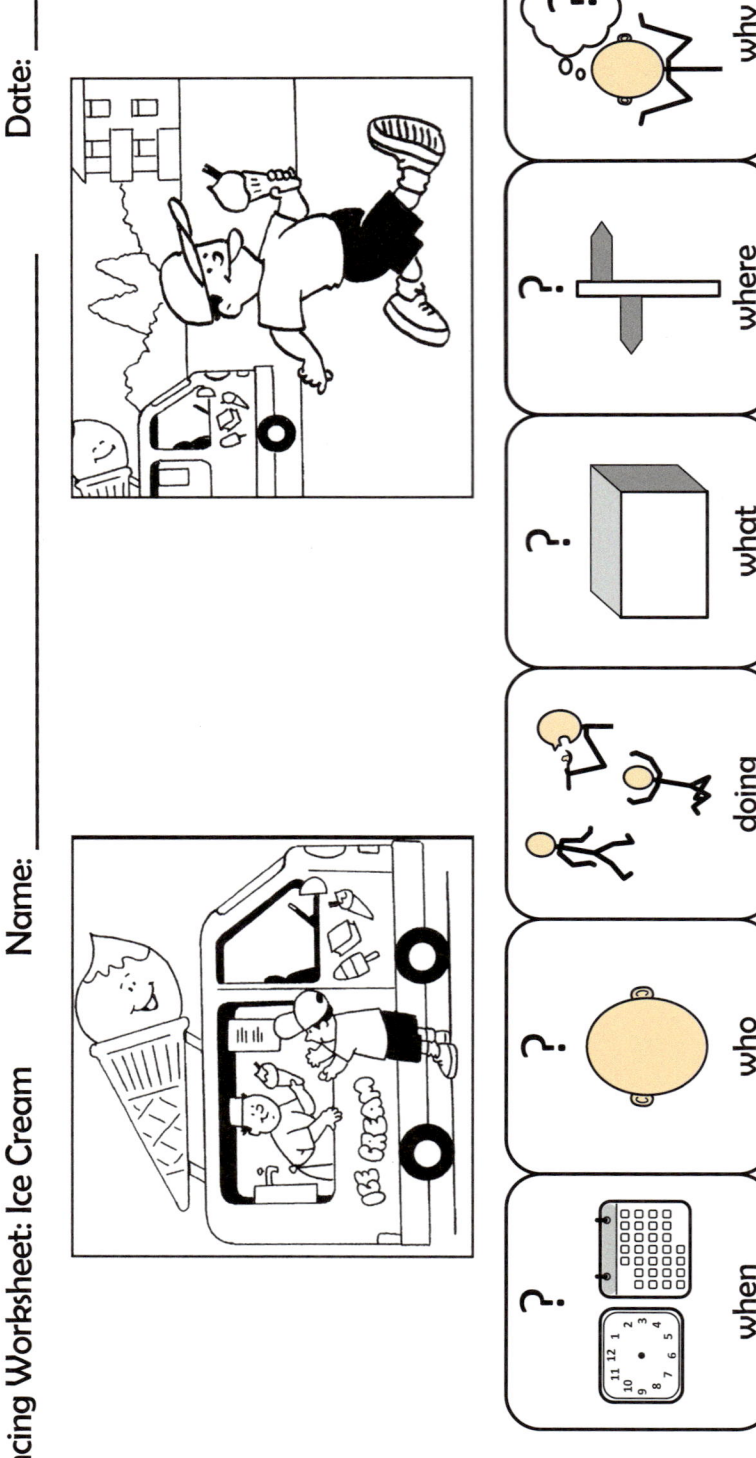

Copyright material from NHS Forth Valley (2020), *Colourful Semantics*, Routledge

Appendix 8
Board games

Copyright material from NHS Forth Valley (2020), *Colourful Semantics*, Routledge

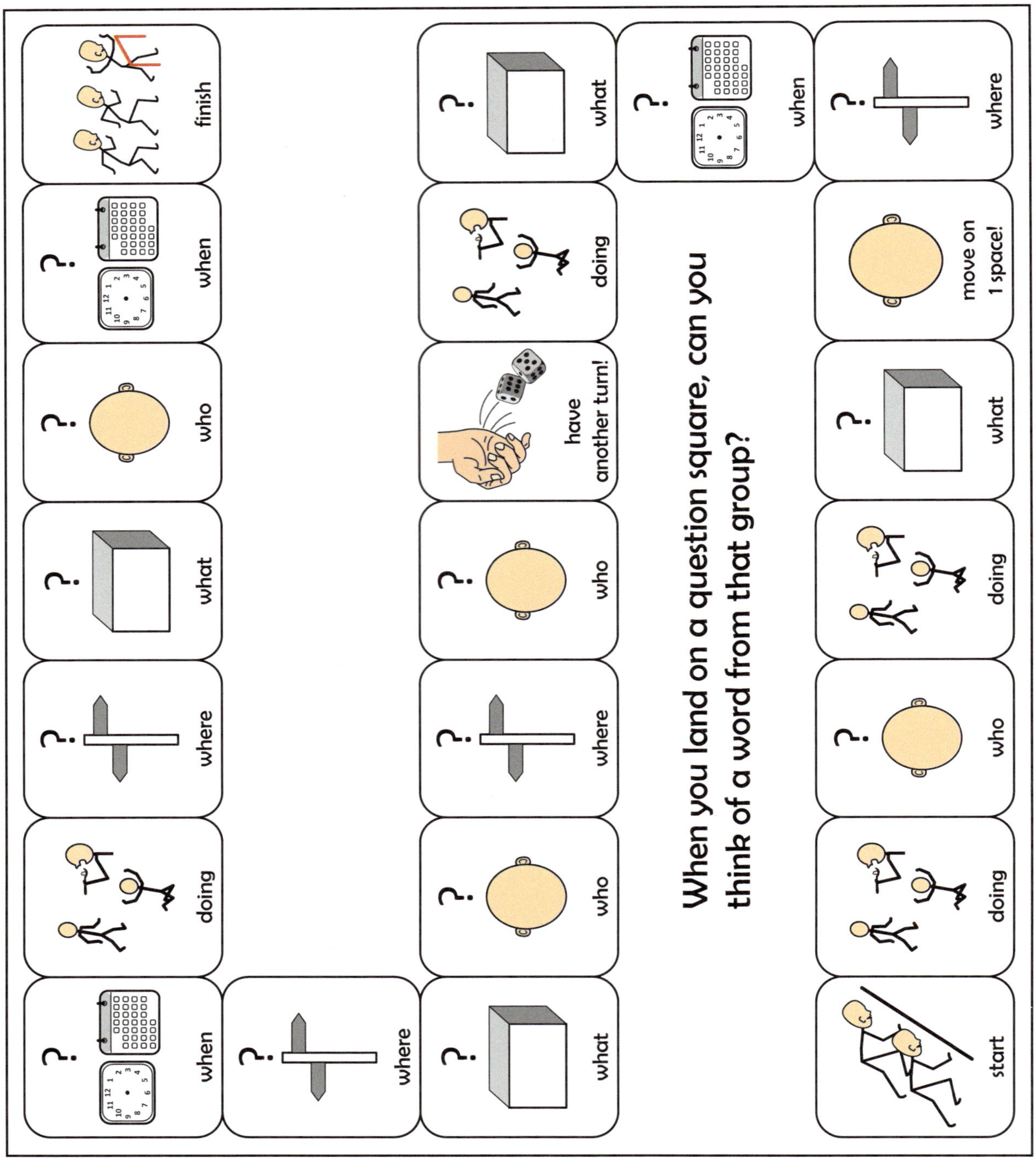

When you land on a question square, can you think of a word from that group?

finish	when	who	what	where	doing	when
what	doing	have another turn!	who	where	who	where	what
where	move on 1 space!	what	doing	who	doing	start

Copyright material from NHS Forth Valley (2020), *Colourful Semantics*, Routledge

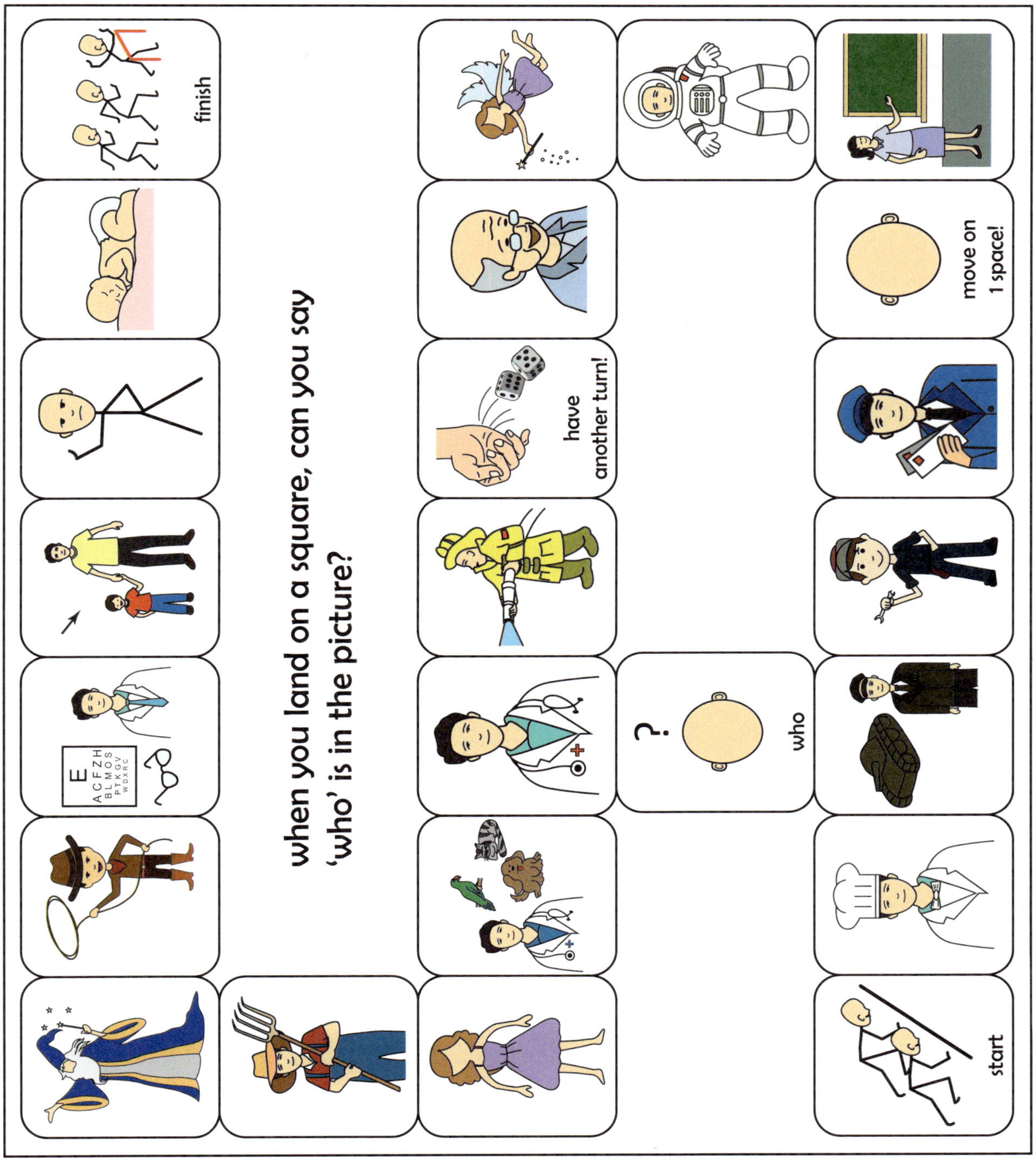

when you land on a square, can you say 'who' is in the picture?

finish

move on 1 space!

have another turn!

who

start

Copyright material from NHS Forth Valley (2020), *Colourful Semantics*, Routledge

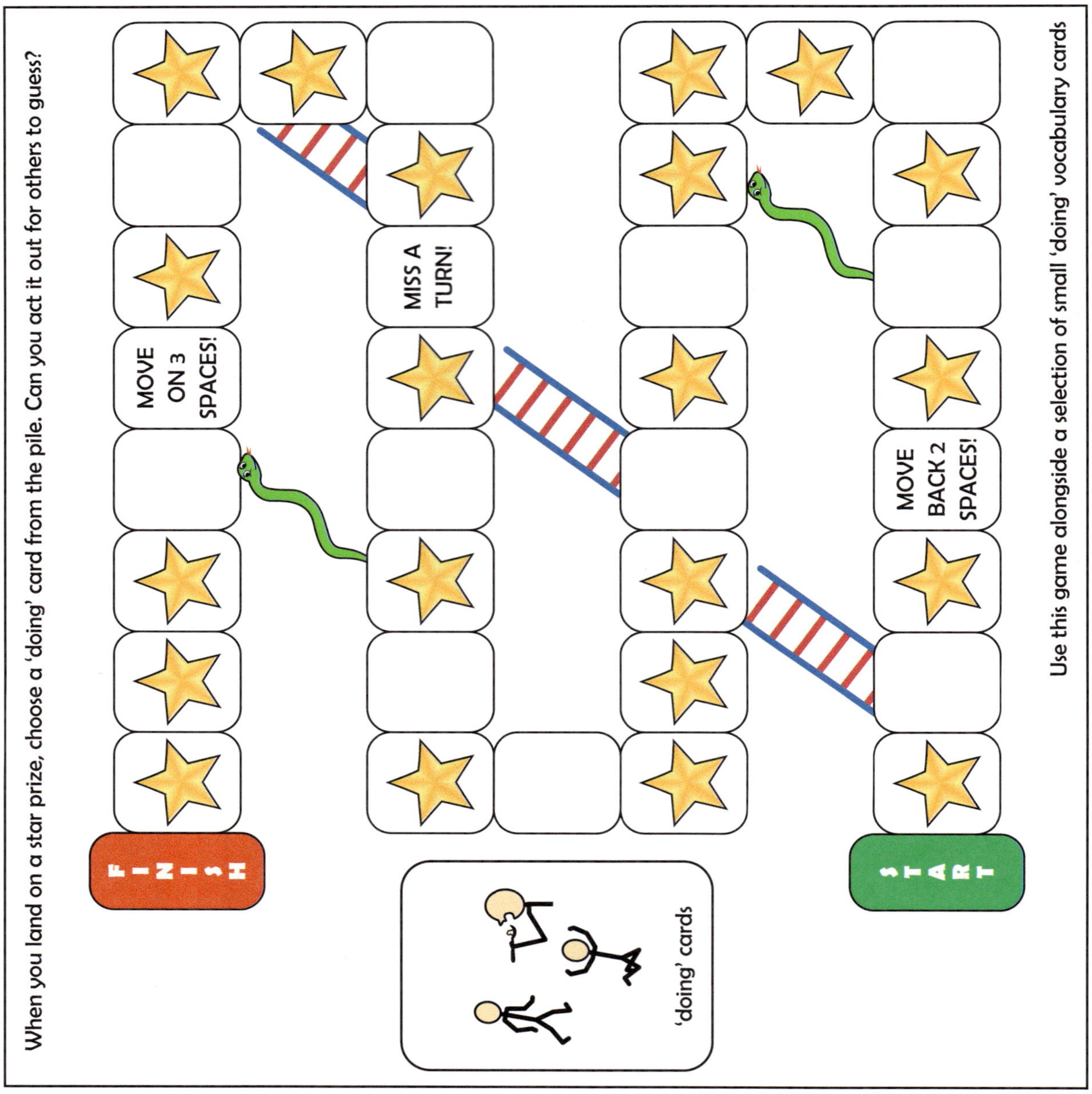

When you land on a star prize, choose a 'doing' card from the pile. Can you act it out for others to guess?

MOVE ON 3 SPACES!

MISS A TURN!

MOVE BACK 2 SPACES!

FINISH

START

'doing' cards

Use this game alongside a selection of small 'doing' vocabulary cards

Copyright material from NHS Forth Valley (2020), *Colourful Semantics*, Routledge

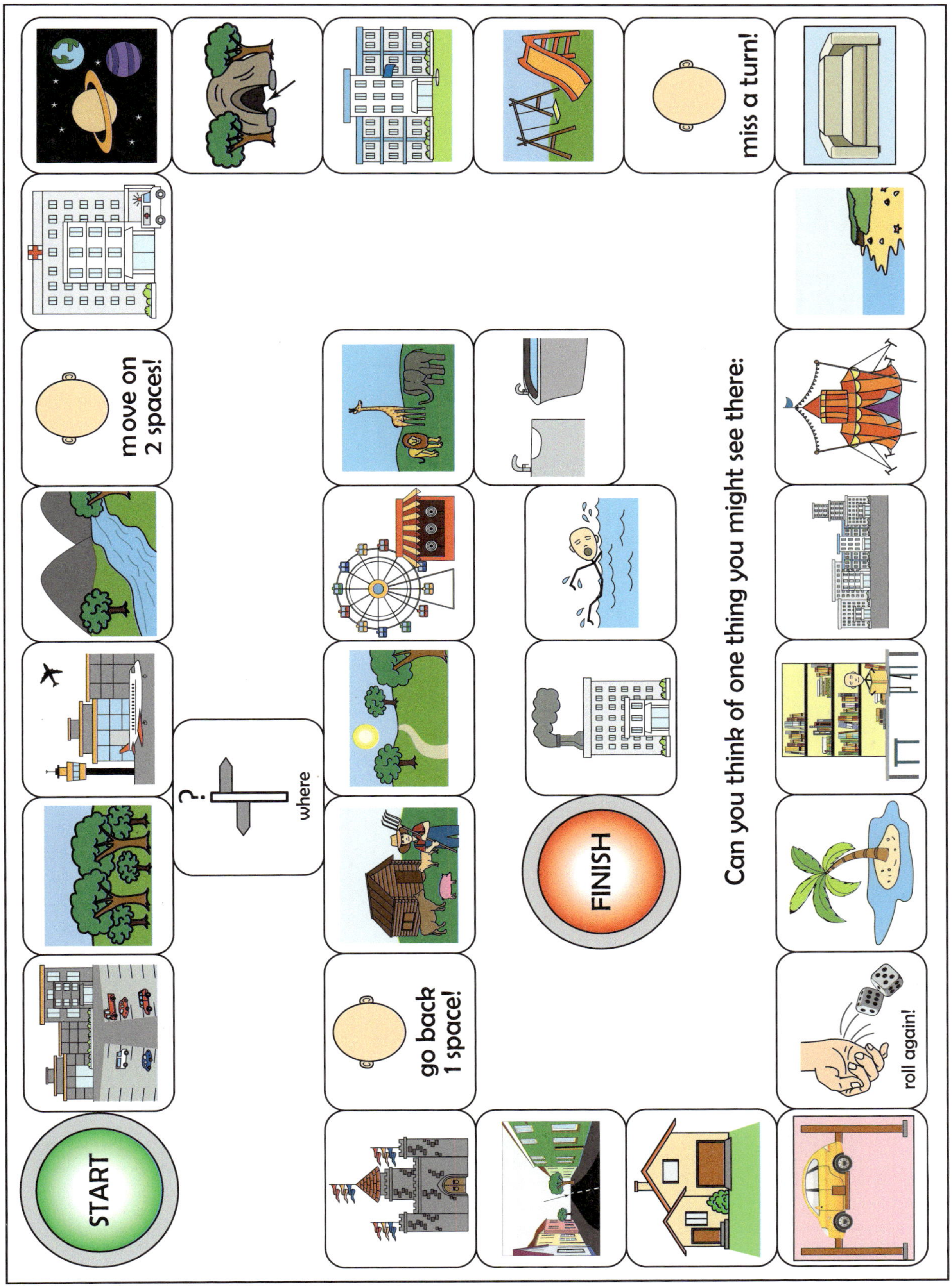

START

FINISH

move on
2 spaces!

miss a turn!

go back
1 space!

roll again!

where ?

Can you think of one thing you might see there:

Copyright material from NHS Forth Valley (2020), *Colourful Semantics*, Routledge

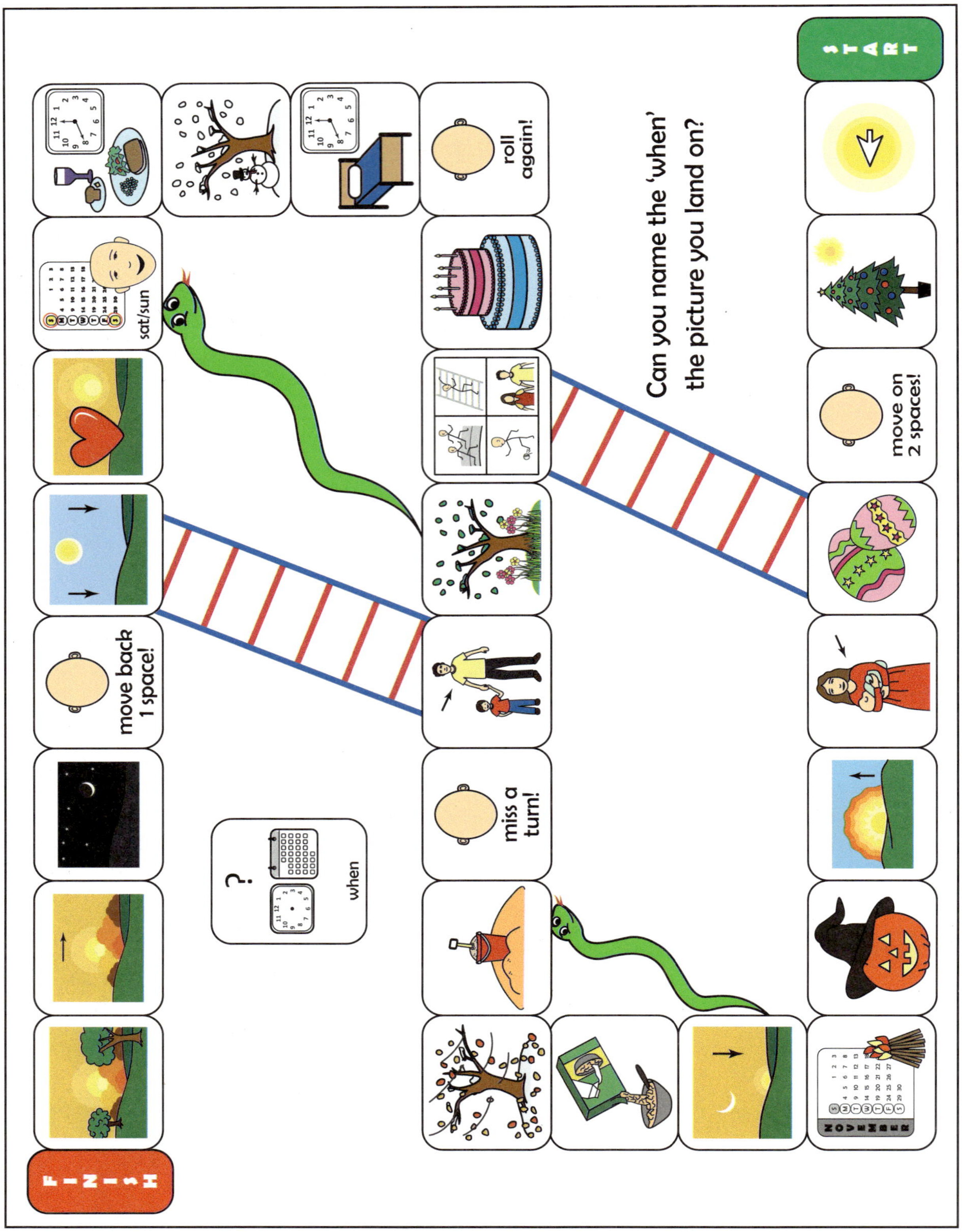

Can you name the 'when' the picture you land on?

START

roll again!

move on 2 spaces!

move back 1 space!

when

miss a turn!

sat/sun

FINISH

Copyright material from NHS Forth Valley (2020), *Colourful Semantics*, Routledge